AINTREE UNIVERSITY NHS
FOUNDATION TRUST
LIVERPOOL
L9 7AL

UNIVERSITY DEPARTMENT OF RADIODIAGNOSIS
2ND FLOOR
JOHNSTON BUILDING
THE QUADRANGLE
PO BOX 147
LIVERPOOL L69 3BX

MRI and CT

ATLAS

OF CORRELATIVE IMAGING IN

OTOLARYNGOLOGY

To my loving husband Koneti for his inspiration and infinite support,
my wonderful children Deepak and Gita
and
to my mother and father for their fathomless love

VMR

To Deborah and my family

AEF

To my wife Robin and my son Michael
and
to my mother and father

BMT

MRI and CT

═══ATLAS═══

OF CORRELATIVE IMAGING IN

OTOLARYNGOLOGY

Vijay M Rao, MD

Professor of Radiology and Otolaryngology
Thomas Jefferson University Hospital and
Jefferson Medical College
Philadelphia, PA, USA

Adam E Flanders, MD

Assistant Professor of Radiology
Thomas Jefferson University Hospital and
Jefferson Medical College
Philadelphia, PA, USA

Barry M Tom, MD

Attending Radiologist
St Joseph's Hospital
Reading, PA, USA

Martin Dunitz

© Martin Dunitz Ltd 1992

First published in the United Kingdom in 1992
by Martin Dunitz Ltd, The Livery House, 7–9 Pratt Street
London NW1 0AE

A CIP catalogue record of this book is available from the
British Library

ISBN 1 85317 037 2

Composition by Scribe Design, Gillingham, Kent
Origination by Adroit Photolitho Ltd, Birmingham
Printed and bound in Singapore by Toppan Printing Company (S) Pte Ltd

CONTENTS

FOREWORD

The growth and development of head and neck imaging in the last decade has been phenomenal. This is, for the most part, due to the introduction, refinement, and technical advances of computed tomography and magnetic resonance imaging. The introduction of gadolinium has further improved our diagnostic recognition and delineation of head and neck lesions.

It is for this reason that a book entitled 'MRI and CT Atlas of Correlative Imaging in Otolaryngology' fulfills a need for many physicians who deal with diseases in otolaryngology. The text is well written and each important finding superbly illustrated. The CT and MRI findings are discussed and illustrated for each entity.

The senior author, Dr Rao, has been prominent in the development and teaching of head and neck radiology and here she draws from her extensive experience over many years. She and her co-authors have accomplished the goal of providing a text that is fluid in style, concise, and highlights the essential CT and MR features of a diverse group of entities in otolaryngologic radiology.

This text atlas should become a helpful addition to radiologists, otolaryngologists and other physicians engaged in the practice of head and neck disease.

Alfred L Weber, MD
Professor of Radiology
Harvard Medical School
Chief of Radiology
Massachusetts Eye and Ear Infirmary
Boston, Massachusetts

PREFACE

Technological advances in imaging techniques have had an impact on many areas of radiology, but few more profoundly than the field of otolaryngology and diseases of the head and neck. Previously, many of the pathologic changes affecting areas such as the skull base, orbital apex, parapharyngeal spaces and deep spaces of the neck were either elusive to adequate visualization or were demonstrable only at advanced stages. CT and, more recently, MRI have become basic tools in the diagnosis of head and neck diseases and have dramatically enhanced our understanding of the anatomic variants and the disease processes in this region.

The rapid evolution of the imaging techniques in this field underscores the pressing need for a text atlas that provides the relevant information pictorially with MRI and CT correlation, accompanied by essential but not excessive text. This book is intended to address the needs of a wide group of individuals involved in the management of diseases of the head and neck including radiologists, otolaryngologists and residents and fellows in these fields. Multiple presentations of several of the more common diseases are shown, the relative merits of MRI and CT scanning are discussed, and imaging strategies to produce optimum examinations are addressed in each chapter.

Vijay M Rao, MD
Adam E Flanders, MD
Barry M Tom, MD

ACKNOWLEDGEMENTS

Our special thanks to JoAnn A Gardner for her diligent and invaluable assistance in the preparation of this atlas. We also thank Pamela A Bittle for help with typing the manuscripts and Saundra Ehrlich for her editorial assistance. Our appreciation is extended to Richard Blob, Ursula Latvys and the CT and MRI technologists who always strive to obtain the best images possible. We thank our residents and fellows who have monitored several of these cases. We acknowledge the assistance of Joseph Hegarty, a senior medical student, for the medical illustrations.

We thank Robert A Zimmerman, MD, at the Children's Hospital of Philadelphia for several cases included in this atlas. We extend deep gratitude to our clinical colleagues in the Department of Otolaryngology and Head and Neck Surgery, Louis D Lowry, MD, Diran O Mikaelian, MD, David A Zwillenberg, MD, David Reiter, MD, Herbert Kean, MD and Gwen Stone, MD, without whose patients such an enormous amount of material could not have been collected. We also thank Jerry Shields, MD, Carol Shields, MD, and Patrick DePotter, MD at the Wills Eye Hospital, Philadelphia, for their collaborative work. We appreciate the support of our colleagues in the department, Carlos Gonzalez, MD, Mark Mishkin, MD, David Friedman, MD, and Lisa Tartaglino, MD.

We wish to acknowledge the invaluable assistance of Mary Banks of Martin Dunitz Publishers who got us started, and to Jacky Alderson who very patiently and effectively completed the task with us. Our thanks to the Production Department of Martin Dunitz Publishers for their diligence in producing illustrations of the highest quality, and to Martin Dunitz himself for his personal involvement.

Finally, we wish to express our deep gratitude to David C Levin, MD, Chairman of the Department of Radiology, Thomas Jefferson University Hospital, for support and encouragement and for creating an environment so highly conducive to such academic endeavors.

VMR
AEF
BMT

CHAPTER 1

PARANASAL SINUSES AND NASAL CAVITY

Introduction

Imaging of paranasal sinus and nasal cavity lesions can be achieved by conventional radiography, computed tomography or more recently, by magnetic resonance imaging. Conventional radiographs offer only limited information because of the overlapping structures and serve as a gross screening examination. With the recent advances in cross-sectional imaging techniques, the radiologists today are better equipped to delineate tumor margins and, therefore, to accurately stage tumors in patients with paranasal sinus and nasal cavity malignancies. The relative roles of computed tomography (CT) and magnetic resonance (MR) in sinonasal imaging are addressed in this chapter. For inflammatory sinus lesions, CT is the preferred modality, while other complications may be better defined by MRI. Because of its ability to differentiate neoplasms from adjacent inflammatory disease by signal characteristics, MR plays an important role in imaging of tumors in the sinuses and nasal cavity.

Normal anatomy

The paranasal sinuses are paired structures and are named according to the bone from which they originate. Maxillary, ethmoid, frontal and sphenoid sinuses collectively form the paranasal sinuses. At birth, only slight aeration of the maxillary sinus and the ethmoid air cells is present. Aeration of the sphenoid sinus becomes apparent by 3 years of age and of the frontal sinus, by 6 years of age.[1] By 10 years of age, all of the paranasal sinuses are developed.

Paranasal sinuses

Maxillary

The maxillary sinuses are usually symmetrical. Septation or hypoplasia of the maxillary sinus is rare. The maxillary sinuses drain into the middle meatus of the nasal cavity along with the anterior ethmoid sinuses and frontal sinus. This entire anterior ethmoid–middle meatus (ostiomeatal complex) is exquisitely demonstrated by computed tomography in a coronal plane and provides a road map to otolaryngologists in endoscopic surgery. The maxillary sinuses are bounded by the nasal cavity medially and the orbits superiorly. The roof of the maxillary sinus also forms the floor of the orbit. The infraorbital nerve, artery and vein lie in the infraorbital groove which continues as the infraorbital canal that exits below the inferior orbital margin as the infraorbital foramen. Inferiorly, the maxillary floor may extend into the alveolar ridge and therefore, dental disease can be considered a source of sinus pathology. Posterior to the sinus and in front of the pterygoid plates is the pterygo-palatine fossa. In the pterygo-palatine fossa lie the spheno-palatine ganglion, branches of the greater and lesser petrosal nerves, branches of the second division of the trigeminal nerve and the internal maxillary artery.

Ethmoid

The ethmoid sinuses are bounded by the orbits laterally and the nasal cavity medially. The ethmoid sinuses consist of multiple air cells, and are divided into an anterior and a posterior portion by the basal lamella. The lamina papyracea is the thin bone that separates the ethmoid sinus from the orbit. The anterior ethmoid air cells are numerous and small in contrast to the posterior air cells which are larger.

The roof of ethmoid sinuses extends on either side of the cribriform plate and forms the floor of the anterior cranial fossa. The cribriform plate is slightly caudal in position relative to the ethmoid roof and lies on either side of crista galli. The anterior ethmoid air cells drain into the anterior aspect of the middle meatus and the posterior ethmoid cells drain into the superior meatus.

Frontal

The frontal sinuses are variable in configuration and are usually asymmetric in the same individual. A bony septum divides the frontal sinuses into right and left sinuses. The posterior wall of the frontal sinus separates it from the anterior cranial fossa. Each frontal sinus drains into the middle meatus via the nasofrontal duct which traverses through the ethmoid labyrinth.

Sphenoid

The sphenoid sinus is highly variable in size and configuration. The septum that divides the sphenoid sinus into two parts is not usually in the midline. The carotid arteries are in close proximity to the sphenoid sinus. The sphenoid sinus pneumatization can extend into the floor of the middle cranial fossa on either side or into the pterygoid plates. The roof of the sphenoid sinus is the planum sphenoidale anteriorly and sella turcica posteriorly. Inferiorly, this sinus is bounded by the nasopharynx. Anteriorly, the sphenoid sinus abuts against the posterior margin of the ethmoid sinus and posteriorly it is bounded by the clivus. The ostium of the sphenoid sinus opens in the spheno-ethmoid recess which is above and behind the superior turbinate.

Nasal cavity

The nasal cavity is triangular in shape. The broad base is formed by the palatal process of the maxilla and the horizontal segment of palatine bone. The apex is at the roof of the nasal cavity which is formed by the cribriform plate. The lateral wall is complex and is formed by parts of the maxilla, lacrimal and ethmoid bones and the perpendicular plate of the palatine bone. There are three projections along the lateral wall, formed by the superior, middle and inferior turbinates or conchae. The nasal septum is formed by the perpendicular plate of the ethmoid bone, the septal cartilage and the vomer bones. The anterior soft portion of the nasal septum is composed of the medial limbs of the U-shaped alar cartilage and the soft tissues between the tip of the nose and anterior nasal spine.

Several important openings are present along the lateral wall of the nasal cavity in the superior, middle and inferior meati which are located below each of the turbinates, respectively. The naso-lacrimal duct opens in the inferior meatus. The middle turbinate extends vertically up to attach to the cribriform plate. Another bony attachment extends via a bony strut termed the basal lamella and separates the anterior ethmoid air cells from the posterior ethmoid cells. The middle meatus receives drainages from the maxillary sinus, anterior ethmoid air cells and the frontal sinus (Fig. 1.1). An aerated middle turbinate is termed concha bullosa, and represents a common normal variant. It is best demonstrated by CT.[2]

Ostiomeatal unit

Because of recent advances in sinus endoscopic surgery, a thorough understanding of the anatomy of the ostiomeatal unit has become essential.[3–5]

The anatomic landmarks of the ostiomeatal unit are the maxillary sinus ostium and infundibulum, ethmoid bulla, uncinate process and hiatus semilunaris. Ethmoid bulla refers to an ethmoid air cell which is located antero-inferiorly and forms the superior lateral boundary of the ethmoid infundibulum. The maxillary sinus ostium and ethmoid infundibulum form the major passage for maxillary sinus into the middle meatus. The ethmoid infundibulum is bordered by the uncinate process medially, the infero-medial orbit laterally, the ethmoid bulla and hiatus semilunaris superiorly and the maxillary sinus inferiorly. The ostiomeatal unit can be best imaged by CT in the coronal plane (Fig. 1.2).

Imaging strategies

Computed tomography

Computed tomography scans are performed in the axial and coronal plane routinely. Axial scans are done parallel to the infraorbital meatal line. Five-millimeter-thick sections from the level of the hard palate to the orbital roof are adequate in the axial plane and from the posterior clinoid to the nasal bone are sufficient in the coronal plane. The use of intravenous contrast is variable. The authors do not use contrast as a routine. In patients with a suspected neoplasm, 100 ml bolus of iodinated contrast is administered followed by a continuous slow infusion drip.

Magnetic resonance imaging

Magnetic resonance examination is performed using a head coil. A sagittal localizer is performed by cephalocaudal orientation. T1- and T2-weighted images are obtained in axial and coronal planes covering the same anatomic regions as described with CT. Usually two averages are sufficient and keep the imaging time short. The advantages of MRI include multiplanar imaging capability, lack of ionizing radiation and superior soft tissue contrast. The artifact secondary to dental fillings is rather localized and does not degrade the entire image, unlike the streaking seen on CT images.

Disadvantages, however, include insensitivity to calcium and inability to detect subtle bone erosions. By MRI, a majority of the sinonasal tumors reveal intermediate signal intensity on T1-weighted and T2-weighted images. Inflammatory changes usually show low signal intensity on T1-weighted and high signal intensity on T2-weighted images. However, there is a considerable overlap of signal intensities. Intravenous administration of 0.1 mmol/kg of gadopentetate dimeglumine (Magnevist, Berlex Inc., Wayne, NJ, USA) can be useful in differentiating mucoceles from neoplasms and in accurately defining the extent of the tumor, particularly intracranial and perineural spread. The assessment of histopathological diagnosis of tumors by MRI as initially anticipated has been rather disappointing.

The normal anatomic landmarks of the nasal cavity and paranasal sinuses on CT and MRI are depicted in axial and coronal planes in Figs 1.2–1.6.

Pathology

Inflammatory disease

Sinusitis may be secondary to infection, allergy, altered immunity, or a combination of the above three factors. The maxillary antrum is the most frequently involved sinus. Sinus opacification and mucosal thickening may be seen with acute or chronic inflammation. Air-fluid levels signify acute infectious sinusitis in absence of other factors such as trauma and antral lavage. The common implicating pathogens are pneumococcus, Hemophilus influenzae and β-hemolytic streptococcus. Multisinus involvement, polypoid mucosal thickening and enlarged turbinates suggest allergic sinusitis.

The normal sinus mucosa is not usually visualized by CT. In the presence of an opacified sinus, contrast-enhanced CT can differentiate infected mucosa from retained secretions. Magnetic resonance imaging is very sensitive in the delineation of inflammatory disease, usually revealing low signal intensity on T1-weighted image and high signal intensity on T2-weighted image. Normal diurnal cyclical changes showing hyperintensity on T2-weighted images limited to the mucosa of the turbinates, nasal cavity and ethmoid sinuses is described.[6] Mucosal thickening in the maxillary sinuses up to 3 mm in asymptomatic patients is a common finding and is of uncertain significance.[7] On the other hand, even minimal disease in the sphenoid sinus should not be casually dismissed, but carefully evaluated in the appropriate clinical context because of the close proximity of the sphenoid sinus to important neurovascular structures such as the optic nerve, the first two divisions of the trigeminal nerve and the carotid artery.[8]

In children under the age of 3 years, the sinuses are usually opaque as a result of redundancy of mucosa. An opacified sinus in childhood does not indicate sinusitis unless there is clinical corroboratory evidence such as local pain, tenderness or discharge from the sinus.[9]

Computed tomography is the modality of choice for imaging inflammatory disease of the paranasal sinuses. Because of better pathophysiologic understanding of mucociliary action and drainage of the sinuses, endoscopic surgery has rapidly become the standard practice. High-resolution CT demonstrates the ostiomeatal complex and thus provides a 'road map' for the surgeons. Computed tomographic characteristics of inflammatory disease include mucosal thickening, air–fluid levels, soft tissue mass, sinus opacification and osseous changes (Fig. 1.6).

By MRI, the inflammatory disease usually reveals high signal intensity on T2-weighted images and low signal on T1-weighted images (Figs 1.7 and 1.8) because of the dominant water component of sinonasal secretions which contain 95% water and 5% proteins. However, in chronically obstructed sinuses, T1 and T2 relaxation times are extremely variable depending upon the protein concentration and the extent of free water resorption (Fig. 1.9). The signal intensity of the sinonasal secretions in an obstructed sinus becomes brighter as the protein content increases up to approximately 25% on T1-weighted images due to free water resorption, while the signal intensity on T2-weighted images remains high. Above 25% protein concentration, a significant cross-linking between protein macromolecules occurs, leading to increased viscosity. The T1- and T2-weighted signal intensities thus decrease, suggesting that these concentrated secretions behave like solid material lacking free mobile protons. The signal void thus may mimic a normal aerated sinus and create a major pitfall in the diagnosis of inflammatory disease.[10,11]

Aggressive inflammatory diseases

Aggressive fungal infections such as mucormycosis, invasive aspergillosis and nocardia usually manifest in debilitated or immune-compromised patients. These infections can invade blood vessels and cause vascular occlusions. Mycetomas and the allergic type of aspergillosis occur in otherwise healthy subjects. Mycetomas are usually associated with single sinus disease while the allergic type of sinusitis involves multiple sinuses. Computed tomography manifestations include soft tissue density in the sinuses often with high density foci and concretions.[12] Bone destruction mimicking carcinoma is seen only with invasive aspergillosis or other mycotic infections (Fig. 1.10). Magnetic resonance imaging characteristically reveals intermediate signal on T1-weighted images and hypointense signal on T2-weighted images. These signal characteristics may be related to the high viscosity of the secretions, high protein and calcium content, and low hydration state. The paramagnetic effect of iron and manganese may also be a contributory factor.[13,14]

Wegener's granulomatosis and midline granuloma

Wegener's granulomatosis is caused by an underlying vasculitis which produces not only diffuse destructive lesions of the nasal cavity and paranasal sinuses, but also lung and kidney involvement. Computed tomography reveals soft tissue nodules and mucosal thickening involving the nasal cavity and septum and subsequently involving the paranasal sinuses (Fig. 1.11). Bony destruction may be visible on CT.[15,16] Midline granuloma is a local aggressive process in the nasal cavity not associated with systemic involvement and vasculitis. The radiographic features are similar to that of Wegener's granulomatosis in the nasal cavity.

Sarcoidosis

Sarcoidosis in the sinonasal region manifests as soft tissue thickening or granuloma formation on the nasal septum and turbinates.[17] The CT and MR findings are nonspecific (Fig. 1.12). Computed tomography reveals nodular soft tissue thickening in the nasal cavity, nasal septum and paranasal sinuses.

Complications of sinusitis

Retention cysts

Mucous retention cysts result from inflammatory obstruction of seromucinous glands. Serous retention cysts form secondary to submucosal accumulation of serous fluid. Retention cysts characteristically are seen as smooth, dome-shaped structures frequently along the inferior aspect of the maxillary sinus. Computed tomography reveals smooth masses of low attenuation. By MRI, retention cysts have low signal on T1-weighted and high signal on T2-weighted images (Fig. 1.13).

Polyps

Nasal and paranasal sinus polyps form as a result of folding and hypertrophy of mucosa with submucosal accumulation of fluid. An association of allergy, inflammation, infection and vasomotor rhinitis with polyp formation is described. Because of similar CT and MRI characteristics, a small polyp in the sinus cannot be differentiated from a retention cyst. Computed tomography reveals a mass of low attenuation and MRI shows low signal on T1-weighted and high signal on T2-weighted images.

Nasal polyps have been associated with intolerance to aspirin. The triad consists of aspirin intolerance, nasal polyposis and bronchial asthma.[18] Allergic type of chronic hypertrophic polypoid rhinosinusitis is associated with multiple polyps which present as expansile masses. Bone erosion due to expanding masses is seen. Longstanding polyps may undergo necrosis or desiccation. The MR appearance of chronic desiccated polyposis and sinusitis may show very low signal or signal void on both T1- and T2-weighted images, mimicking aerated sinuses (Fig. 1.14).[10,11]

Antrochoanal polyp

Antrochoanal polyps are benign, solitary polypoid lesions that arise in the maxillary sinus and grow until they cause complete opacification of the antrum. These subsequently extend through the ostium into the nasal cavity and through the posterior choana into the nasopharynx.[19] Occasionally, these polyps may be purely choanal or arise in the sphenoid sinus (sphenochoanal).[20] Tracing the polyps to their origin is easily done by CT or MRI and is essential for complete surgical resection of these polyps.[21] Acute sinusitis with edematous redundant mucosa may prolapse through the ostiomeatal complex and mimic an antrochoanal polyp (Figs 1.15 and 1.16).[22]

Mucocele

Mucoceles are expansile lesions of the sinuses resulting from ostial obstruction, which is usually secondary to inflammatory scarring and occasionally caused by trauma or tumor. The frontal sinuses are most frequently involved (65%), followed by the ethmoid sinus (25%). Less than 10% of mucoceles occur in the maxillary sinuses and sphenoid sinus mucoceles are rare. Computed tomography reveals a non-enhancing, low attenuation expansile mass in the sinus.[23–25] The bony margins may be thinned and eroded due to pressure erosion. This is in contrast to the aggressive destruction seen in squamous cell carcinoma.

Magnetic resonance imaging demonstrates mucoceles as well-defined, expansile masses with variable signal intensities using spin-echo techniques (Figs 1.17–1.20). The signal intensity on T1-weighted images may be isointense, low or higher than that of muscle. A similar variation in the signal intensity of mucocele is found on T2-weighted images. The two most frequently observed patterns include moderate to marked hyperintense signal on both T1- and T2-weighted images, and moderate to marked low signal on both T1- and T2-weighted images.[26–28] The marked variation in signal intensity depends primarily upon the state of hydration, protein content and viscosity of the contents of mucoceles.

Regional and intracranial complications

These include periorbital and orbital cellulitis, subperiosteal orbital abscess, superior orbital fissure syndrome, subdural empyema, brain abscess, osteomyelitis, meningitis and venous sinus thrombosis. The orbital complications most commonly result from ethmoid sinusitis spreading through the thin lamina papryacea, or through the emissary veins. The frontal sinusitis is often implicated in intracranial complications. These potential complications of sinusitis are easily diagnosed by CT or MRI (Figs 1.21 and 1.22).[29,30]

Malignant tumors

Squamous cell carcinoma

Squamous cell carcinoma is the most common malignant tumor of the paranasal sinuses and nasal cavity and accounts for 80–90% of all neoplasms. There is a 2:1 male predominance, and 95% of patients are over 40 years of age. Eighty per cent of the squamous cell carcinomas arising from the sinuses occur in the maxillary sinus and 10–20% occur in the ethmoid sinuses. The frontal and sphenoid sinuses are rarely involved by carcinoma. An association of sinus carcinoma with exposure to mustard gas, chromium, isopropyl alcohol and radium is described.[31] Squamous cell carcinoma is often associated with pre-existing chronic sinusitis. The tumor mass may further obstruct the ostium and cause secondary sinusitis. Thus, differentiation of tumor from coexistent inflammatory disease becomes important (Figs 1.23–1.26).

Computed tomography reveals a soft tissue mass in the sinus, usually with aggressive bone destruction. The lack of bone expansion in squamous cell carcinoma is emphasized which differentiates it from other maxillary malignancies.[32] However, in our experience, and also described by other investigators,[33] no significant difference in the proportion of bone expansion between squamous cell carcinoma and other malignancies was found.

These carcinomas enhance minimally following intravenous contrast administration, making differentiation between the tumor mass and obstructed sinus difficult. Magnetic resonance imaging is superior to CT in mapping tumors.[34,35] T2-weighted MR images can be extremely useful because of the inherent differences in signal intensity of the tumor and inflammatory sinus disease. The sinonasal carcinomas usually reveal homogeneous intermediate signal intensity on both T1- and T2-weighted images, because of their uniform cellular pattern.[34] However, tumor necrosis and hemorrhage may cause inhomogeneity. Foci of necrosis show focal areas of low signal on T1-weighted images that become hyperintense on T2-weighted images. Foci of hemorrhage show variable signal intensities depending upon the nature of the hemorrhagic products. The pattern of enhancement with gadolinium administration can further aid in differentiating mucoceles from neoplasms; mucoceles show ring-like enhancement while the tumors enhance diffusely and often homogeneously. While bone erosion is often considered to be a hallmark of malignancy, it may occur with histologically benign lesions such as longstanding chronic polyps and mucoceles at the skull base. Magnetic resonance imaging can help separate such benign lesions from malignant tumors, by the morphology and signal characteristics.[36]

Adenocarcinoma

Adenocarcinoma most commonly occurs in the ethmoid sinuses. Woodworkers in the hardwood furniture industry have a higher incidence of ethmoid adenocarcinoma. Males between the ages of 55 and 65 years are affected more frequently. Computed tomography usually demonstrates a soft tissue mass which enhances only slightly with contrast. Bone erosion and intracranial extension are common. The signal intensity on T1- and T2-weighted MR images is variable and slight enhancement with gadolinium administration is usually observed (Fig. 1.27). The usual pattern includes intermediate signal on T1-weighted and intermediate to high signal on T2-weighted images.

Adenoid cystic carcinoma

Adenoid cystic carcinoma (cylindroma) arises from the accessory salivary glands. There is no sex predilection and peak incidence is in the fourth decade. The growth rate is variable. These tumors have a propensity for perineural invasion; distant metastases occur in 20–30% of patients.[37] The salivary gland carcinomas typically reveal low signal on both T1- and T2-weighted images while the benign tumors such as pleomorphic adenomas are bright on T2-weighted images. Magnetic resonance imaging is superior in tumor mapping and also in its ability to demonstrate perineural extension of tumor with gadolinium enhancement (Fig. 1.28).

Lymphoma

Lymphomas arising in the sinonasal region are almost always non-Hodgkin's lymphomas (NHL). Non-Hodgkin's lymphomas can be further divided by location into (1) nodal; (2) extranodal, lymphatic (Waldeyer's Ring); and (3) extranodal, extralymphatic (sinonasal, orbit, face, parotids, skin).[38] Hodgkin's disease in the extranodal, extralymphatic site is extremely rare.[39] Lymphoma usually presents as bulky soft tissue masses that insinuate from one anatomic space into the next with relatively little bone erosion. Computed tomography reveals bulky homogeneous soft tissue masses. The nodal NHL usually reveals enlarged homogeneous nodes with relative absence of central necrosis. Extranodal, lymphatic NHL in the Waldeyer's Ring may be indistinguishable from other malignancies. Extranodal, extralymphatic NHL in the sinonasal region may demonstrate expansile masses with permeative bone involvement.[40] However, infiltration and destruction similar to squamous cell carcinoma is also described.[38] Magnetic resonance imaging demonstrates intermediate signal intensity on both T1- and T2-weighted sequences (Figs 1.29 and 1.30).

Melanoma

In the sinonasal tract, malignant melanomas arise from melanocytes within the nasal mucosa over the turbinates and septum and account for 1% of all melanomas. Metastatic melanoma is rare in this location. Computed tomography reveals an expansile, homogeneously enhancing mass. Magnetic resonance imaging shows a homogeneous mass with intermediate or high signal intensity on T1-weighted image and intermediate or low signal intensity on T2-weighted image (Figs 1.31 and 1.32). Melanotic melanomas have a characteristic intensity pattern on MR images unlike any other tumor; hyperintense on T1- and hypointense on T2-weighted images. This pattern is attributed to the paramagnetic effect of melanin, which is also dependent on the field strength of the magnet.[41] The paramagnetic effect of the associated products of hemorrhage is also contributory.[42] About one-fourth of the melanomas are amelanotic and reveal signal intensities similar to those of other sinonasal tumors.

Esthesioneuroblastoma

Esthesioneuroblastoma arises from the basal layer of olfactory epithelium high in the nasal cavity. Its peak incidence is in the second and third decades with a slight male predominance. These tumors are locally invasive and recurrences are common. Distant metastases are seen only in 10–20%. Histologic appearance is easily confused with anaplastic carcinoma, melanoma, plasmacytoma or histiocytic lymphoma. Secretory catecholamine granules seen by electron microscopy confirm the diagnosis.[37] Computed tomography reveals an expansile nasal mass which often extends into the ethmoid sinuses or cranial cavity (Fig. 1.33). Exuberant bony proliferation can be seen rarely.[43] Magnetic resonance characteristics include intermediate signal intensity on both T1- and T2-weighted images (Fig. 1.34).[44]

Extramedullary plasmacytoma

Extramedullary plasmacytoma accounts for about 3–4% of sinonasal tumors. This tumor is more common in men than women and usually occurs above 40 years of age. The majority of the extramedullary plasmacytomas occur in the upper respiratory tract. Although only about 20% of these patients initially show accompanying multiple myeloma, up to 50% eventually develop disseminated disease. Computed tomography reveals expansile masses which usually enhance homogeneously. Bone erosion is either minimal or absent.[45] Magnetic resonance imaging reveals intermediate signal on T1- and T2-weighted images (Fig. 1.35).

Malignant fibrous histiocytoma

Fibrous histiocytoma is a neoplasm composed of fibroblasts and histiocytes, often occurring in the retroperitoneum, abdomen, extremities or sinonasal region. Most of the fibrous histiocytomas in the head and neck region are malignant. There is a predilection for men. Computed tomography reveals homogeneous soft tissue masses which may cause bone destruction. Magnetic resonance imaging usually shows intermediate signal intensity on T1- and T2-weighted images (Fig. 1.36).[46]

Osteosarcoma

An estimated 10% of all osteosarcomas occur in the head and neck region, predominantly in the mandible and maxilla. Conversely, these tumors comprise less than 1% of all head and neck tumors. Although most osteosarcomas in the sinonasal region arise in the alveolar ridge of the maxilla, a subgroup arising primarily within the nasal cavity and paranasal sinuses is described.[47] Computed tomography reveals soft tissue masses with aggressive bone destruction. Although new tumor bone formation occurs in only 20–30% of the cases, when seen, this appearance clinches the diagnosis (Fig. 1.37). These tumors can be purely lytic. Magnetic resonance imaging may reveal low to intermediate signal on both T1- and T2-weighted images (Fig. 1.38).

Benign tumors

Osteoma

Osteomas most commonly occur in the frontal sinus and are of little clinical significance unless they block the sinus drainage. They are seen as dense, well-circumscribed masses (Fig. 1.39). In the maxillary sinuses, osteomas may mimic dental tumors.

Papilloma

Papillomas account for 4% of sinonasal tumors and are the most common benign tumors. Squamous papillomas usually occur along the nasal septum as solitary masses. There is no known malignant potential. Inverted papillomas characteristically arise along the lateral nasal wall and are so called because the surface epithelium inverts into the stroma on histology. They are locally invasive and may grow into the ipsilateral maxillary sinus or ethmoid sinus. Men are more frequently affected, usually above the age of 40 years. An associated malignancy, usually squamous cell carcinoma, is reported in 10–15% of patients with inverted papilloma.[37] Computed tomography reveals polypoid expansile masses in the nasal cavity which may remodel or erode bone.[48,49] Calcification may occur occasionally, especially in recurrent tumors (Figs 1.40 and 1.41). Magnetic resonance imaging is not sensitive in the detection of calcification. The signal characteristics include low to intermediate signal on all pulse sequences.

Hemangioma

Hemangiomas most frequently occur in the vertebral bodies and calvaria. Hemangiomas arising in the sinuses are rare. When confined to bone, CT shows an expansile mass with a radiating trabecular pattern.[50] However, these lesions can expand into the sinus and present as large masses with bone destruction (Fig. 1.42).[51] Preoperative diagnosis lowers the risk of exsanguination accompanying biopsy or surgery. By MRI, hemangiomas reveal low signal on T1- and high signal on T2-weighted images (Fig. 1.43).[51]

Pleomorphic adenoma (benign mixed tumor)

These tumors arise from minor salivary glands, usually occur along the palate and can expand into the nasal cavity or sinuses. Occasionally, these tumors can arise along the septum in the nasal cavity. Computed tomography shows inhomogeneous masses that remodel bone. Magnetic resonance imaging reveals high signal intensity on T2-weighted images (Fig. 1.44).

Neurogenic tumors

Neurinomas in the nasal cavity or paranasal sinuses are rare. They may also secondarily extend into the sinuses from the parapharyngeal space and infratemporal fossa or arise from the 5th, 9th, 10th, 11th or 12th cranial nerves. Computed tomography reveals expansile masses which enhance inhomogeneously (Fig. 1.45). These tumors demonstrate low signal intensity on T1-weighted images and variable signal (usually high) intensity on T2-weighted images.

Secondary tumors

Odontogenic cysts and tumors

A large variety of odontogenic cysts and tumors occur in the mandible and maxilla. Only common lesions that may expand into the maxillary sinuses are presented.

Ameloblastoma

Ameloblastoma is a benign epithelial odontogenic tumor and accounts for about 1% of all tumors and cysts in the jaw. Ameloblastomas occur more commonly in the mandible than in the maxilla. Radiographically, they can present as unilocular or multilocular radiolucent lesions.[37] The size of the lesion varies from a small cyst confined to the bone to large expansile and erosive lesion. Ameloblastomas that grow into the maxillary sinus from the maxilla present as large expansile antral lesions. Magnetic resonance imaging may reveal intermediate signal intensity on both T1- and T2-weighted images. Enhancement with gadolinium may be inhomogeneous (Fig. 1.46).

Dentigerous cyst

Dentigerous cysts arise from the enamel organ after amelogenesis has been completed and are associated with an unerupted tooth. These occur in the mandible more frequently than the maxilla. These cysts usually manifest in the second decade. Radiographically, they present as unilocular cystic lesions that can expand bone and grow into the sinus if they arise in the maxilla (Fig. 1.47). Dentigerous cysts have the potential to develop into ameloblastoma.[37]

Pituitary tumors

Pituitary tumors are classified as expanding adenoma, invasive adenoma or carcinoma based on the biologic behavior. Invasive adenomas, although histologically benign, locally invade the adjacent regions. Magnetic resonance imaging may show intense enhancement with gadolinium (Fig. 1.48). Extension of tumor into the suprasellar cistern should raise the index of suspicion for pituitary origin.

Nasopharyngeal tumors

Nasopharyngeal angiofibroma and nasopharyngeal carcinoma can invade the paranasal sinuses. These tumors are discussed in detail in Chapter 4.

Metastatic tumors

Although uncommon, metastases to the sinuses and nasal cavity from distant primary tumors such as renal, breast and lung carcinomas are reported.

Computed tomography reveals soft tissue masses with bone destruction which enhance minimally and are similar to the primary squamous cell carcinoma (Fig. 1.49). Vascular metastases from renal cell carcinoma or melanoma may also show moderate to marked enhancement. In 8% of patients, metastatic tumor in the sinonasal region may be the presenting mass with a silent primary tumor.[52]

Miscellaneous

Fibrous dysplasia

Fibrous dysplasia is a disease of unknown pathogenesis in which the medullary cavity is replaced by fibrous tissue with the potential for new bone formation by osseous metaplasia. Three radiographic patterns seen by plain films and CT are described: sclerotic, cystic and pagetoid.[53,54] The sclerotic type is common in the maxilla and reveals diffuse increased homogeneous density which expands the bone. The cystic type is more common in the mandible and demonstrates a cystic area with sharp and sclerotic margins. The pagetoid form reveals marked expansion of the bone with alternating areas of radiolucency and radiodensity; it resembles Paget's disease. Magnetic resonance imaging reveals predominantly low signal intensity on T1- and T2-weighted images with the sclerotic type of fibrous dysplasia. Cystic types may reveal variable signal intensity on T1- and T2-weighted images (Fig. 1.50).

Fat ablation of frontal sinuses

Following fat ablation of frontal sinuses, CT reveals soft tissue of low attenuation similar to that of subcutaneous fat. Magnetic resonance demonstrates high signal on T1-weighted images and intermediate signal on T2-weighted images. This appearance should not be mistaken for blood products or mucoproteinaceous secretions in the sinus (Fig. 1.51).

Polymethylmethacrylate cranioplasty

Polymethylmethacrylate is commonly used to repair craniotomy or craniectomy defects. These cranioplasty plates on CT characteristically show multiple gas bubbles within the prosthesis (Fig. 1.52). The gas bubbles result from rapid mixing of the liquid and solid components of the plastic to ensure homogeneity. This appearance should not be confused with infection and abscess formation. The surface density of the plates is similar to that of soft tissue or brain. However, premanufactured, pressure-cured plates do not contain bubbles.[55]

References

1 MARESH MM, Paranasal sinuses from birth to adolescence, *Am J Dis Child* (1940) **60**:58.

2 ZINREICH SJ, MATTOX DE, KENNEDY DW et al, Concha bullosa: CT evaluation, *J Comput Assist Tomogr* (1988) **12**:778–84.

3 KENNEDY DW, ZINREICH SJ, ROSENBAUM AE et al, Functional endoscopic sinus surgery: theory and diagnostic evaluation, *Arch Otolaryngol* (1985) **111**:576–82.

4 ZINREICH SJ, KENNEDY DW, ROSENBAUM AE et al, Paranasal sinuses: CT imaging requirements for endoscopic surgery, *Radiology* (1987) **163**:769–75.

5 TERRIER F, WEBER W, RUEFENACHT D et al, Anatomy of the ethmoid: CT, endoscopic and macroscopic, *AJNR* (1985) **6**:77–84.

6 ZINREICH SJ, KENNEDY DW, KUMAR AJ et al, MR imaging of normal nasal cycle: comparison with sinus pathology, *J Comput Assist Tomogr* (1988) **12**:1014–19.

7 RAK KM, NEWELL JD II, YAKES WF et al, Paranasal sinuses on MR images of the brain: significance of mucosal thickening. *AJNR* (1990) **11**:1211–14.

8 DIGRE KB, MAXNER CE, CRAWFORD S et al, Significance of CT and MR findings in sphenoid sinus disease, *AJNR* (1989) **10**:603–6.

9 TOWBIN R, DUNBAR JS, The paranasal sinuses in childhood, *Radiographics* (1982) **2**:253–79.

10 SOM PM, DILLON WP, FULLERTON GD et al, Chronically obstructed sinonasal secretions: observations on T1 and T2 shortening, *Radiology* (1989) **172**:515–20.

11 DILLON WP, SOM PM, FULLERTON GD, Hypointense MR signal in chronically inspissated sinonasal secretions, *Radiology* (1990) **174**:73–8.

12 KOPP W, FOTER R, STEINER H et al, Aspergillosis of the paranasal sinuses, *Radiology* (1985) **156**:715.

13 SOM PM, DILLON WP, CURTIN HD et al, Hypointense paranasal sinus foci: differential diagnosis with MR imaging and relation to CT findings, *Radiology* (1990) **176**:777–81.

14 ZINREICH SJ, KENNEDY DW, MALAT J et al, Fungal sinusitis: diagnosis with CT and MR imaging, *Radiology* (1988) **169**:439–44.

15 PALING MR, ROBERTS RL, FAUCI AS, Paranasal sinus obliteration in Wegener granulomatosis, *Radiology* (1982) **144**:539.

16 SIMMONS JT, LEAVITT R, KORNBLUT AD et al, CT of paranasal sinuses and orbits in patients with Wegener's granulomatosis, *Ear, Nose Throat* (1987) **66**:134–40.

17 MAILLARD AAJ, GEOPFERT H, Nasal and paranasal sarcoidosis, *Arch Otolaryngol* (1978) **104**:197–201.

18 MOLONEY JR, Nasal polyps, nasal polypectomy, asthma and aspirin sensitivity: their association in 445 cases of nasal polyps, *J Laryngol Otol* (1977) **91**:837.

19 TOWBIN R, DUNBAR JS, BOVE K, Antrochoanal polyps, *AJR* (1979) **132**:27–31.

20 HAYES E, LAVELLE W, Sphenochoanal polyp: CT findings, *J Comput Assist Tomogr* (1989) **13**:365–6.

21 WEISSMAN JL, TABOR EK, CURTIN HD, Sphenochoanal polyps: evaluation with CT and MR imaging, *Radiology* (1991) **178**:145–8.

22 NINO-MURCIA M, RAO VM, MIKAELIAN DO et al, Acute sinusitis mimicking antrochoanal polyp, *AJNR* (1986) **7**:513.

23 HESSELINK JR, WEBER AL, NEW PJ et al, Evaluation of mucoceles of the paranasal sinuses with computed tomography, *Radiology* (1979) **133**:397–400.

24 CHUI MC, BRIANT TDR, GRAY T et al, Computed tomography of sphenoid sinus mucocele, *J Otolaryngol* (1983) **12**:263–9.

25 PERUGINI S, PASQUINI U, MENICHELLI F et al, Mucoceles in the paranasal sinuses involving the orbit: CT signs in 43 cases, *Neuroradiology* (1982) **23**:133–9.

26 VAN TASSEL P, LEE YY, JIN BS et al, Mucoceles of the paranasal sinuses: MR imaging with CT correlation, *AJNR* (1989) **10**:607–12.

27 FLANDERS AE, RAO VM, Paranasal sinus mucocele: unusual MR manifestations at 1.5 T, *Magn Reson Imaging* (1989) **7**:333–7.

28 DAWSON RC, HORTON JA, MR imaging of mucoceles of the sphenoid sinus, *AJNR* (1989) **10**:613–14.

29 ZIMMERMAN RA, BILANIUK LT, CT of orbital infection and its cerebral complications, *AJR* (1980) **134**:45.

30 BILANIUK LT, ZIMMERMAN RA, Computer assisted tomography: sinus lesions with orbital involvement, *Head Neck Surg* (1980) **2**:293.

31 SOM P, BERGERON RT (eds) Tumor and tumor-like conditions. In: *Head and Neck Imaging* (Mosby: St Louis 1991) 169–227.

32 SOM PM, SHUGAN JMA, Significance of bone expansion associated with the diagnosis of malignant tumors of the paranasal sinuses, *Radiology* (1980) **136**:97–100.

33 SILVER AJ, BAREDES S, BELLO JA et al, Opacified maxillary sinus: CT findings in chronic sinusitis and malignant tumors, *Radiology* (1987) **163**:205–10.

34 SHAPIRO MD, SOM PM, MRI of the paranasal sinuses and nasal cavity, *Radiol Clin North Am* (1989) **27**:447–75.

35 CRAWFORD SC, HARNSBERGER HR, LUFKIN RB et al, The role of gadolinium in the evaluation of extracranial head and neck mass lesions, *Radiol Clin North Am* (1989) **27**:219–42.

36 SOM PM, DILLON WP, SZE G et al, Benign and malignant sinonasal lesions with intracranial extension: differentiating with MR imaging, *Radiology* (1989) **172**:763–6.

37 BATSAKIS JG (ed), *Tumors of the Head and Neck. Clinical and Pathological Considerations* (Williams and Wilkins: Baltimore 1979) 130–76.

38 HARNSBERGER HR, BRAGG DG, OSBORN AG et al, Non-Hodgkin's lymphoma of the head and neck: CT evaluation of nodal and extranodal sites, *AJNR* (1987) **8**:673–9.

39 SHLANSKY-GOLDBERG RD, RAO VM, CHOI HY et al, Hodgkin disease of the maxillary sinus, *J Comput Assist Tomogr* (1988) **12**:507–9.

40 KONDO M, HASHIMOTO T, SHINGA H et al, Computed tomography of sinonasal non-Hodgkin's lymphoma, *J Comput Assist Tomogr* (1984) **8**:216–19.

41 HAMMERSMITH SM, TERK MR, JEFFREY PB et al, Magnetic resonance imaging of nasopharyngeal and paranasal sinus melanoma, *Magn Reson Imaging* (1990) **8**:245–53.

42 GOMORI JM, GROSSMAN RE, SHIELDS JA et al, Choroidal melanomas: correlation of NMR spectroscopy and MR imaging, *Radiology* (1986) **158**:443–512.

43 REGENBOGEN VS, ZINREICH SJ, KIM KS et al, Hyperostotic esthesioneuroblastoma: CT and MR findings, *J Comput Assist Tomogr* (1988) **12**:52–6.

44 ROSENGREN JE, JING B, WALLACE S et al, Radiographic features of olfactory neuroblastoma, *AJR* (1979) **132**:945–8.

45 KONDO M, HASHIMOTO S, INUYAMA Y et al, Extramedullary plasmacytoma of the sinonasal cavities: CT evaluation, *J Comput Assist Tomogr* (1986) **10**: 841–4.

46 MERRICK RE, RHONE DP, CHILIS TJ, Malignant fibrous histiocytoma of the maxillary sinus, *Arch Otolaryngol* (1980) **106**:365.

47 OOT RF, PARIZEL PM, WEBER AL, Computed tomography of osteogenic sarcoma of nasal cavity and paranasal sinuses, *J Comput Assist Tomogr* (1986) **10**:409.

48 MOMOSE KJ, WEBER AL, GOODMAN M et al, Radiological aspects of inverted papilloma, *Radiology* (1980) **134**:73–9.

49 WILSON WR, CARROLL ED, BENTKOVER SH et al, Inverted papilloma, *Arch Otolaryngol* (1980) **106**:54–61.

50 STASSI J, RAO VM, LOWRY L, Hemangioma of bone arising in the maxilla, *Skeletal Radiol* (1984) **12**:187–91.

51 KULKARNI MV, BONNER FM, ABDOG J, Maxillary sinus hemangioma: MR and CT studies, *J Comput Assist Tomogr* (1989) **13**:340–2.

52 SOM PM, NORTON KI, SHUGAR JMA et al, Metastatic hypernephroma to the head and neck, *AJNR* (1987) **8**:1103.

53 FRIES JW, The roentgen features of fibrous dysplasia of the skull and facial bones, *AJR* (1957) **77**:71.

54 SHERMAN NH, RAO VM, BRENNAN RE et al, Fibrous dysplasia of the facial bones and mandible, *Skeletal Radiol* (1982) **8**:141–3.

55 MASON TO, ROSE BS, GOODMAN JH, Gas bubbles in polymethylmethacrylate cranioplasty simulating abscesses: CT appearance, *AJNR* (1986) **7**:829–31.

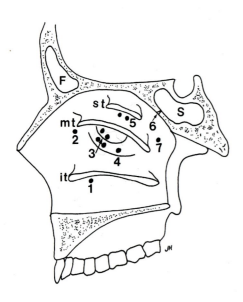

FIGURE 1.1

Drawing of the lateral wall of the nose depicting sinus ostia. The cut surfaces of the superior (st), middle (mt) and inferior (it) turbinates are depicted. F, frontal sinus: S, sphenoid sinus. The inferior meatus shows the opening of the nasolacrimal duct (1). The middle meatus contains the openings of the frontal sinus (2), anterior and middle ethmoid air cells (3), and the maxillary sinus (4). The superior meatus contains multiple ostia of the posterior ethmoid air cells (5). The sphenoid sinus drains into the sphenoethmoid recess (6). The sphenopalatine foramen (7) provides the connection between the nasal cavity medially and the pterygopalatine fossa laterally.

A

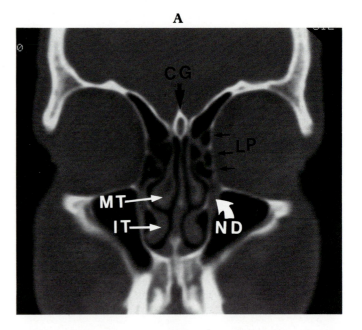

B

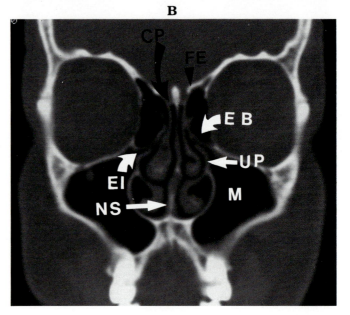

FIGURE 1.2

Normal CT anatomy in coronal plane: sections A – F (from anterior to posterior direction). (**A**) CT sections extends through the anterior aspect of the maxillary sinuses and anterior ethmoid. Inferior and middle turbinates (concha) are visualized on either side of the nasal septum. ND, nasolacrimal duct; IT, inferior turbinate; MT, middle turbinate; LP, lamina papyracea; CG, crista galli. (**B**) CT section through the ostiomeatal complex. UP, uncinate process; EI,

continued

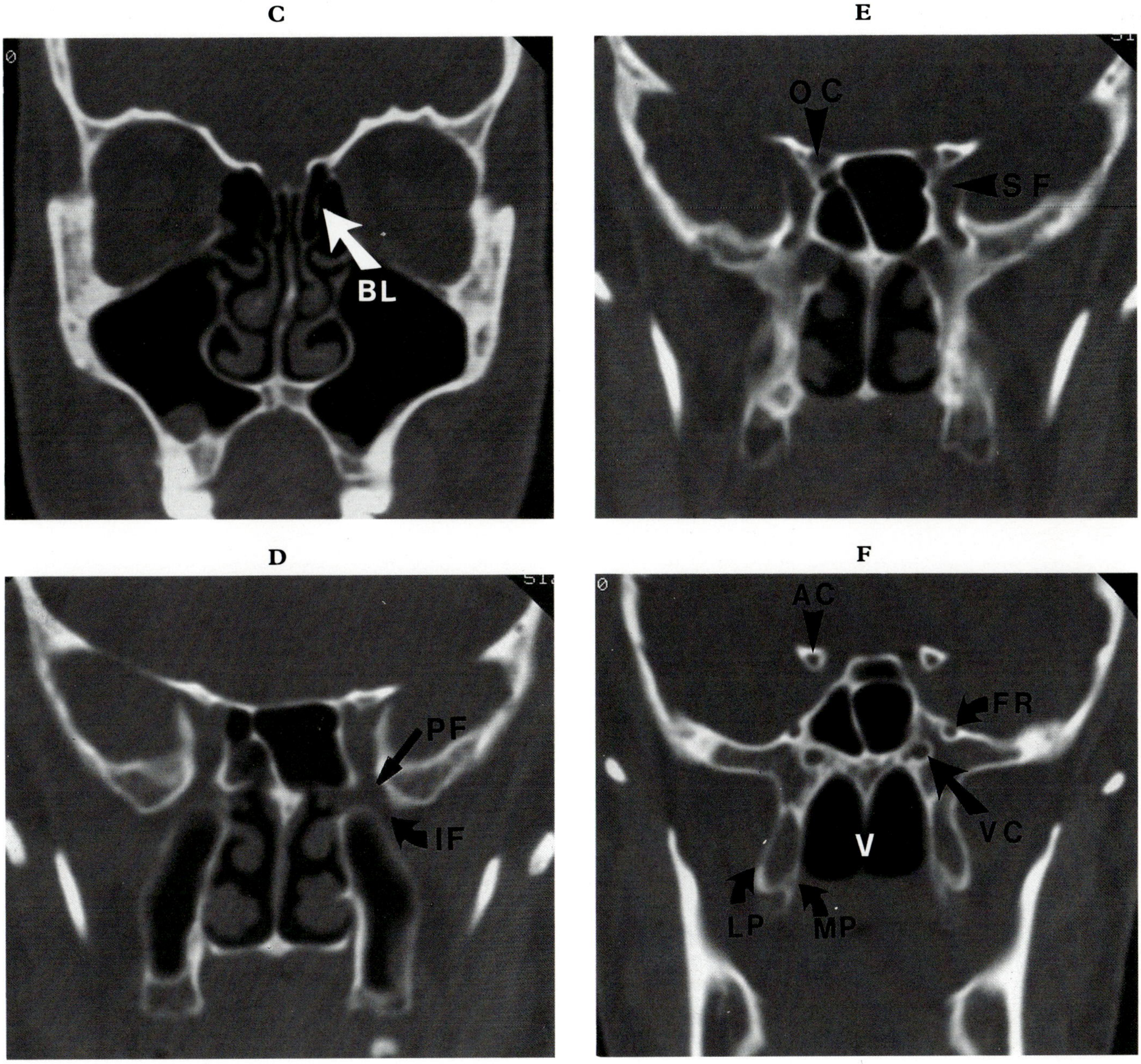

FIGURE 1.2 *(continued)*

ethmoid infundibulum; EB, ethmoid bulla; CP, cribriform plate; FE, fovea ethmoidalis; NS, nasal septum; M, maxillary sinus. (**C**) CT section through the middle of the maxillary sinuses and orbits. The basal lamella (BL) demarcates the anterior ethmoid cells from the posterior ethmoid cells. (**D**) CT section through the sphenoid sinus and close to the orbital apex. The pterygopalatine fossa (PF) and inferior orbital fissure (IF) are visualized.

(**E**) CT section demonstrates optic canal (OC) and superior orbital fissure (SF). (**F**) CT section shows foramen rotundum (FR) and vidian canal (VC). Vomer bone (V) forming posterior portion of the nasal septum and posterior choana are also in this plane. MP and LP, medial and lateral pterygoid plates are behind the maxillary sinus; AC, anterior clinoid.

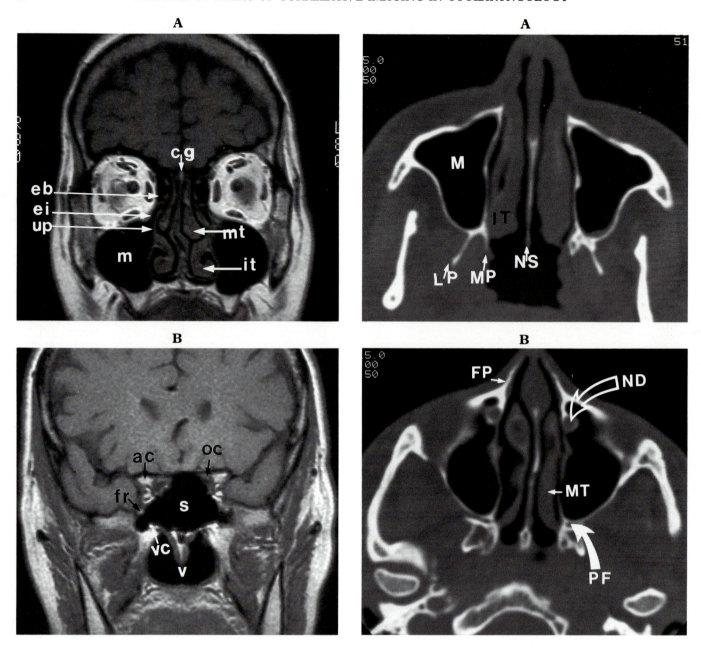

FIGURE 1.3

Normal MR anatomy in coronal plane. (**A**) T1-weighted spin echo (SE) (repetition time TR = 800 ms, echo delay time TE = 20 ms) MR image through the ostiomeatal unit. m, maxillary sinus; mt, middle turbinate; it, inferior turbinate; eb, ethmoid bulla; ei, ethmoid infundibulum; up, uncinate process; cg, crista galli. (**B**) T1-weighted SE (TR = 800 ms, TE = 20 ms) MR images through the sphenoid sinus (s). v, vomer; vc, vidian canal; fr, foramen rotundum; oc, optic canal; ac, anterior clinoid.

FIGURE 1.4

Normal CT anatomy in axial plane from inferior to superior direction. (**A**) Section through the lower maxillary sinuses (M). IT, inferior turbinate; NS, nasal septum; MP, medial pterygoid plate; LP, lateral pterygoid plate. (**B**) Section through middle of the maxillary sinuses. ND, nasolacrimal duct; MT, middle turbinate; FP, frontal process of maxilla; PF, pterygopalatine fossa.

continued

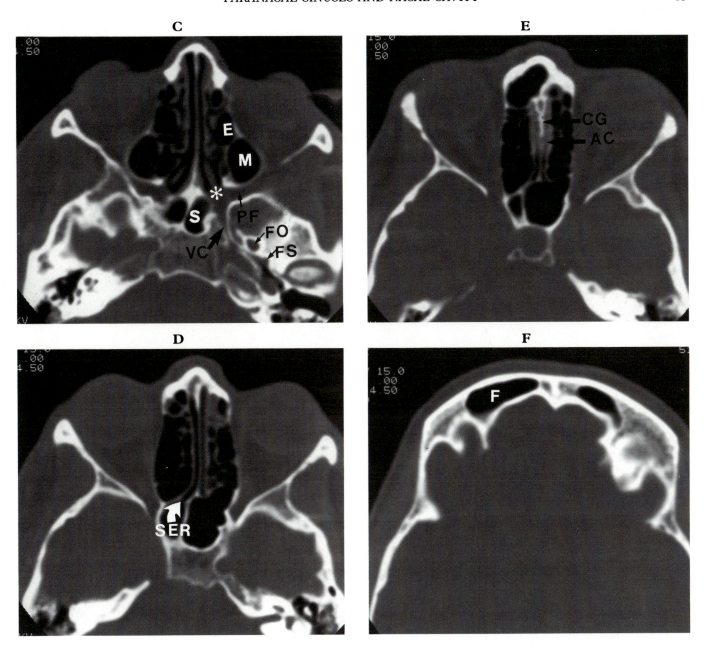

FIGURE 1.4 *(continued)*

(**C**) Section through the ethmoid (E), sphenoid (S), sinuses and the apex of maxillary sinus (M). PF, pterygopalatine fossa; *, sphenopalatine foramen; VC, vidian canal; FO, foramen ovale; FS, foramen spinosum. (**D**) Section through the sphenoethmoid recess (SER). (**E**) Section through the crista galli (CG). Note the soft tissue density of the anterior cranial fossa (AC) which should not be confused with ethmoid disease. (**F**) Section through the frontal sinuses (F).

A

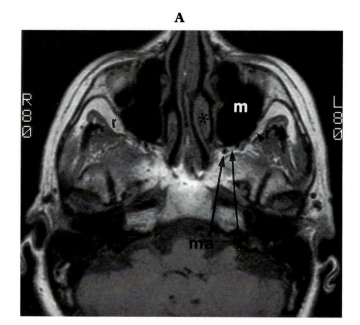

C

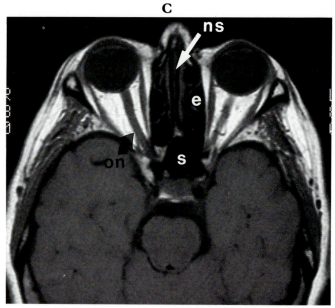

B

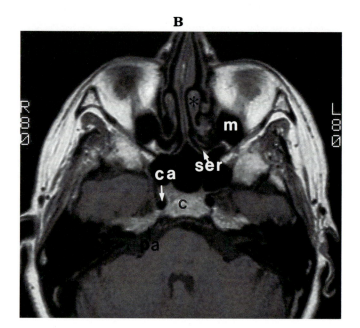

FIGURE 1.5

T1-weighted SE MR images depicting normal MR anatomy in axial plane. (**A**) Section through the mid maxillary sinus. The pterygopalatine fossa contains fat (pf). Note the signal void from internal maxillary artery (ma). Note fat in retroantral region (r). *, middle turbinate; m, maxillary sinuses. (**B**) Section through the apex of maxillary sinuses (m). The carotid artery (ca) does not reveal any signal. The clivus (c) and petrous apex (pa) show high signal

continued

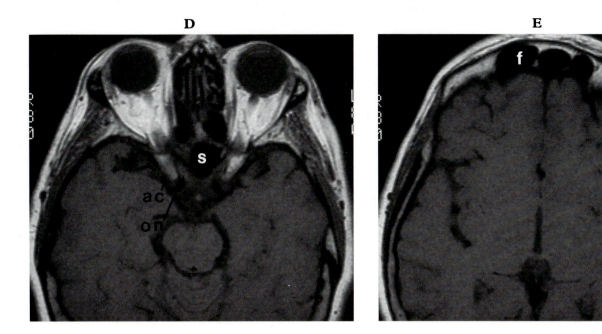

FIGURE 1.5 *(continued)*

from the marrow. The sphenoid sinus drains into the sphenoethmoid recess (ser). *, middle turbinate. (**C**) Section through the ethmoid (e) and sphenoid (s) sinuses. ns, nasal septum; on, optic nerve. (**D**) Section through the optic canal showing the optic nerve (on). ac, anterior clinoid; s, sphenoid sinus. (**E**) Section through the frontal sinuses (f).

A

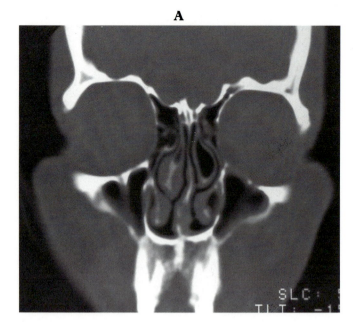

C

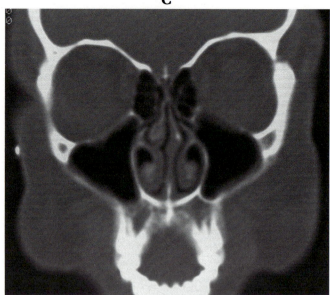

B

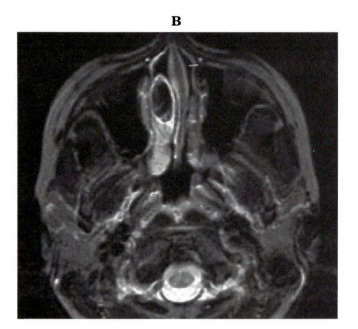

FIGURE 1.6

Normal variants. (**A,B**) Concha bullosa: an aerated middle turbinate is termed concha bullosa. It is demonstrated by both CT (**A**) and T2-weighted MR image (**B**). (**C**) Absent middle turbinate. The middle turbinate is absent on the left. The ostiomeatal unit is well visualized.

continued

D

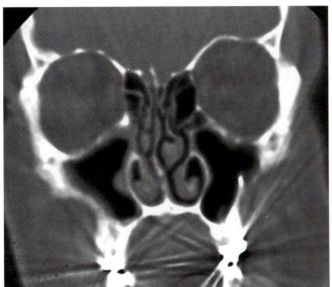

E

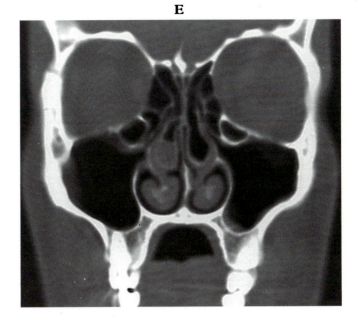

F

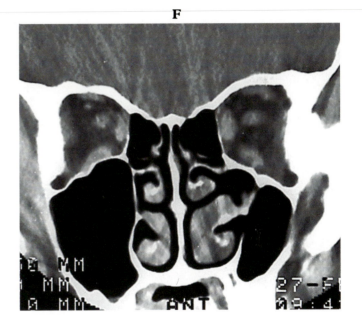

FIGURE 1.6 *(continued)*

(**D**) paradoxical middle turbinate. The left middle turbinate curves paradoxically towards the midline. (**E**) Halle cells. Coronal CT scan. Note air cells extending to the orbital floor from the ethmoid cells known as Halle or Haller cells. Also note bilateral concha bullosa with an air-fluid level on the right side. (**F**) Hypoplastic sinus: coronal CT scan reveals hypoplasia of the left maxillary sinus. Note lateral bowing of the ipsilateral orbital floor.

A

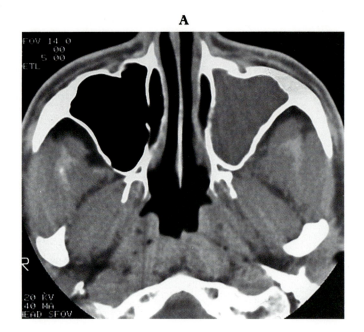

B

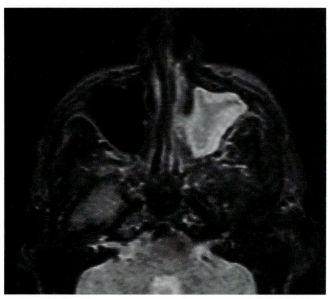

FIGURE 1.7

Sinusitis. (**A**) Axial CT section reveals opacification of the left maxillary sinus. (**B**) Axial T2-weighted MR image (TR = 2000 ms, TE = 80 ms) in the same patient. There is a peripheral zone of high signal intensity representing thickened mucosa with submucosal fluid. The central zone reveals slightly lower signal intensity. The mucoproteinaceous secretions show variable signal depending on the protein content.

A

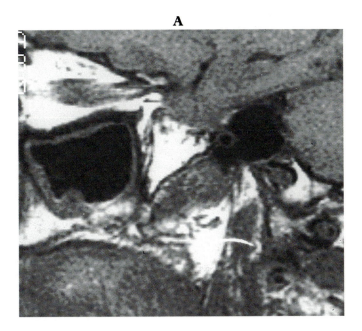

B

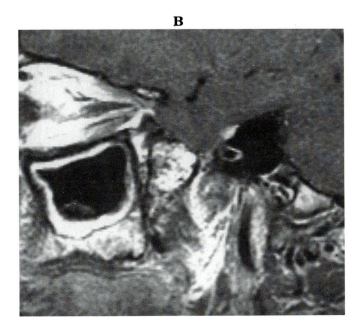

C

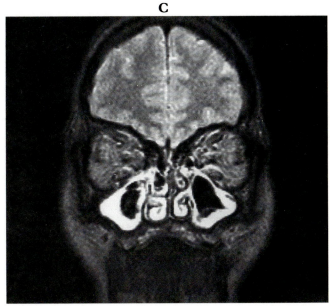

FIGURE 1.8

Sinusitis. (**A**) Sagittal T1-weighted images show soft tissue with intermediate signal intensity in the maxillary sinus. (**B**) Sagittal T1-weighted images following gadolinium administration demonstrate enhancement of the mucosa. (**C**) T2-weighted images show markedly high signal of the thickened mucosa bilaterally, consistent with inflammatory disease. Also note the normal high signal intensity of the nasal turbinates.

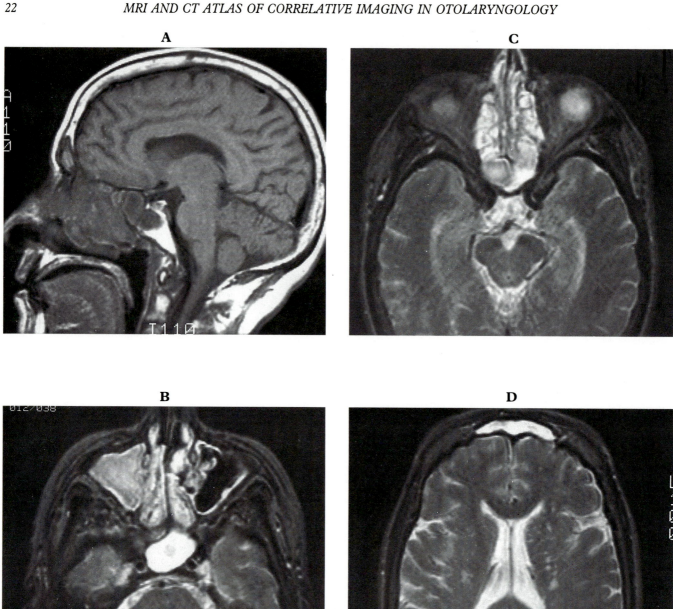

FIGURE 1.9

Pansinusitis. (**A**) Sagittal T1-weighted MR scan (TR = 800 ms, TE = 16 ms). Opacification of the frontal, sphenoid and ethmoid sinuses is noted. The soft tissue reveals intermediate signal intensity with a few foci of high signal. (**B,C,D**) Axial T2-weighted MR images (TR = 2500 ms, TE = 90 ms) show inhomogeneous and variable signal intensity in the sinuses. The signal intensity of the sinonasal secretions vary depending on their proteinaceous content.

A

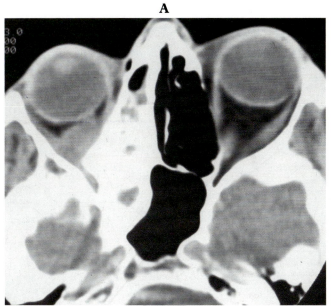

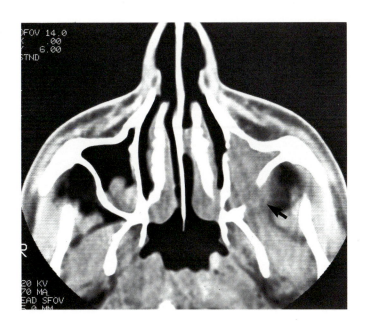

FIGURE 1.10

Mucormycosis. Axial CT scan demonstrates soft tissue density filling the left maxillary sinus with extension into the retroantral fat (arrow). Note the bone erosion along the lateral wall.

B

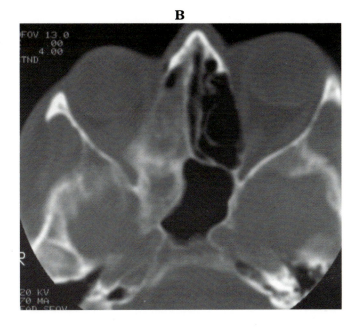

FIGURE 1.11

Wegener's granulomatosis. Axial CT scans (**A,B**) at soft tissue and bone window settings reveal opacification of right ethmoid and sphenoid sinuses with adjacent bony sclerosis. Note the soft tissue mass at the right orbital apex.

A

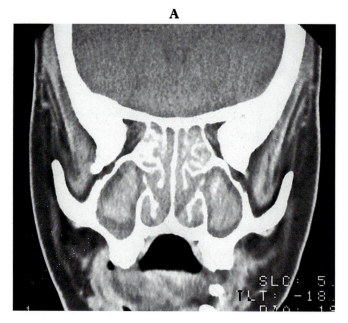

A

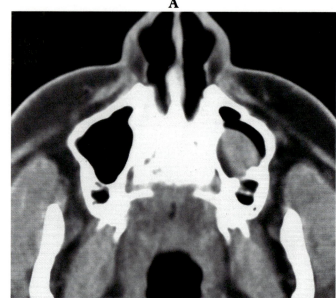

B

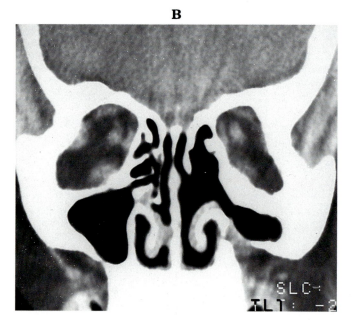

B

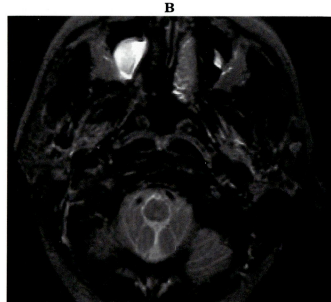

FIGURE 1.12

FIGURE 1.13

Sarcoid rhinosinusitis. (**A**) Coronal CT scan reveals complete opacification of all paranasal sinuses. Note central increased density with surrounding low attenuation. No bone erosion is present. (**B**) Coronal CT scan following treatment shows improvement. Note thickening of left maxillary sinus wall and residual soft tissue density. There has been a left ethmoidectomy.

Retention cyst. (**A**) Axial CT scan reveals well-defined mass along the inferior aspect of the right maxillary sinus. (**B**) The retention cyst is seen as a hyperintense mass on this axial T2-weighted MR image (TR = 2000 ms, TE = 80 ms).

A

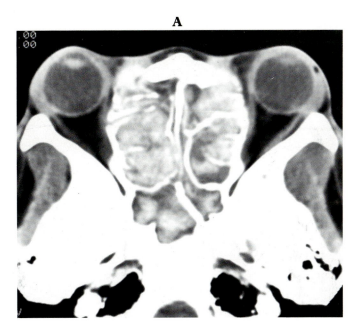

C

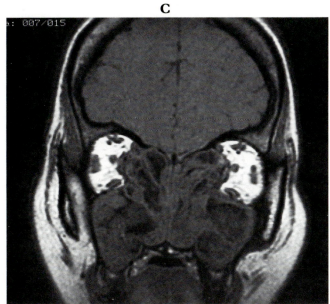

B

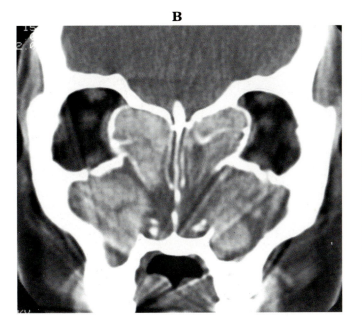

D

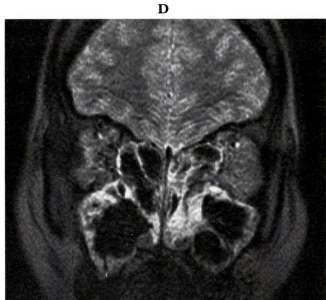

FIGURE 1.14

Chronic hypertrophic polypoid rhinosinusitis. Axial
(**A**) and coronal (**B**) CT scans show pansinusitis
with marked expansion of the ethmoids bilaterally.
Note the central foci of high attenuation surrounded
by a peripheral zone of low attenuation in the
sinuses. The nasal cavity is also totally filled with
soft tissue density. Coronal MR T1-weighted
(TR = 800 ms, TE = 20 ms) image (**C**) shows
inhomogeneous soft tissue filling the sinuses and
nasal cavity with intermediate or low signal. Coronal
T2-weighted (TR = 2700 ms, TE = 80 ms) SE
image (**D**) reveals high signal intensity along the
periphery of the sinuses. The central regions lack
signal mimicking aerated sinus. The absent signal is
in fact due to desiccated polyps and sinonasal
secretions with high protein content.

continued

E

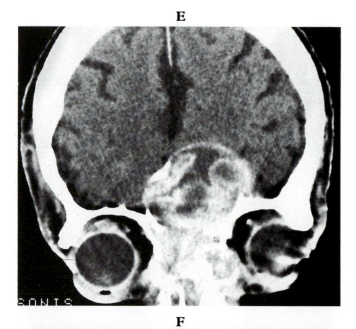

F

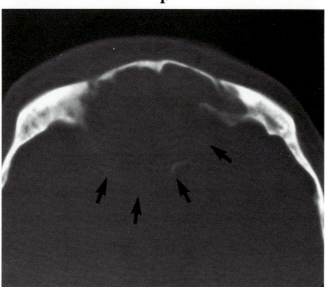

FIGURE 1.14 *(continued)*

(**E,F**) 40-year-old man with extensive polyposis.
Coronal and axial CT scans reveal multiple
inhomogeneously enhancing masses which have
expanded intracranially. Bone windows reveal a thin
expansile bony margin (arrows).

A

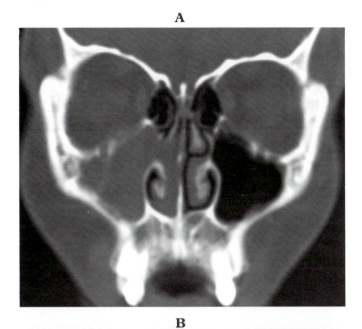

B

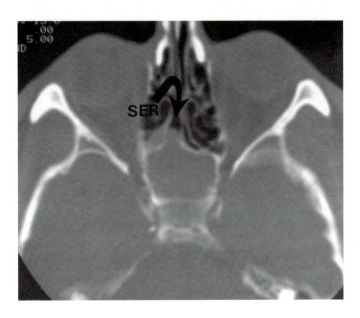

C

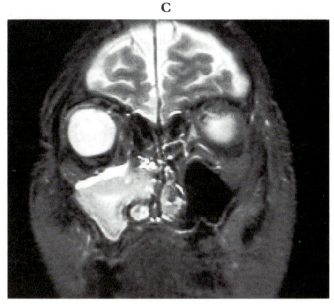

FIGURE 1.15

Antrochoanal polyp. (**A**) Coronal CT scan demonstrates a soft tissue mass occupying the entire right maxillary sinus and protruding into the ipsilateral nasal cavity through a widened maxillary ostium. (**B,C**) Coronal double echo T2-weighted MR scans (TR = 2000 ms, TE = 20, 90 ms). The mass is inhomogeneous but hyperintense due to high free water content.

FIGURE 1.16

Sphenochoanal polyp. Axial CT scan shows soft tissue mass opacifying the sphenoid sinus. Note the widening of the sphenoethmoid recess (SER).

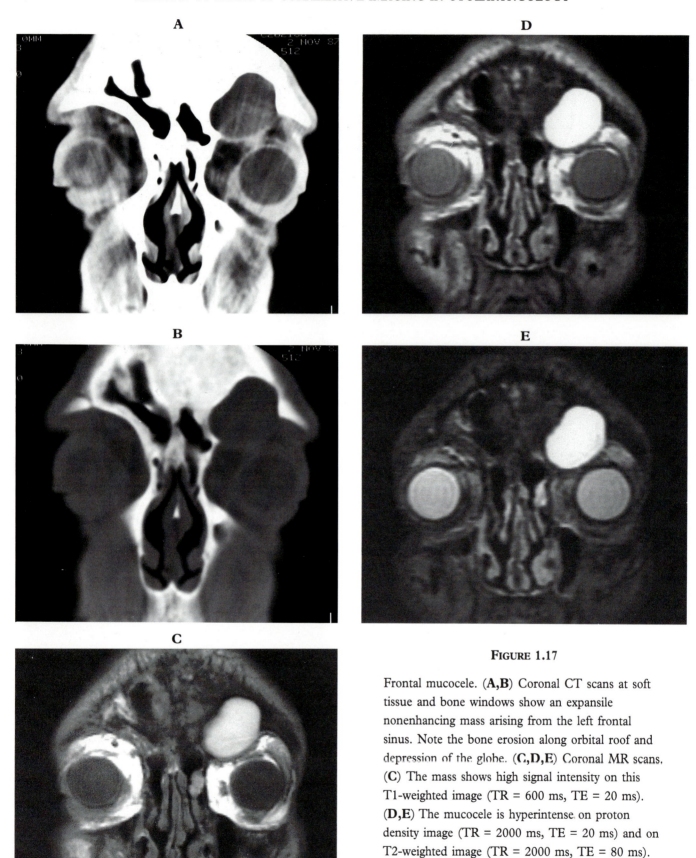

A

D

B

E

C

FIGURE 1.17

Frontal mucocele. (**A,B**) Coronal CT scans at soft tissue and bone windows show an expansile nonenhancing mass arising from the left frontal sinus. Note the bone erosion along orbital roof and depression of the globe. (**C,D,E**) Coronal MR scans. (**C**) The mass shows high signal intensity on this T1-weighted image (TR = 600 ms, TE = 20 ms). (**D,E**) The mucocele is hyperintense on proton density image (TR = 2000 ms, TE = 20 ms) and on T2-weighted image (TR = 2000 ms, TE = 80 ms).

A

C

B

D

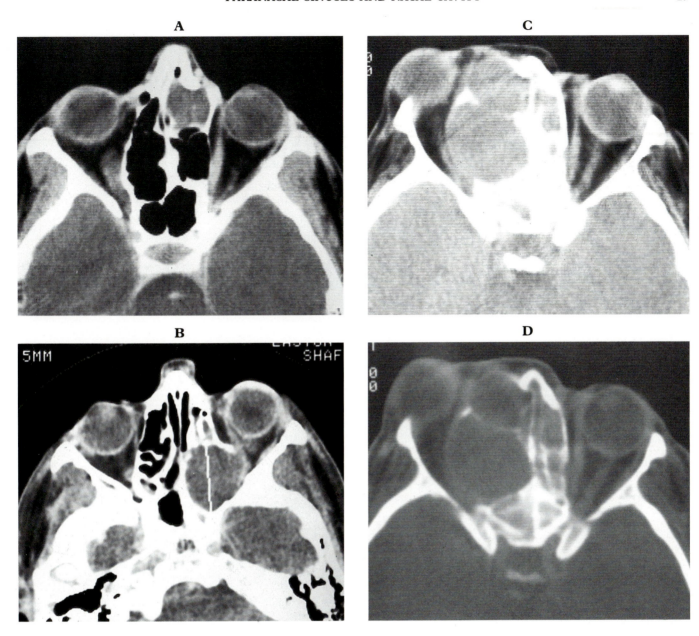

FIGURE 1.18

Ethmoid mucocele. (**A**) Axial contrast enhanced CT scan shows an expansile mass in the left anterior ethmoid sinus. The mass does not demonstrate enhancement. (**B**) Axial CT scan reveals an expansile nonenhancing mass in the left posterior ethmoid sinus. The cursor is measuring the antero- posterior dimension of the mass. (**C,D**) Axial CT scans at soft tissue and bone windows demonstrate markedly expansile masses in both the anterior and posterior right ethmoids. Also note opacification of left ethmoid air cells and sphenoid sinus.

A

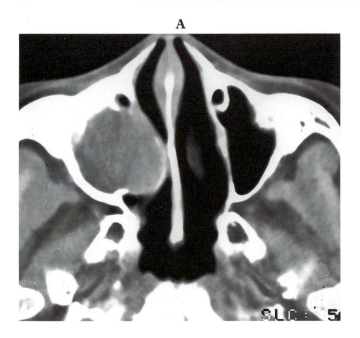

C

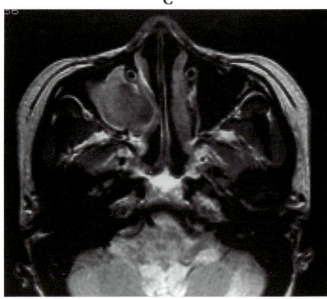

B

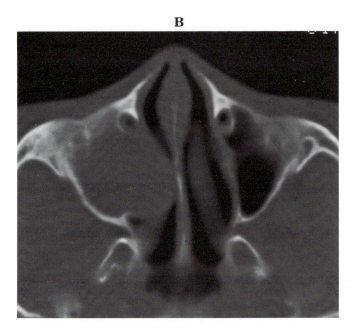

D

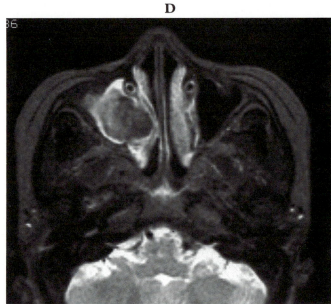

FIGURE 1.19

Maxillary mucocele. (**A,B**) Axial CT scans at soft tissue and bone window settings reveal expansile mass in the right maxillary sinus. (**C,D**) Axial MR scans. Proton density image (TR = 2400 ms, TE = 20 ms) reveals an inhomogeneous mass in the right maxillary sinus with intermediate and low signal intensity. The mass shows persistent low signal on T2-weighted SE image (TR = 2400 ms, TE = 80 ms). The mucosal thickening surrounding the mass is bright.

A

C

B

D

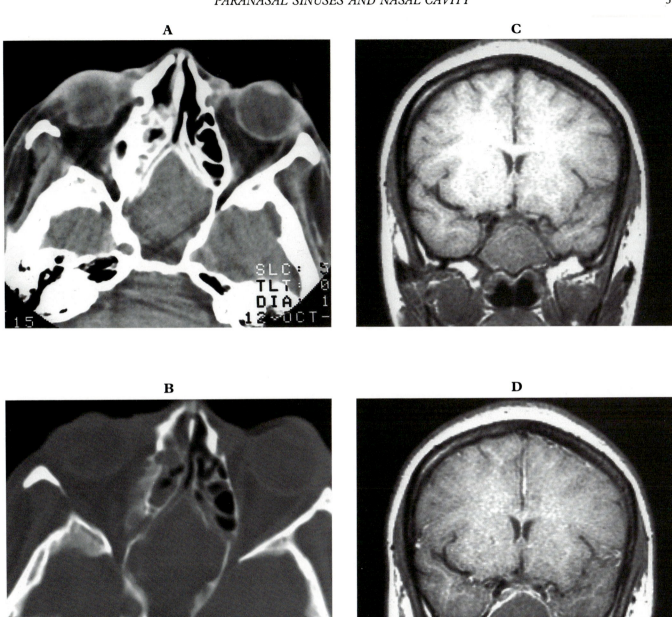

FIGURE 1.20

Sphenoid mucocele. (**A,B**) Axial CT scans. An expansile mass is noted in the sphenoid sinus. (**C,D**) Coronal MR scans. T1-weighted SE MR image (TR = 700 ms, TE = 20 ms) reveals an expansile mass in the sphenoid sinus of intermediate signal intensity. Following gadolinium administration (**D**), a rim of peripheral enhancement is noted.

A

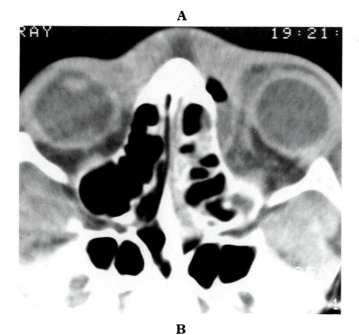

C

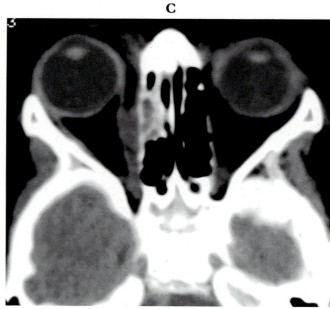

B

FIGURE 1.21

Subperiosteal abscess. Axial (**A**) and coronal (**B**) CT scans in a 17-year-old man with left eye proptosis. There is left periorbital soft tissue swelling and a subperiosteal abscess with an air-fluid level. Note sinusitis involving left anterior ethmoid air cells and maxillary sinus. (**C**) Axial CT scan in a 21-year-old reveals a subperiosteal abscess involving the right orbit. Note ethmoid sinusitis.

A

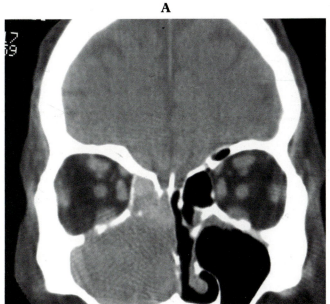

B

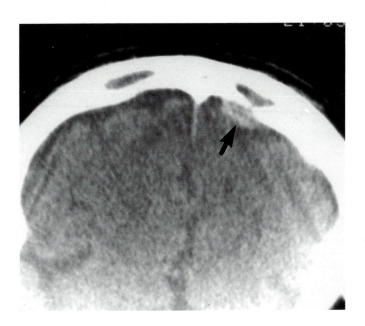

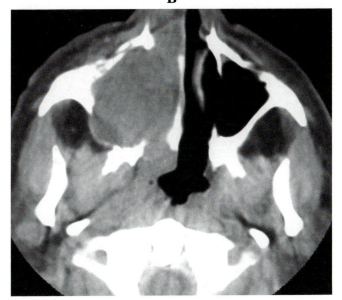

FIGURE 1.22

Epidural abscess. Axial CT scan in a 67-year-old shows bifrontal sinusitis and a left epidural abscess (arrow). There is dehiscence of the posterior margin of the left frontal sinus.

FIGURE 1.23

Squamous cell carcinoma. Axial and coronal CT scans (**A,B**) show a soft tissue mass expanding the right maxillary sinus with bone erosion. The mass extends into the ipsilateral nasal cavity and ethmoid sinus. The sphenoid sinus is also opacified.

A

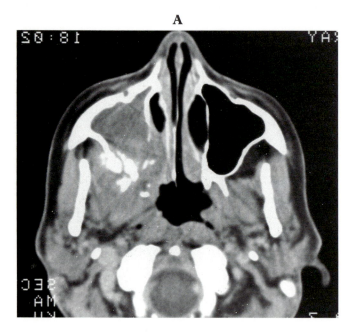

A

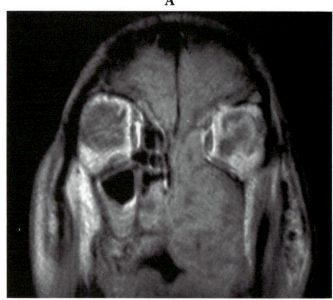

B

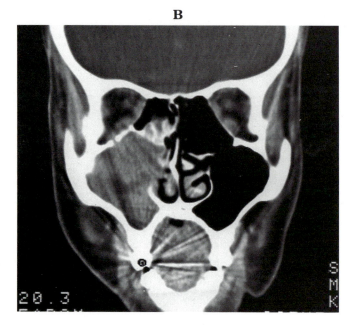

B

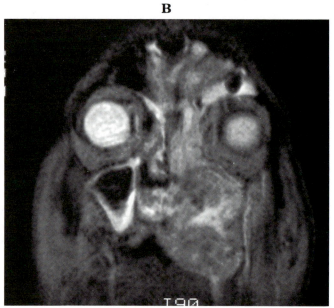

FIGURE 1.24

Squamous cell carcinoma. Axial (**A**) and coronal (**B**) CT scans show soft tissue mass opacifying the right maxillary sinus. The mass extends into the nasal cavity, pterygopalatine fossa, nasopharynx and infratemporal fossa. Note bone erosion involving the maxillary sinus and pterygoid plates.

FIGURE 1.25

Squamous cell carcinoma. (**Λ,B**) Proton density and T2-weighted SE MR images in coronal plane demonstrate a large mass expanding and eroding the left maxillary sinus. The mass shows intermediate signal intensity with a few foci of high signal on T2-weighted image. Note that the inflammatory mucosal thickening of the right maxillary sinus and both frontal sinuses show very high signal and is easily differentiated from tumor on the T2-weighted images.

A

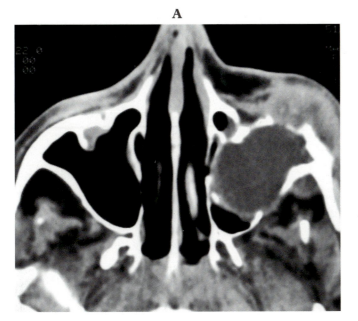

C

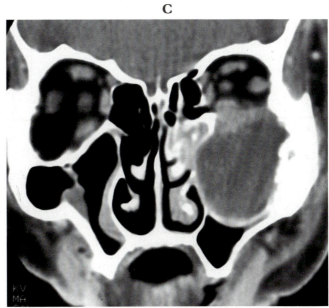

B

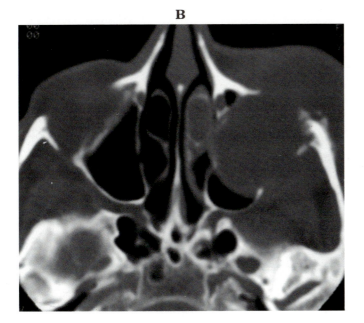

D

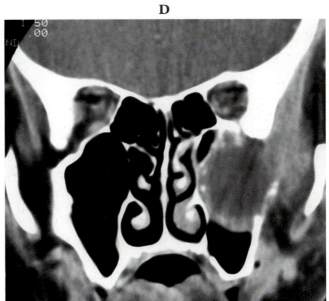

FIGURE 1.26

Squamous cell carcinoma. Axial CT scans (**A,B**) reveal a mucocele in a septated sinus with an associated squamous cell carcinoma. Note the irregular bone destruction and the large soft tissue mass in the soft tissues of the left cheek. Coronal CT scans (**C,D**) demonstrate upward bowing and erosion of the orbital floor. The posterolateral margin of the maxillary sinus is destroyed with direct extension of the mass into the infratemporal fossa.

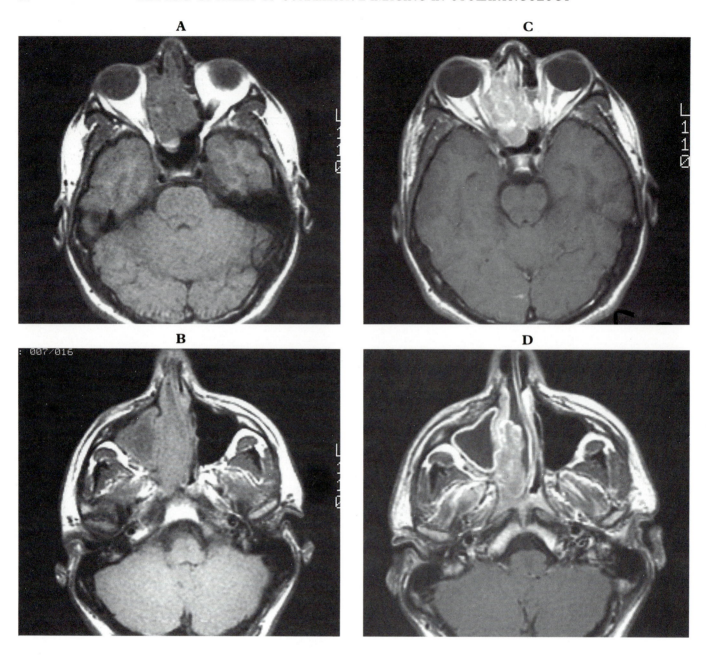

FIGURE 1.27

Adenocarcinoma. 18-year-old male with nasal stuffiness. T1-weighted (TR − 600 ms, TE = 20 ms) axial MR images (**A,B**) show a soft tissue mass in the ethmoid sinuses and nasal cavity. The signal intensity of the mass is slightly higher than that of the adjacent muscles. Note the lower signal intensity of the right maxillary sinus opacification.

(**C,D**) T1-weighted MR images following gadolinium enhancement show slight enhancement of the tumor mass. The tumor extends into the ethmoid and sphenoid sinuses. Note the peripheral mucosal enhancement of the obstructed right maxillary sinus.

continued

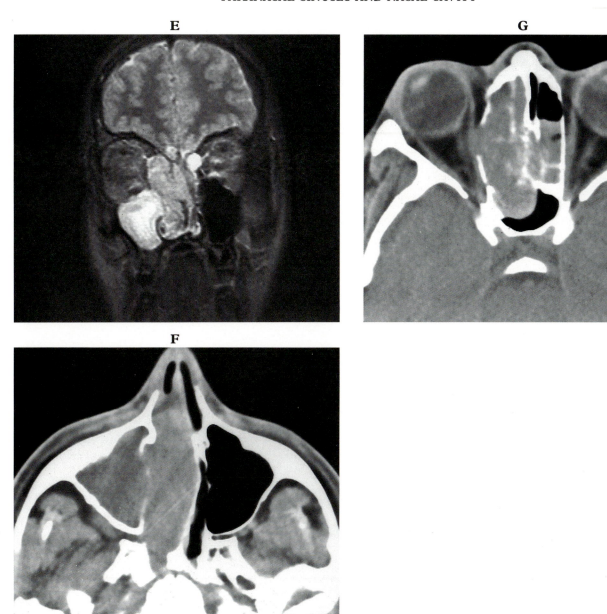

FIGURE 1.27 *(continued)*

(**E**) Coronal T2-weighted SE image (TR = 2700 ms, TE = 80 ms) reveals differential signal intensities of the malignant neoplasm, and inflammatory sinus disease. The tumor mass shows intermediate signal intensity while the inflammatory disease in the maxillary and left ethmoid sinus show high signal intensity. (**F,G**) Axial unenhanced CT scans. A soft tissue mass is seen in the nasal cavity, ethmoid sinus and right sphenoid with erosion of the ethmoid septae, lamina papyracea and anterior wall of the sphenoid sinus. The maxillary sinus is opacified. No differential attenuation is noted between the tumor and the maxillary sinus disease.

A

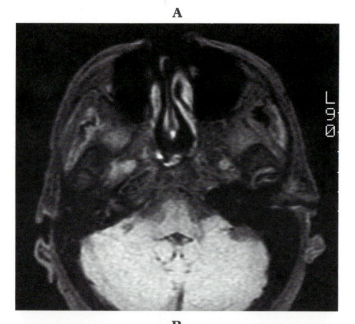

C

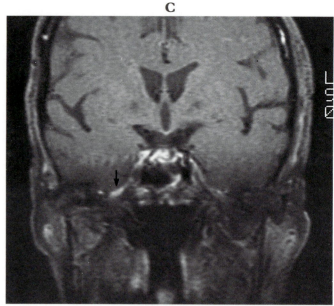

B

FIGURE 1.28

Perineural spread of carcinoma along the 5th cranial nerve. Primary tumor: adenoid cystic carcinoma. Axial T1-weighted images (**A,B**) (TR = 700 ms, TE = 20 ms) pre- and post-gadolinium enhancement with fat suppression. Note the enhancing tumor at the right skull base (arrow) and at the level of the foramen ovale (curved arrow). Tumor is also seen along V3 in the coronal plane (**C**) in this T1-weighted SE image following gadolinium enhancement and with fat suppression (small arrow).

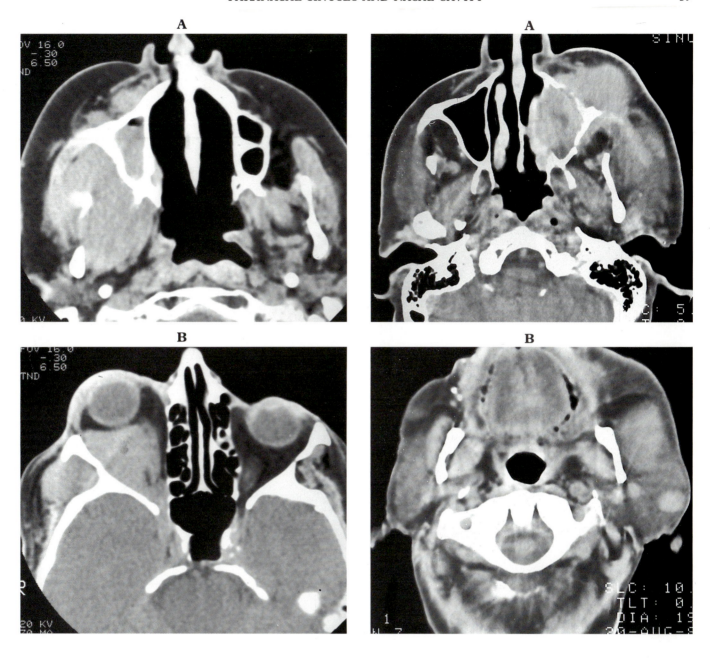

FIGURE 1.29

Lymphoma. Axial CT scans (**A,B**) reveal a large bulky soft tissue mass in the right maxillary sinus, masticator space, and orbit consistent with extranodal, extralymphatic non-Hodgkin's lymphoma. The mass is homogeneous. The globe is displaced anteriorly. Note the relative lack of bone erosion.

FIGURE 1.30

Hodgkin's disease. Axial CT scans (**A,B**) demonstrate a mass opacifying the left maxillary sinus with direct extension into the soft tissues anteriorly. Also note a large mass involving the left masseter muscle and an intraparotid node.

A

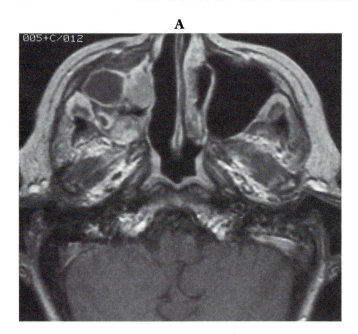

C

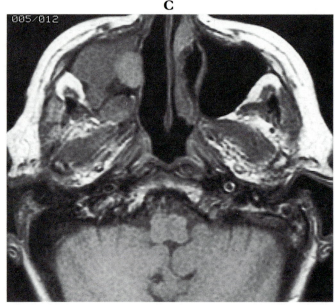

B

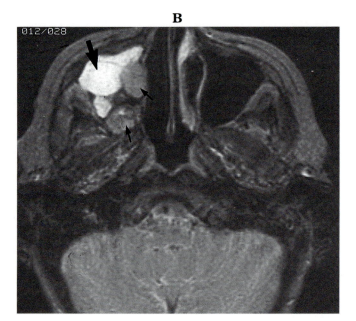

D

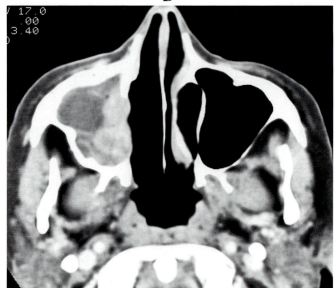

FIGURE 1.31

Malignant melanoma. (**A**) Axial T1-weighted SE MR image (TR = 800 ms, TE = 30 ms). The right maxillary sinus is filled with soft tissue of intermediate signal. Along the medial border note a nodular mass with higher signal intensity. (**B**) Axial T2-weighted MR image (TR = 2000 ms, TE = 80 ms). The two tumor nodules (small arrows) reveal intermediate signal intensity. Along the lateral aspect, the inflammatory component shows high signal intensity (large arrow).

(**C**) Axial T1-weighted MR image following gadolinium administration shows slight enhancement of the tumor masses. Note rim enhancement of the inflammatory component. (**D**) Contrast enhanced axial CT scan. The tumor nodules show enhancement while the inflammatory component demonstrates low attenuation.

continued

E

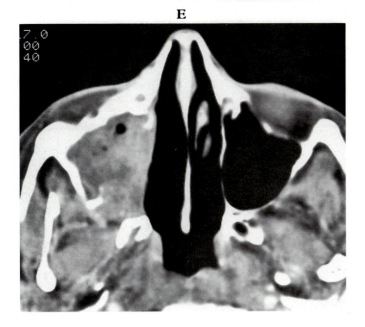

F

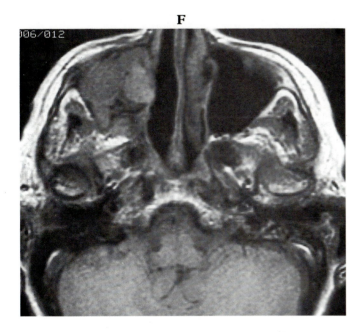

FIGURE 1.31 *(continued)*

(**E**) CT scan through the superior aspect of the
maxillary sinus shows bone erosion along the
posterior aspect of the sinus with tumor extension
into the pterygo-palatine fossa. (**F**) Axial T1-
weighted MR image at the same level. Bone erosion
is not as well delineated by MR in comparison to
the CT scan.

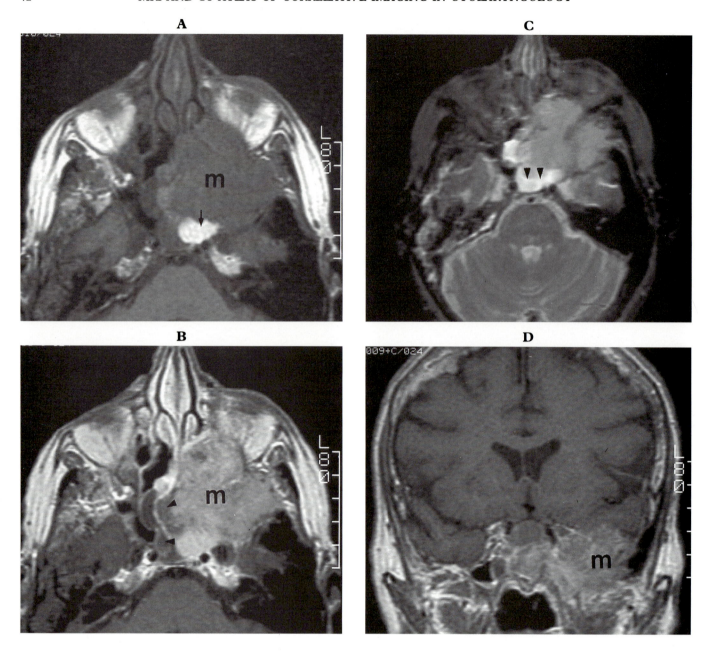

FIGURE 1.32

Malignant melanoma. (**A,B**) Axial T1-weighted MR images pre and post gadolinium administration reveal a large enhancing mass (m) in the left maxillary sinus with extension into the ethmoid and sphenoid sinus and into the masticator space. High signal represents hemorrhage into the tumor (arrow). The inflammatory component in the sphenoid sinus has low signal intensity with rim enhancement (arrowheads).

(**C**) Axial T2-weighted image (TR = 3000 ms, TE = 80 ms) reveals high signal of the inflammatory component (arrowheads). The tumor mass shows intermediate signal. (**D**) Coronal T1-weighted MR image with gadolinium demonstrates intradural extension of melanoma in the left middle cranial fossa (m). Tumor also extends into the cavernous sinus.

continued

E

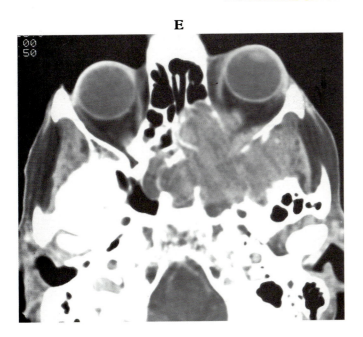

FIGURE 1.32 *(continued)*

(E) Axial contrast enhanced CT scan shows extensive skull base destruction. The associated inflammatory component is not as well demonstrated by CT.

A

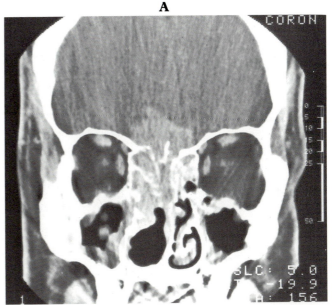

B

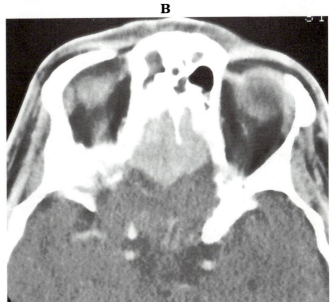

FIGURE 1.33

Esthesioneuroblastoma. 37-year-old man with a history of nasal polyps. (A,B) Coronal and axial contrast-enhanced CT scans reveal an enhancing mass in the nasal cavity and ethmoid sinuses with intracranial extension. Mucosal thickening is noted in both the maxillary sinuses. Note the postsurgical changes in the right nasal cavity from polypectomy and turbinectomy.

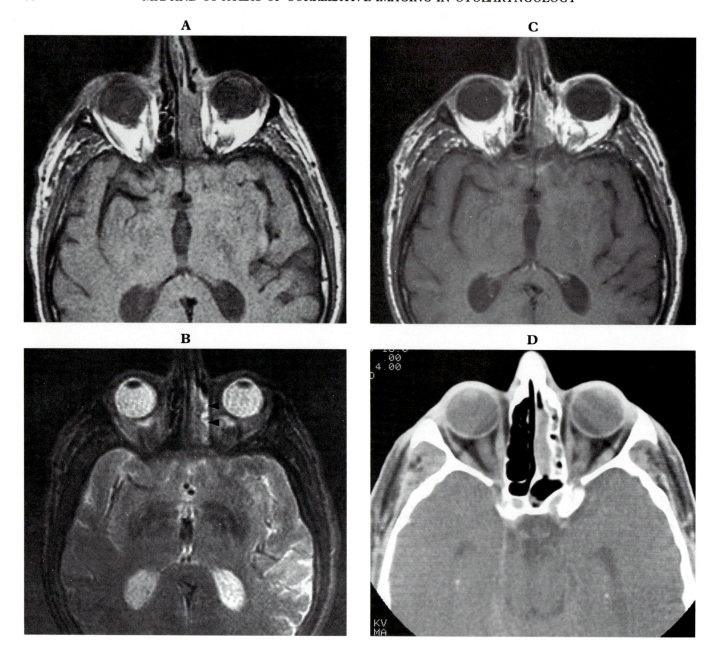

FIGURE 1.34

Esthesioneuroblastoma. (**A,B**) Axial T1- and T2-weighted MR images. An expansile mass in the left nasal cavity reveals intermediate signal intensity on both the T1- and T2-weighted images. Note inflammatory changes in the left ethmoid air cells which show a high signal on the T2-weighted image (arrowheads).

(**C**) Following gadolinium administration, there is slight enhancement of the tumor and greater enhancement of the mucosal thickening in the ethmoid air cells. (**D**) Axial CT. The mass is isodense with the extraocular muscles. The left ethmoid air cells reveal mucosal thickening.

A

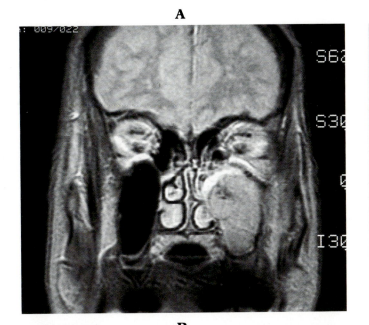

C

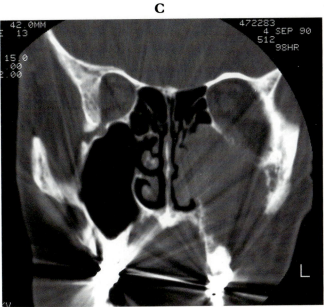

B

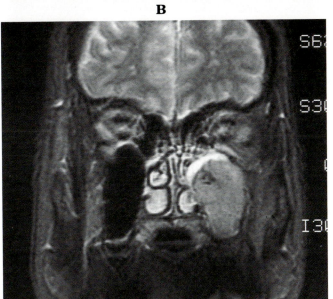

FIGURE 1.35

Plasmacytoma. 69-year-old man with progressive facial swelling for 6 months. (**A,B**) Axial proton density and T2-weighted MR images (TR = 2600 ms, TE = 40, 80 ms) reveal an expansile mass opacifying the left maxillary sinus with intermediate signal intensity. Note the crescentic inflammatory changes with high signal intensity along the superior and medial aspect of the mass. (**C**) Axial CT scan pictured at bone window setting shows an expansile mass in the left maxillary sinus with extensive bone erosion along the lateral margin and orbital floor. Bone erosion is not apparent on the MR images. Streaking artifact from metallic dental fillings degrades the image quality of CT. On MR images, this artifact does not affect the entire image but leads to drop out of signal only locally.

A

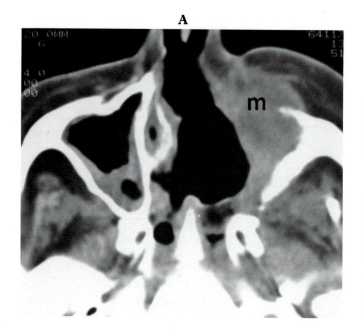

C

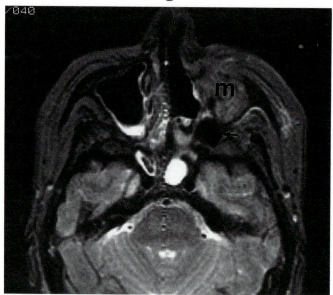

B

FIGURE 1.36

Recurrent malignant fibrous histiocytoma (MFH). 61-year-old woman. 10 months post partial left maxillectomy for MFH. (**A**) Axial CT shows a bulky homogeneous mass (m) in the postoperative bed. (**B,C**) Axial T1- and T2-weighted SE MR images (TR = 600 ms, TE = 20 ms and TR = 2000 ms, TE = 80 ms). The recurrent MFH (m) demonstrates intermediate signal intensity. The inflammatory disease in the right maxillary and sphenoid sinuses reveal very high signal on the T2-weighted image. Halo of signal drop out in the region of the left pterygopalatine fossa (arrow) is noted due to surgical clips.

A

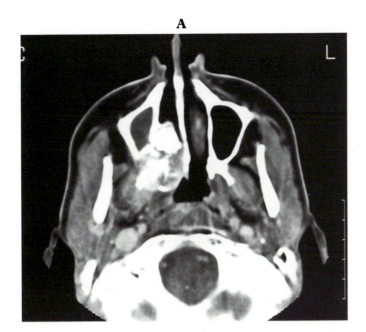

FIGURE 1.37

Osteosarcoma. A 28-year-old woman with a history of nasal obstruction. Axial CT scans (**A,B**) show a destructive mass arising from the pterygoid plates with erosion of the posterior wall of the maxillary sinus. The mass extends into the ipsilateral nasal cavity. The tumor new bone formation suggests the diagnosis.

B

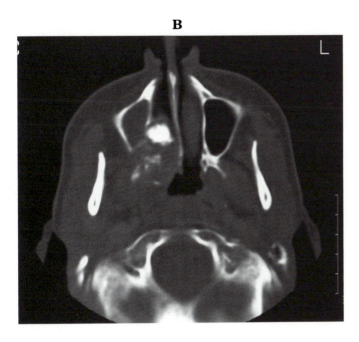

A

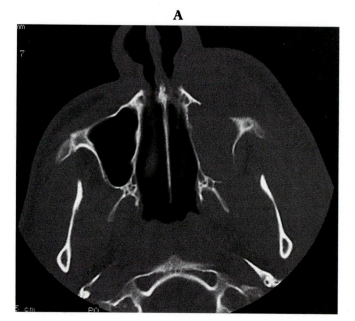

B

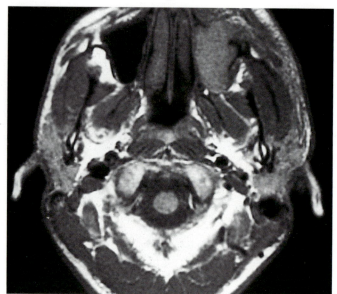

FIGURE 1.38

Osteosarcoma. 18-year-old male underwent right orbital exenteration and left orbital radiation for bilateral retinoblastomas at the age of 3 years, now presents with a postradiation osteosarcoma in the left maxillary sinus. (**A**) Axial CT shows a large mass filling the left maxillary sinus with bone destruction and tumor extension into the soft tissues anteriorly and in the retroantral region.

C

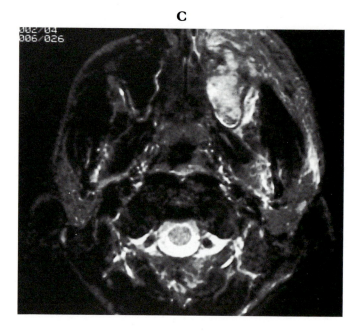

(**B,C**) Axial T1- and T2-weighted MR images (TR = 600 ms, TE = 20 ms and TR = 2000 ms, TE = 90 ms). The signal intensity of the mass is higher than that of muscle on the T1-weighted image and very high on the T2-weighted images.

continued

D

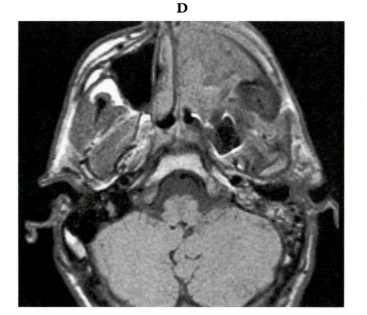

F

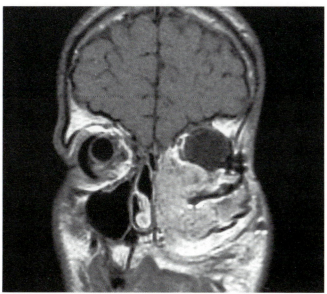

E

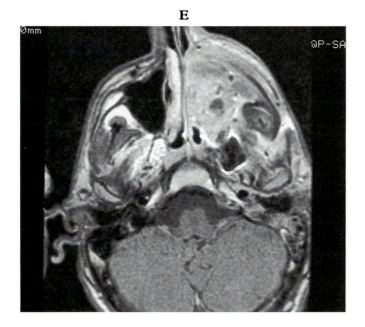

(**F**) The tumor extends into the ipsilateral orbit and ethmoids in this coronal image. Note the right orbital prosthesis.

FIGURE 1.38 *(continued)*

(**D,E**) Axial MR images obtained 1 month later reveal rapid growth of the tumor. T1-weighted image (**D**) shows marked expansion and erosion of the left maxillary sinus. Note tumor extension into the nasal cavity, the pterygopalatine fossa and up to the skull base. Gadolinium administration (**E**) demonstrated inhomogeneous, patchy but diffuse, enhancement of the tumor.

A

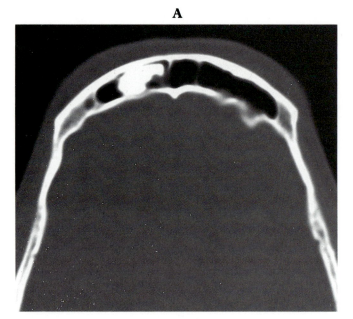

A

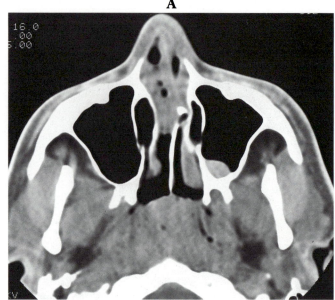

B

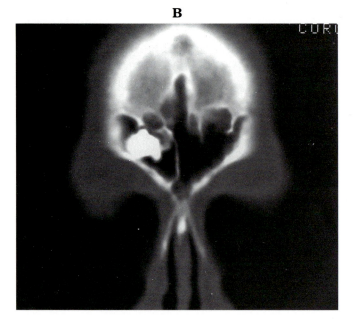

B

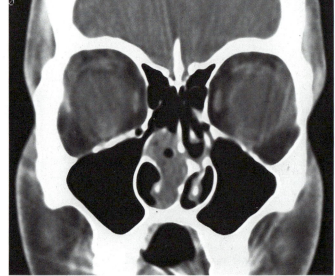

FIGURE 1.39

Osteoma. (**A,B**) Axial and coronal CT scans reveal a dense osteoma in the right frontal sinus as an incidental finding. No associated sinusitis is present.

FIGURE 1.40

Inverted papilloma. (**A,B**) Axial and coronal CT scans show a mass in the middle meatus along the lateral nasal wall.

A

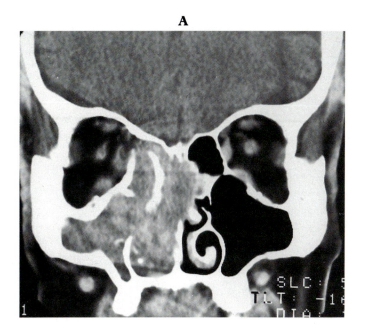

B

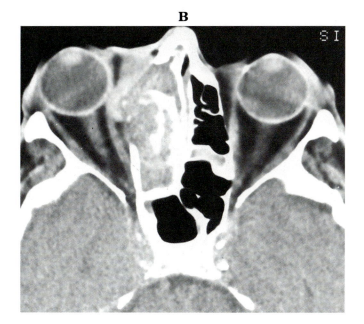

FIGURE 1.41

Recurrent inverted papilloma associated with squamous cell carcinoma. 75-year-old man with several prior resections of inverted papilloma. (**A,B**) Coronal and axial CT scans show a large mass in the nasal cavity, right maxillary sinus and ethmoid sinus with calcification. There is frank destruction of lamina papyracea and tumor extension into the ipsilateral orbit.

A

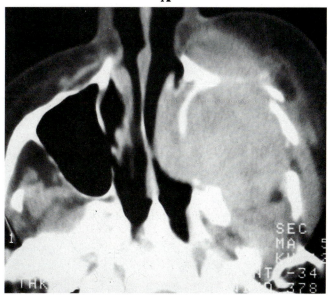

B

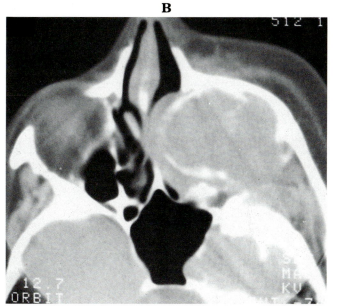

FIGURE 1.42

Hemangioma. 60-year-old woman with slowly enlarging left facial mass. Axial CT scans (**A,B**) show a large expansile mass in the left maxillary sinus with bony erosion. The mass extends into the soft tissues of the face anteriorly and into the infratemporal fossa.

A

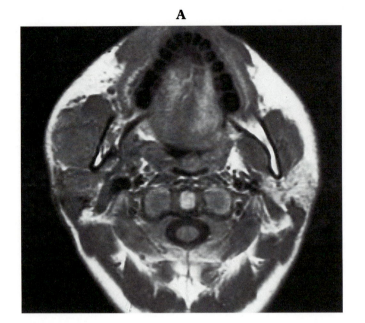

B

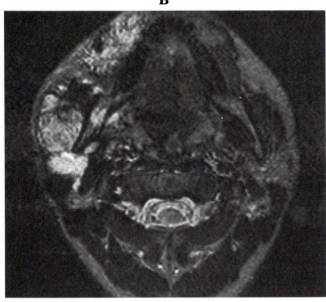

FIGURE 1.43

Invasive hemangioma. 29-year-old man with recurrent hemangioma in the right parotid bed and masticator space. Axial T1- and T2-weighted MR images (**A,B**) reveal a large soft tissue mass in the masticator space with infiltration into the masseter muscle. The mass is isointense with the muscle on the T1-weighted image and hyperintense on the T2-weighted image. The mass also infiltrates into the mandible through the alveolar canal.

A

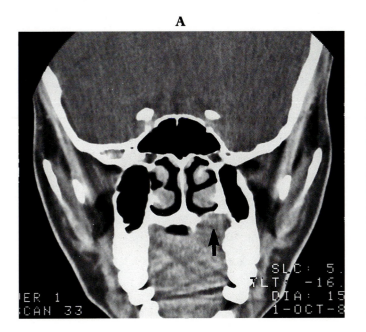

A

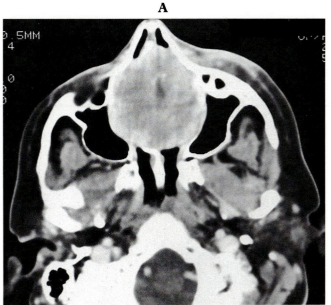

B

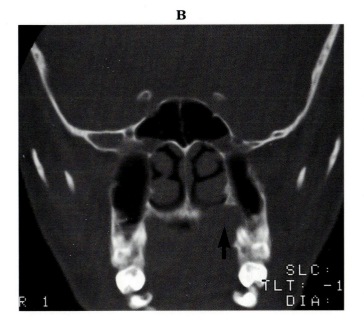

B

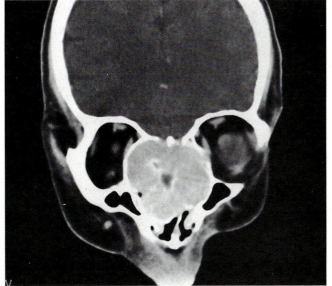

FIGURE 1.44

Pleomorphic adenoma. Coronal CT scans (**A,B**) reveal an expansile mass along the left hard palate (arrow). The maxillary sinus is normal.

FIGURE 1.45

Schwannoma. Axial and coronal CT scans (**A,B**) demonstrate a large, expansile, midline enhancing mass in the nasal cavity with a few central foci of low attenuation. No intracranial extension is seen.

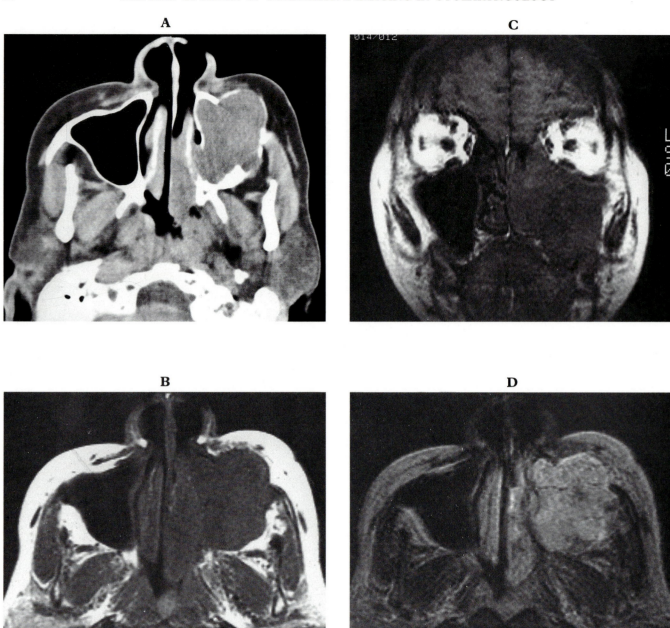

FIGURE 1.46

Ameloblastoma. (**A**) Axial CT scan shows an expansile mass involving the left maxillary sinus. Axial (**B**) and coronal (**C**) T1-weighted MR images (TR = 500 ms, TE = 20 ms) reveal an expansile mass of intermediate signal intensity. Soft tissue is also noted in the ipsilateral nasal cavity and ethmoid sinus. (**D**) T2-weighted image (TR = 2000 ms, TE = 80 ms) shows the mass to be of high signal intensity.

continued

E

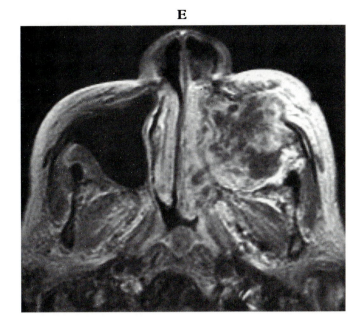

A

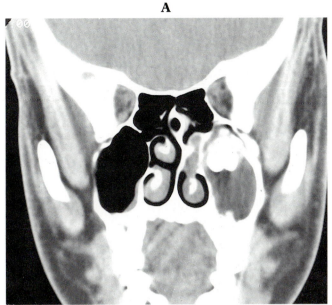

FIGURE 1.46 *(continued)*

(**E**) T1-weighted image following gadolinium administration shows diffuse but patchy enhancement of the tumor.

B

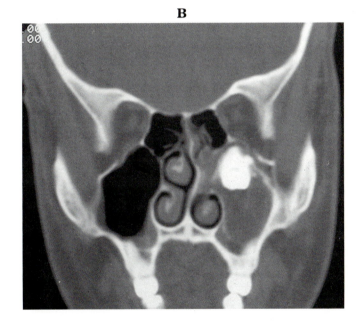

FIGURE 1.47

Dentigerous cyst. (**A,B**) Coronal CT scans reveal a mass of low attenuation growing into the left maxillary sinus from the alveolar ridge. Note the associated unerupted tooth. Minimal mucosal thickening is present along the inferior margin of the right maxillary sinus.

A

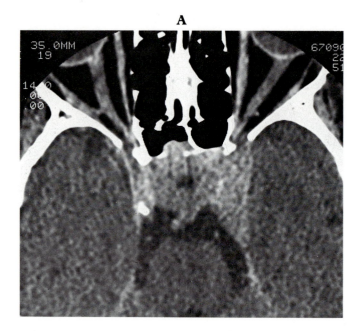

C

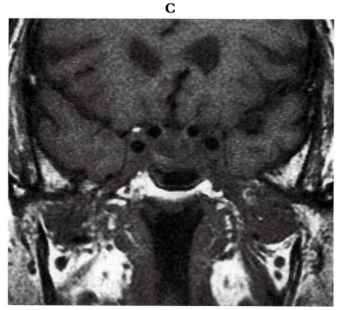

B

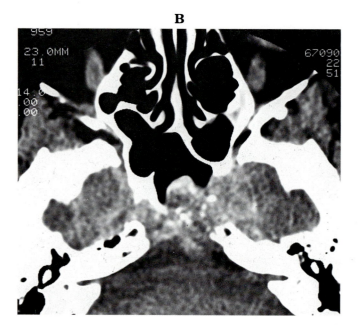

D

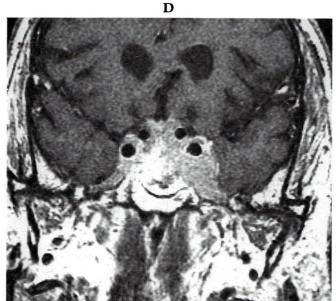

FIGURE 1.48

Invasive pituitary adenoma. (**A,B**) Contrast-enhanced axial CT scans. A large enhancing suprasellar mass extending into the sphenoid sinus and both cavernous sinuses is seen.

(**C**) Coronal T1-weighted MR scan reveals encasement of the carotid arteries bilaterally. The pituitary adenoma is isointense with the brain. (**D**) Coronal T1-weighted image following administration of gadolinium shows intense enhancement of the adenoma.

continued

E

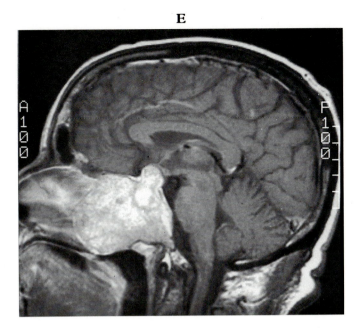

A

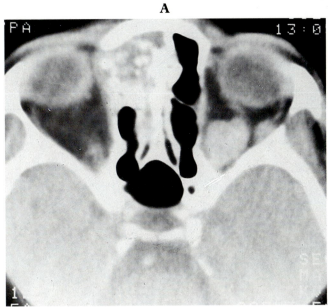

B

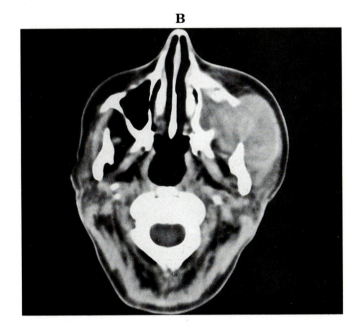

FIGURE 1.48 *(continued)*

(**E**) 61-year-old man with invasive pituitary adenoma. Sagittal T1-weighted image following gadolinium administration shows enhancing mass replacing the body of the sphenoid with extension in the nasal cavity. The suprasellar component is suggestive of the diagnosis.

FIGURE 1.49

Metastatic carcinoma. (**A**) 60-year-old woman with breast carcinoma. Axial CT scan shows metastatic carcinoma in the right anterior ethmoid sinus with erosion of the lamina papyracea. Metastatic tumor is also seen in the left orbit. (**B**) 47-year-old woman with breast carcinoma. Axial CT scan reveals a large destructive mass in the left maxillary sinus and the masticator space.

A

C

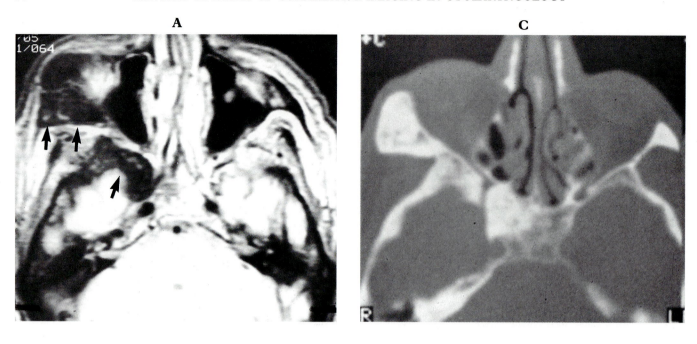

B

D

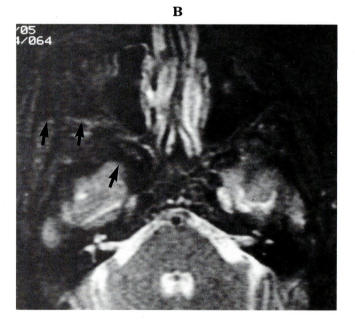

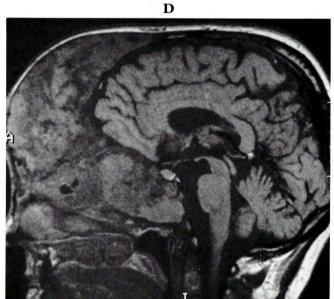

FIGURE 1.50

Fibrous dysplasia. (**A,B**) Axial proton density and T2-weighted MR images of the skull base reveal bony expansion of the right zygoma and skull base with markedly low signal (arrows). The axial CT scan (**C**) shows increased density and expansion of the bones. This is consistent with a sclerotic type of fibrous dysplasia. (**D**) 24-year-old woman. Sagittal T1-weighted MR image shows extensive fibrous dysplasia involving the calvarium, skull base and facial skeleton. All of the paranasal sinuses are totally obliterated.

A

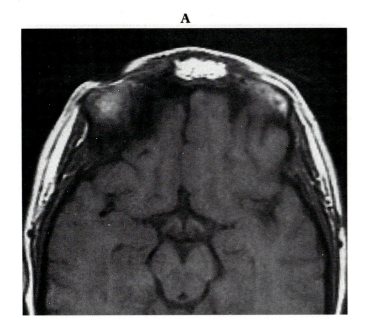

FIGURE 1.51

Fat ablation of frontal sinus. Axial T1-weighted (**A**) and T2-weighted (**B**) MR images reveal soft tissue in the left frontal sinus. The signal intensity is high on the T1-weighted and intermediate on the T2-weighted images similar to that of the subcutaneous fat.

B

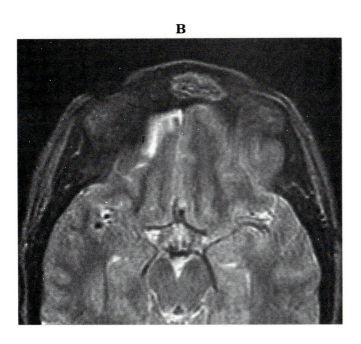

A

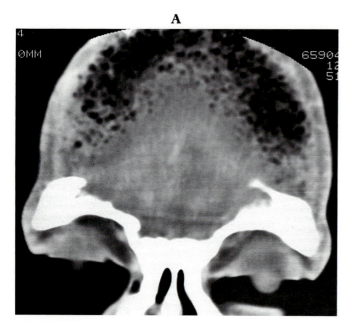

C

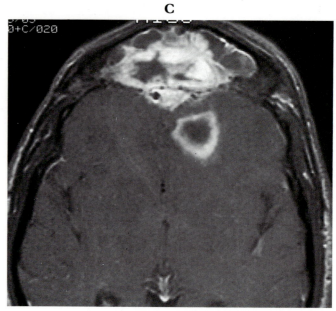

B

FIGURE 1.52

Polymethylmethacrylate (PMMA) cranioplasty plate.
(**A**) Coronal CT scan. The PMMA plate prosthesis
following frontal craniectomy. Note multiple rounded
lucencies which should not be confused with
subcutaneous air. (**B**) Axial contrast-enhanced CT
scan 6 months later reveals a fluid collection and an
infection of the prosthetic plate. (**C**) Axial T1-
weighted MR image post gadolinium administration
reveals enhancing inflammatory debris and a fluid
collection in the infected prosthesis. Also note the
epidural extension and brain abscess.

CHAPTER 2

PARAPHARYNGEAL SPACE

Introduction

A wide variety of tumors occur within the parapharyngeal space (PPS), many of which are characterized by slow insidious growth. Painless mass is the most frequent clinical presentation. Masses of the PPS are clinically apparent only when they become large enough to medially bow the lateral pharyngeal wall or cause parotid enlargement. Less frequent presentations include trismus, conductive hearing loss (subsequent to eustachian tube blockage and middle ear effusion), syndrome of Vernet (deficits of 9th, 10th and 11th cranial nerves with resultant speech and swallowing dysfunction) and Horner's syndrome.

Prior to the advent of computed tomography (CT) and magnetic resonance imaging (MRI), preoperative diagnosis was only speculatively based on angiography and sialography. In the late 1970s CT provided direct visualization of the PPS. Using modern CT techniques, preoperative diagnosis can be made in approximately 85% of patients. The recent development of MR imaging has greatly enhanced the preoperative evaluation of PPS tumors. Improved soft tissue contrast and direct multiplanar imaging are significant MRI advantages. With modern MRI techniques in combination with the clinical information, preoperative diagnosis can be established in more than 90% of patients.[1]

Normal anatomy

The parapharyngeal space is located in the deep soft tissues of the face. It is shaped like an 'inverted pyramid' extending from the skull base superiorly to the greater cornu of the hyoid bone inferiorly. Bilateral symmetry is a persistent feature of the parapharyngeal spaces and any asymmetry should suggest pathology. Each is a fat-filled (loose areolar tissue) triangular space located deep to the mandibular ramus and parotid gland.

The PPS is bordered laterally by the parotid space and the masticator space which contain the parotid gland and muscles of mastication, respectively. The posterior border is formed by the paravertebral musculature and the vertebral column. Medially, the superior pharyngeal constrictor muscles, the tonsillar fossa and the soft palate border the PPS.[2,3] Inferiorly, at the level of the hyoid, the PPS is in direct communication with the submandibular space.

The boundaries of the PPS are predominantly rigid with the exception of the medial wall and a portion of the lateral wall. Because the medial wall is the most pliable, medial bowing of the lateral nasopharyngeal and oropharyngeal wall and downward displacement of the soft palate can be produced by PPS lesions of 1.5 cm or greater.[1] The retromandibular portion of the lateral wall is also relatively pliable and composed primarily of parotid tissue. Fullness near the angle of the mandible may be produced by intraparotid or extraparotid PPS masses.

It is useful to separate the PPS into prestyloid and poststyloid compartments based on the relationship to the styloid process and muscles arising from the styloid process. The prestyloid compartment constitutes the large compartment anterior to the styloid process. The poststyloid compartment or the posterior PPS is in fact the carotid space and contains the internal carotid artery, internal jugular vein, cervical sympathetic chain, lymph nodes and the 9th–12th cranial nerves. The carotid space continues beyond the hyoid bone into the infrahyoid neck.

The PPS lies between several layers of the deep cervical fascia. Laterally, the PPS abuts the medial slip of the superficial layer of the deep cervical fascia as it curves around the medial surfaces of the parotid gland and muscles of mastication. The middle layer of the deep cervical fascia (buccopharyngeal fascia) lines the medial extent of the PPS. Posteriorly, the PPS is continuous with the structures of the carotid space. The pharyngobasilar fascia is a tough membrane which separates the PPS from the nasopharynx. This fascial membrane extends from the skull base superiorly to the pharyngeal constrictors inferiorly (Figs 2.1 and 2.2).

Imaging strategies

Angiography and sialography

Prior to CT and MRI, sialography and angiography were the primary modes of preoperative evaluation in suspected PPS pathology. If the tumor had a characteristic vascularity consistent with a paraganglioma, or if there was a specific sialographic appearance suggestive of intraparotid origin, a preoperative diagnosis could be offered.[4–17] Sialography and angiography provided accurate preoperative diagnosis in only 20–40% of cases.

Computed tomography

Computed tomography gained wide utilization in head and neck imaging in the late 1970s and early 1980s. At approximately the same time, the surgical philosophy regarding PPS masses was undergoing change. If the surgeon knew preoperatively that a PPS mass was extraparotid in origin, then surgical removal could be performed by a transcervical or transoral approach, thereby avoiding facial nerve manipulation.[15] Computed tomography provided information which led to the development of criteria to separate intraparotid from extraparotid masses. The most reliable CT finding of an extraparotid mass is a PPS fat plane between the mass and the adjacent parotid gland. Computed tomography also provides information in differentiating solid from cystic pathology. Contrast enhancement provides additional information in hypervascular lesions such as paraganglioma. Several prior investgators have analyzed the dynamic enhancement curves of the major primary PPS tumors.[10,18–24]

Computed tomography of the PPS is routinely performed following intravenous contrast administration. Contiguous 5 mm axial images are obtained from the skull base to the hyoid bone. Coronal images can be obtained at 5 mm increments from the midmaxillary sinus to the anterior cervical spine. Coronal images are most helpful in demonstrating skull base invasion and erosion. Additional information regarding intra- versus extra-parotid origin can be gained in the coronal plane. Utilizing conventional CT techniques, preoperative diagnosis can be achieved in approximately 85% of patients.

Magnetic resonance imaging

Magnetic resonance imaging has several distinct advantages over CT in the preoperative evaluation of PPS pathology. Magnetic resonance imaging is superior to CT for the following reasons: (1) superior soft tissue contrast; (2) direct multiplanar imaging; (3) demonstration of vascular structures without the use of iodinated contrast material; and (4) lack of ionizing radiation. The major disadvantage of MRI is its inability to demonstrate calcification and subtle osseous changes.

Magnetic resonance imaging of the PPS can be performed utilizing the head coil or the anterior neck coil. Initially a sagittal T1-weighted (repetition time TR = 600 ms, echo delay time TE = 20 ms) localizer is obtained. T1- and T2-weighted (TR = 2000 ms, TE = 20/80 ms) images are then obtained in the axial and coronal planes.

In a recent report, Robinson et al reviewed the utility of gadolinium-DTPA enhanced MRI in the evaluation of head and neck tumors. In their experience, gadolinium-DTPA enhancement was useful in differentiating paranasal sinus tumors from inflammatory disease. Gadolinium also aids the demonstration of perineural involvement and intracranial extent.[25]

Pathology

Exquisite symmetry is a persistent feature of normal parapharyngeal spaces. Lesions may arise either within the parapharyngeal space or they may arise in tissues adjacent to the PPS. Displacement of PPS fat and/or the internal carotid artery are helpful in determining the origin of a mass; displacement also aids in narrowing the differential diagnosis. With a large or frankly invasive mass, it may be impossible to determine the site of origin.

Salivary gland tumors

The vast majority of PPS lesions are salivary gland tumors arising from the parotid gland or from salivary gland rests within the PPS. Salivary gland tumors account for approximately 45% of all PPS lesions. Between 80 and 90% of salivary gland tumors which arise in the PPS are benign pleomorphic adenomas. Salivary gland malignancies are less common and the majority of these include mucoepidermoid carcinoma, adenoid cystic carcinoma or acinic cell carcinoma.[12,14,16,17,20,26–29]

Pleomorphic adenoma (benign mixed tumor)

Pleomorphic adenoma is the most common prestyloid PPS tumor (Figs 2.3 and 2.4). It is most commonly found in the parotid gland where it comprises 65% of all tumors of that gland. Although the majority of patients are in the fifth decade of life, these tumors are more common in women and have been reported in all age groups. Mixed tumors of minor salivary gland origin usually occur in patients over 50 years old. Patients present with a smooth, freely moveable and nontender mass. Medial pharyngeal bowing may be appreciated at physical examination with sufficiently large tumors. Slow insidious growth is a feature of these tumors.

Computed tomography of mixed tumors, small to moderate in size, demonstrates homogeneous attenuation and contrast enhancement. Larger tumors may become inhomogeneous as areas of hemorrhage and necrosis develop. Dystrophic calcification is highly suggestive of a pleomorphic adenoma.

The MRI appearance is nonspecific. Typically these tumors exhibit intermediate signal intensity on both T1-weighted and proton density weighted images, and intermediate to high signal intensity on T2-weighted images. Large tumors will displace the internal carotid artery posterolaterally. Lobulated contour is suggestive of the diagnosis and is best demonstrated by MR.[30] Lesions arising from the deep portion of the parotid gland often assume a 'dumb-bell' configuration on axial images. This configuration is produced by constriction at the stylomandibular tunnel as the tumor grows medially into the parapharyngeal space.[31,32]

Careful attention must be paid to the interface between a PPS tumor and the parotid gland. If fat is seen in this interface on all of the images throughout the tumor, the lesion is not of parotid origin. If no fat is seen on these images, then the tumor either arises from, abuts, or infiltrates the parotid gland.[1] Parapharyngeal space tumors arising from the parotid gland may be pedunculated with only a narrow isthmus connecting the mass to the gland. It is therefore essential to appreciate the fatty interface on all images to accurately determine intra-from extra-parotid origin. This distinction is often crucial in determining the surgical approach. Exquisite soft tissue detail and contrast make MRI superior to CT in detecting this fatty interface.[20,30]

Malignant salivary gland tumors

Salivary gland malignancies of the PPS are rare. Parotid malignancies are most often mucoepidermoid carcinomas and minor salivary gland malignancies are most often adenoid cystic carcinomas.

The CT appearance of malignant lesions is variable. Smaller tumors may be homogeneous and demonstrate enhancement. Larger tumors become inhomogeneous due to hemorrhage and necrosis.[30,33] It is difficult to predict malignancy by CT unless frank soft tissue invasion or bony destruction is present. Facial nerve paralysis often heralds the presence of malignancy.

Although malignant tumors may lack conspicuous T2 hyperintensity, T1- and T2-weighted MR relaxation times are not particularly useful in distinguishing benign from malignant neoplasm. The appearance of the tumor margin seems to be the most sensitive indicator of malignancy. Benign tumors usually demonstrate well-defined borders whereas malignant lesions may demonstrate ill-defined borders and direct invasion of the adjacent soft tissues and skull base.

Neurogenic tumors

Neurogenic tumors are the most common retrostyloid PPS lesions and the second most common prestyloid PPS lesions (Fig. 2.5). They comprise approximately 20% of all PPS tumors and they most commonly arise from the vagus nerve.[12,14,16,17,20,26–29] Less commonly, neuromas may arise from the superior sympathetic chain. Multiplicity and an overall homogeneous appearance are characteristic features. These tumors are almost always benign. Neuromas of the PPS are not uncommon manifestations of the neurofibromatosis syndrome.

On contrast-enhanced CT scans, approximately 30% of the neuromas will densely enhance and therefore may simulate a paraganglioma. This distinction can be made at angiography where the neuroma will exhibit few if any tumor vessels.[18,34] Larger tumors will contain foci of hemorrhage, necrosis, fibrosis, cystic degeneration and calcification.[20] These changes are probably responsible for the inhomogeneous appearance on MRI. Anterior and medial displacement of the internal carotid artery is frequently present with large tumors and is highly suggestive of origin in the retrostyloid compartment.

Paragangliomas

Paragangliomas (glomus tumors) are hypervascular lesions that arise from the cells of chemoreceptor bodies. These include carotid body tumor, glomus tympanicum, glomus vagale and glomus jugulare. Paragangliomas account for 10–15% of all parapharyngeal space tumors (Figs 2.6–2.8).

Glomus vagale is the most common paraganglioma to affect the PPS. This tumor accounts for 3% of all paragangliomas[35] and arises from the paraganglionic cells of the nodose ganglion. Glomus jugulare tumors, which arise from the paraganglioma cells around the jugular bulb, may spread below the skull base to involve the PPS. Skull base erosion and intracranial extent help to distinguish this tumor from glomus vagale lesions. Infrequently, carotid body tumors become large enough to involve the PPS. Although paragangliomas are bilateral in only 2.8% of cases, the bilaterality may be as high as 26% in patients who show a familial tendency.[36]

Contrast-enhanced CT demonstrates a densely enhancing PPS mass. Anterior and medial bowing of the internal carotid artery may be present. Skull base erosion may be seen with glomus jugulare tumors.

The dominant MR findings are serpentine or channel-like areas of signal void within the tumor. This feature is present on all spin-echo pulse sequences. These channel voids are vascular flow voids produced by the dominantly vascular make-up of glomus tumors.

Miscellaneous lesions

Cysts, adjacent infections, and infiltrating neoplasms from the masticator and pharyngeal spaces comprise the remainder of PPS lesions.

Cystic lesions

Cystic lesions of the PPS include branchial cleft cyst (Fig. 2.9), abscess collections (Fig. 2.13), lymphangioma (Figs 2.11 and 2.12) and deep lobe parotid cysts (Fig. 2.10). These lesions demonstrate decreased attenuation on CT scans and may or may not demonstrate wall enhancement. Typical MR characteristics of a cyst include prolonged T1- and T2-relaxation times, although this is not always the case. Occasionally a cystic lesion will appear solid on MR images with increased T1-weighted signal intensity. This is usually the result of sequestration of proteins which causes shortening of the T1 relaxation time. In general, the CT appearance of a cystic lesion is more specific than MRI.

Cystic hygromas are most often encountered in the pediatric population although cases have been reported in adults. These hygromas typically arise in the posterior triangle of the neck and, if sufficiently large, they may extend into the PPS. These lesions may be very large and are characterized by their multiloculated appearance.

PPS abscess is usually the result of spread from an adjacent source. The most frequent seeding source is the palatine tonsil.[1] Odontogenic infection spreading to the masticator space may also involve the adjacent PPS.

Finally, cystic lesions of the parotid gland may bulge into the PPS. The most common cyst of the parotid gland is a retention cyst followed by branchial cleft cyst.

Infiltrating neoplasms

Neoplasms which infiltrate the PPS may arise from any of the adjacent compartments. Most commonly, an infiltrating neoplasm will arise from the medially placed pharyngeal surface. Nearly all of these tumors are carcinomas, predominantly squamous cell carcinomas by histology (Figs 2.14 and 2.15).[18,37,38] Less frequently occurring malignancies of the pharynx are minor salivary gland lesions (adenoid cystic and mucoepidermoid carcinomas), non-Hodgkin's lymphoma (Fig. 2.16) and sarcomas.[39,40] Rarely, juvenile angiofibromas attain sufficient size to infiltrate the PPS.

Tumors of the masticator space may involve the PPS. These are most commonly squamous cell carcinomas or minor salivary gland tumors which arise in the oral cavity. Primary sarcomas are much less common.

References

1 SOM PM, BERGERON MD, Parapharyngeal space. In: *Head and neck imaging*, 2nd edn (CV Mosby: St Louis 1991) 467–96.

2 SHOSS SM, DONOVAN DT, ALFORD BR, Tumors of the parapharyngeal space, *Arch Otolaryngol* (1985) 111:753–7.

3 MARAN AGD, MACKENZIE IJ, MURRAY JAM, The parapharyngeal space, *J Laryn Otol* (1984) 98:371–80.

4 EINSTEIN RAJ, Sialography in the differential diagnosis of parotid masses, *Surg Gynecol Obstet* (1966) 122:1079–83.

5 MEINE FJ, WOLOSHEN HJ, Radiologic diagnosis of salivary gland tumors, *Radiol Clin North Am* (1970) 8:475–85.

6 WHITE IL, Sialoangiographic x-ray visualization of major salivary glands, *Laryngoscope* (1972) 82:2032–48.

7 POTTER GD, Sialography and the salivary glands, *Otolaryngol Clin North Am* (1973) 6:509–15.

8 CALCATERRA TC, HEMENWAY WG, HANSEN GC et al, The value of sialography in the diagnosis of parotid tumors, *Arch Otolaryngol* (1977) 103:727–9.

9 WORK WP, JOHNS ME, Symposium on salivary gland diseases, *Otolaryngol Clin North Am* (1977) 10:261–426.

10 SOM PM, BILLER HF, The combined CT-sialogram, *Radiology* (1980) 135:387–90.

11 TSAI FY, GOLDSTEIN JC, PARHAD IM, Angiographic features of lateral neck masses, *J Otorhinolaryngol Relat Spec* (1977) 84:840–50.

12 WORK WP, Tumors of the parapharyngel space, *Trans Am Acad Ophthalmol Otolaryngol* (1969) 73:389–94.

13 BAKER D, CONLEY J, Surgical approach to retromandibular parotid tumors, *Ann Plast Surg* (1979) 3:304–14.

14 WORK WP, HYBELS R, A study of tumors of the parapharyngeal space, *Laryngoscope* (1974) 84:1748–55.

15 MCLEAN WC, Differential diagnosis and management of deep lobe parotid tumors, *Laryngoscope* (1976) 86:28–35.

16 LAWSON V, Unusual parapharyngeal lesions, *J Otolaryngol* (1979) 8:241–9.

17 HEENEMAN H, MARAN A, Parapharyngeal space tumors, *Clin Otolaryngol* (1979) 4:57–66.

18 SOM PM, BILLER HF, LAWSON W et al, Parapharyngeal space masses: an updated protocol based upon 104 cases, *Radiology* (1984) 153:149–56.

19 LLOYD GAS, PHELPS PD, The demonstration of tumors of the parapharyngeal space by MRI, *Br J Radiol* (1986) 59:675–83.

20 SOM PM, BRAUN IF, SHAPIRO MD et al, Tumors of the parapharyngeal space and upper neck: MRI characteristics, *Radiology* (1987) 64:823–9.

21 SOM PM, BILLER HF, The combined CT-sialogram: a technique to differentiate deep lobe parotid tumors from extraparotid pharyngomaxillary space tumors, *Ann Otolaryngol* (1979) 88:590–5.

22 SOM PM, BILLER HF, LAWSON W, Tumors of the parapharyngeal space: preoperative evaluation, diagnosis and surgical approaches, *Ann Otol, Rhino, Laryngol* (1981) 90(Suppl. 80, Part 4):3–15.

23 CARTER BL, HAMMERSCHLAG SB, WOLPERT SM, Computerized scanning in otorhinolaryngology, *Adv Otorhinolaryngol* (1978) 24:21–3.

24 SHUGAR MA, MAFEE MF, Diagnosis of carotid body tumors in dynamic computerized tomography, *Head Neck Surg* (1982) 4:518–21.

25 ROBINSON JD, CRAWFORD SC, LOUIS MT et al, Extracranial lesions of the head and neck: preliminary experience with Gd-DTPA enhanced MR imaging, *Radiology* (1989) 172:165–70.

26 HEENEMAN H, GILBERT IJ, ROOD SR, The parapharyngeal space: anatomy and pathologic conditions with emphasis on neurogenous tumors, Alexandria VA, 1980, *Am Acad Otolaryngol*.

27 MCILRATH DC, REMINE WH, DEVINE KD et al, Tumors of the parapharyngeal region, *Surg Gynecol Obstet* (1963) 116:88–93.

28 BATSAKIS JG, *Tumors of the head and neck: clinical and pathological considerations*, 2nd edn (Williams and Wilkins: Baltimore 1979) 1–75.

29 PEEL RZ, GNEPP DR, Diseases of salivary glands. In: Barnes L, ed *Surgical pathology of the head and neck*, Vol I (Marcel Dekker Inc: New York 1985) 533–645.

30 SOM PM, SACHER M, STOLLMAN AL et al, Common tumors of the parapharyngeal space: refined imaging diagnosis, *Radiology* (1988) **169**:81–5.

31 BERGERON RJ, OSBORN AG, SOM PM, *Head and neck imaging excluding the brain* (CV Mosby: St Louis 1984) 235–374.

32 SILVER AJ, MAWARD ME, HILAL SK et al, Computed tomography of the carotid and related spaces: Part I Anatomy, *Radiology* (1984) **150**:723–8.

33 MADELBLATT SM, BRAUN IF, PARIS PC et al, Parotid masses: MR imaging, *Radiology* (1987) **163**:411–14.

34 KUMAR AJ, KUHAJDA FP, MARTINEZ CR et al, Computed tomography of extracranial nerve sheath tumors with pathological correlation, *J Comput Assist Tomogr* (1983) 7:857–65.

35 OLSON JR, ABELL MR, Non-functional non-chromaffin paragangliomas of the retroperitoneum, *Cancer* (1969) **23**:1358–67.

36 COOK RL, Bilateral chemodectomas in the neck, *J Laryngol* (1977) **91**:611–16.

37 HARDIN CW, HARNSBERGER HR, OSBORN AG et al, Infection and tumor of the masticator space: CT evaluation, *Radiology* (1985) **157**:413–17.

38 SMOKER WRK, GENTRY LR, Computed tomography of the nasopharynx and related spaces, *Seminars Ultrasound, CT, MR* (1986) 7:107–11.

39 DILLON WP, *Nasopharynx and skull base*, presented at the New York Univ Med Center Post-Graduate course in Neuroradiology, CT and MR. Course Syllabus 1988, p. 10.

40 MANCUSO AA, HANAFEE WN, *Computed tomography and magnetic resonance imaging of the head and neck* (Williams and Wilkins: Baltimore 1985) 428–42.

A

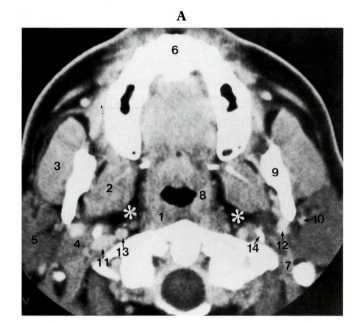

B

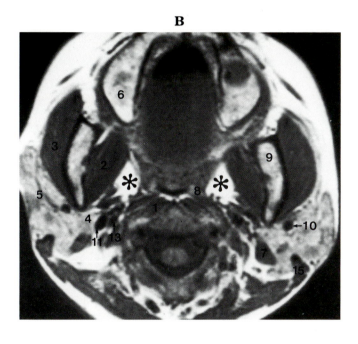

FIGURE 2.1

(**A,B**) Normal axial anatomy demonstrated by computed tomography and T1-weighted MR images (TR = 600 ms, TE = 20 ms). Key: *, parapharyngeal spaces; 1, longus coli muscle; 2, medial pterygoid muscle; 3, masseter muscle; 4, parotid gland deep lobe; 5, parotid gland superficial lobe; 6, alveolar ridge of maxilla; 7, posterior belly digastric muscle; 8, palatal muscles; 9, mandible; 10, retromandibular vein; 11, internal jugular vein; 12, external carotid artery; 13, internal carotid artery; 14, styloid process; 15, sternocleidomastoid muscle.

A

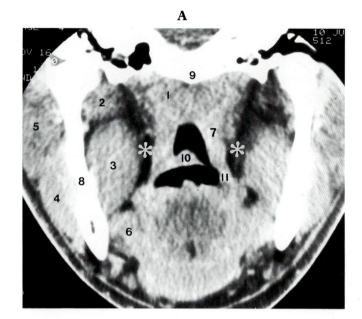

B

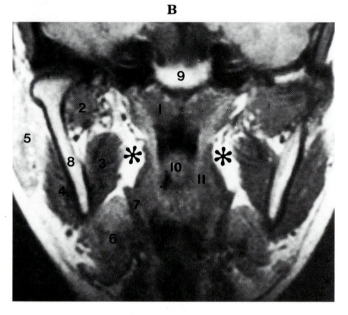

FIGURE 2.2

(**A,B**) Normal coronal anatomy demonstrated by computed tomography and T1-weighted MR images (TR = 600 ms, TE = 20 ms). Key: *, parapharyngeal spaces; 1, longus coli muscle; 2, lateral pterygoid muscle; 3, medial pterygoid muscle; 4, masseter muscle; 5, parotid gland superficial lobe; 6, submandibular gland; 7, pharyngeal musculature; 8, mandible; 9, clivus; 10, uvula; 11, tonsillar pillar.

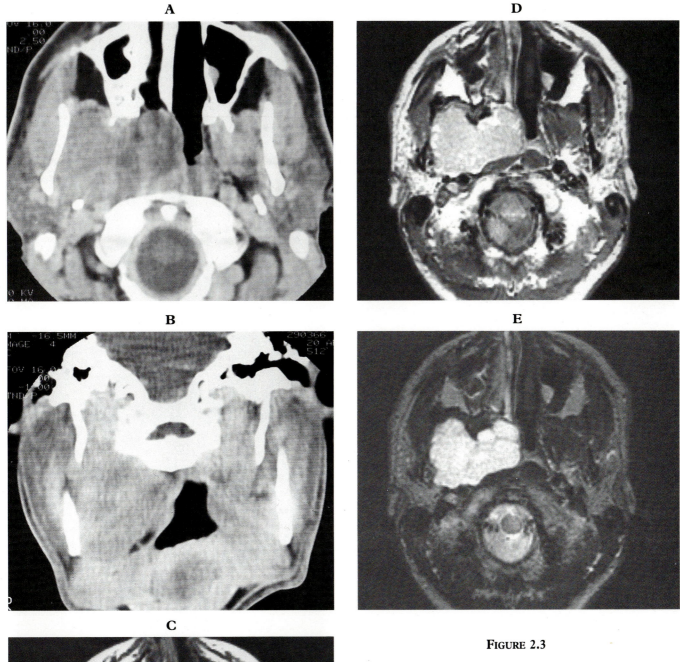

A

B

C

D

E

FIGURE 2.3

Benign pleomorphic adenoma arising from the deep lobe of the parotid gland. (**A,B**) Axial and coronal contrast-enhanced CT images. There is a large irregularly enhancing right PPS mass. No definite fat plane of separation is present between the mass and the deep lobe of the parotid gland. (**C – E**) Axial T1-weighted (TR = 600 ms, TE = 20 ms) and T2-weighted (TR = 2000 ms, TE = 20/80 ms) images demonstrate a relatively homogeneous, lobulated PPS mass which is inseparable from the adjacent parotid gland. Note the high T2 signal intensity exhibited by this tumor.

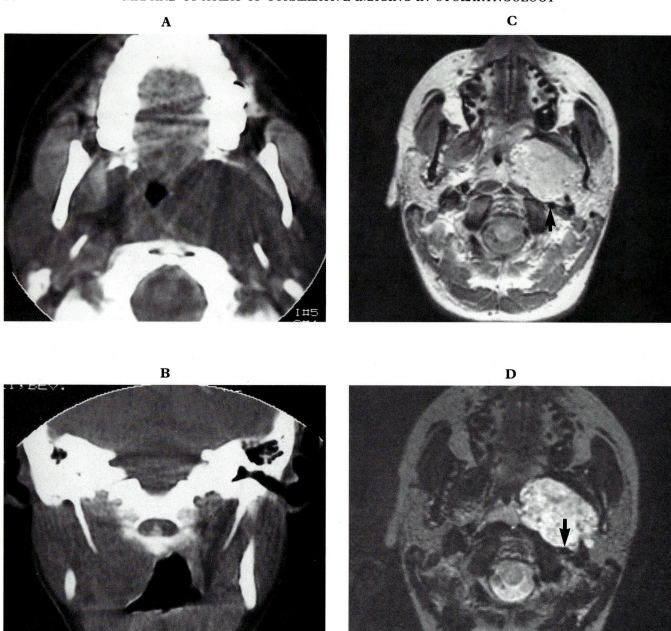

FIGURE 2.4

Benign pleomorphic adenoma left PPS. (**A,B**) Axial and coronal CT images demonstrate a large left PPS mass. There is medial bowing of the lateral pharyngeal margin.

(**C – F**) Axial and coronal T2-weighted MR images (TR = 2400 ms, TE = 20/80 ms). There is posterior and lateral displacement of the internal carotid artery (arrow) consistent with a prestyloid PPS mass. The

continued

E

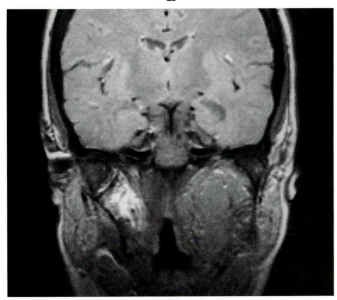

F

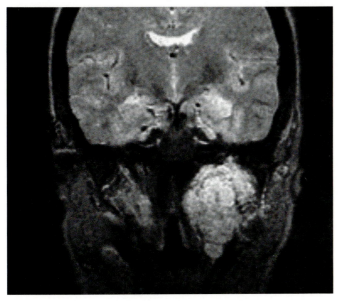

FIGURE 2.4 *(continued)*

mass exhibits slightly hyperintense and markedly
hyperintense signal intensity of proton density and
T2-weighted images.

A

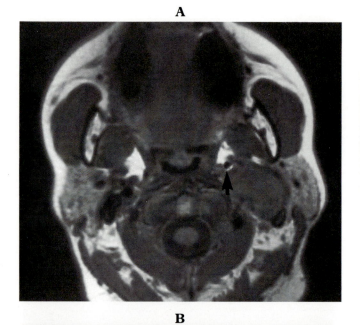

C

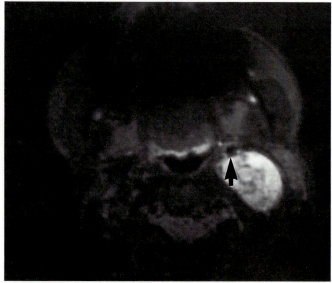

B

FIGURE 2.5

Schwannoma of the 9th cranial nerve. (**A – C**) Axial T1-weighted (TR = 600 ms, TE = 20 ms) and T2-weighted (TR = 2000 ms, TE = 20/80 ms) MR images. There is anterior and medial displacement of the left internal carotid artery (arrow) produced by the left retrostyloid PPS mass. The signal characteristics of this mass are nonspecific, however, the retrostyloid PPS origin and the lack of 'channel-voids' make neuroma a likely diagnosis.

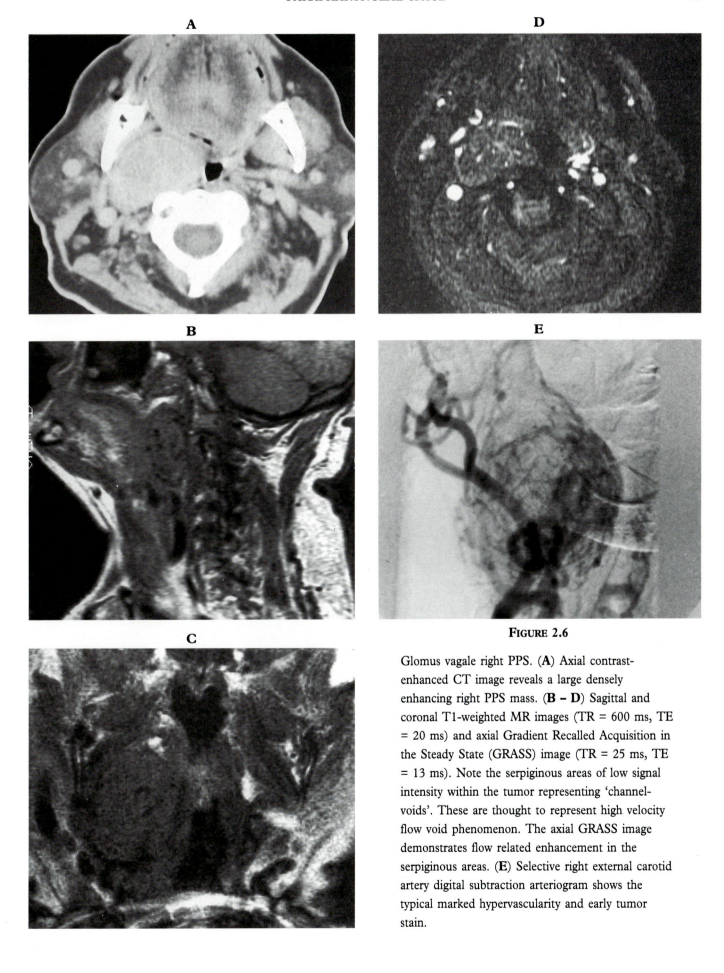

FIGURE 2.6

Glomus vagale right PPS. (**A**) Axial contrast-enhanced CT image reveals a large densely enhancing right PPS mass. (**B – D**) Sagittal and coronal T1-weighted MR images (TR = 600 ms, TE = 20 ms) and axial Gradient Recalled Acquisition in the Steady State (GRASS) image (TR = 25 ms, TE = 13 ms). Note the serpiginous areas of low signal intensity within the tumor representing 'channel-voids'. These are thought to represent high velocity flow void phenomenon. The axial GRASS image demonstrates flow related enhancement in the serpiginous areas. (**E**) Selective right external carotid artery digital subtraction arteriogram shows the typical marked hypervascularity and early tumor stain.

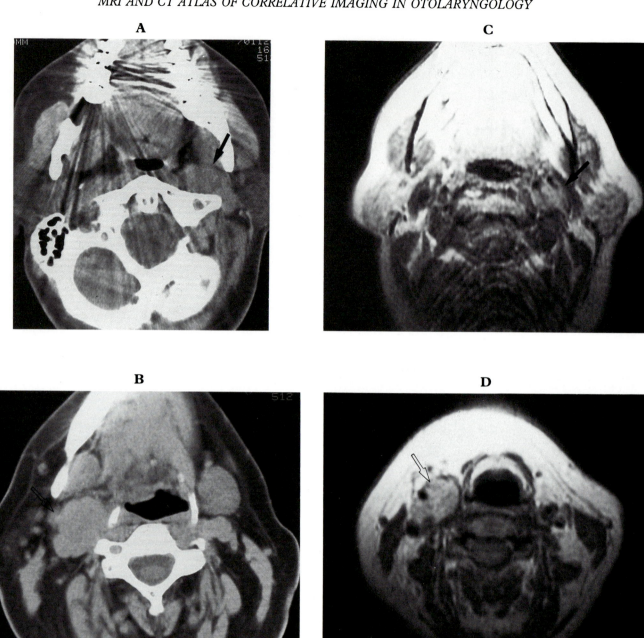

FIGURE 2.7

Bilateral paragangliomas. (**A,B**) Axial noncontrast CT images. There is a soft tissue mass deforming the posterior and lateral boundaries of the left PPS (solid arrow). A second mass is present at the level of the hyoid bone (open arrow). This mass displaces the right submandibular gland anteriorly.

(**C,D**) Proton density MR images (TR = 2000 ms, TE = 30 ms). The masses are well demarcated and homogeneous. The left PPS mass (solid arrow) is a glomus vagale and the mass in the right neck (open arrow) is a carotid body tumor.

A

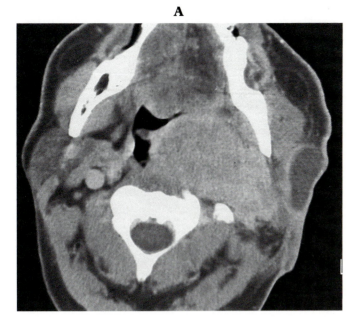

C

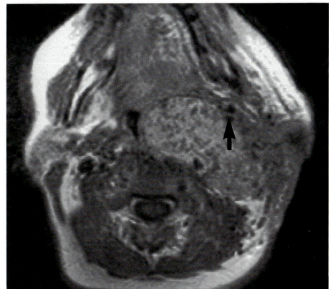

B

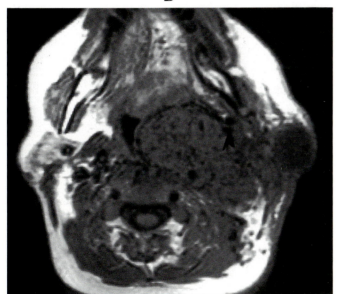

FIGURE 2.8

Glomus vagale left PPS. (**A**) Axial contrast-enhanced CT image. There is a large enhancing left PPS mass. The overlying left subcutaneous structure is an incidental finding unrelated to the mass. (**B,C**) Axial T1-weighted MR images (TR = 600 ms, TE = 16 ms) pre- and post-gadolinium infusion. There is anterior displacement of the carotid artery (arrow) as well as multiple 'channel-voids' within the tumor. The mass demonstrates moderate contrast enhancement.

continued

D

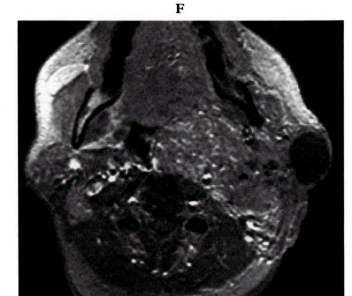

E

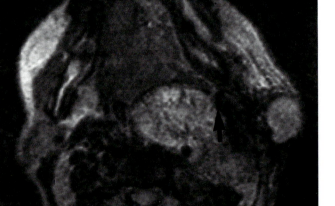

FIGURE 2.8 *(continued)*

(**D,E**) T2-weighted MR images (TR = 2000 ms, TE = 20/80 ms). Again note the anterior displacement of the carotid artery placing the mass in the retrostyloid PPS (arrow). (**F**) Axial spoiled GRASS (TR = 50 ms, TE = 5 ms, flip angle = 45°). Note the flow-related enhancement within the mass.

A

D

B

E

C

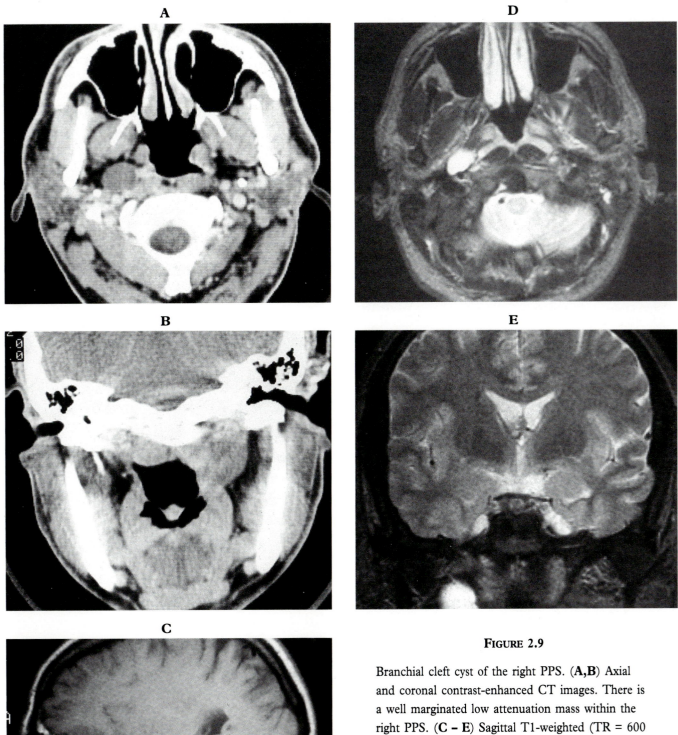

FIGURE 2.9

Branchial cleft cyst of the right PPS. (**A,B**) Axial and coronal contrast-enhanced CT images. There is a well marginated low attenuation mass within the right PPS. (**C – E**) Sagittal T1-weighted (TR = 600 ms, TE = 20 ms) and axial and coronal T2-weighted (TR = 2500 ms, TE = 80 ms) MR images. The shortened T1 relaxation time with resultant increase in T1 signal intensity may be produced by high protein content. On the T2-weighted pulse sequence, the mass demonstrates high signal intensity. This is a branchial cleft remnant of the second branchial pouch.

A

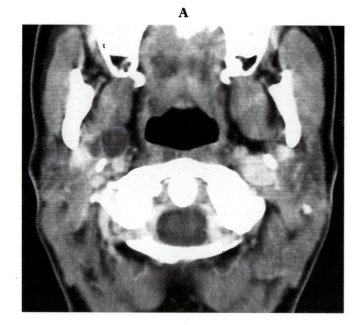

B

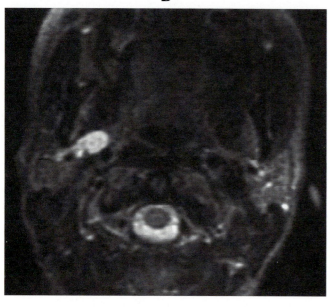

FIGURE 2.10

Retention cyst of the deep lobe of the parotid gland. (**A**) Axial contrast-enhanced CT image reveals a 2 cm low attenuation cystic-appearing mass in the region of the right PPS. (**B**) Axial T2-weighted MR image (TR = 2400 ms, TE = 80 ms). The mass exhibits high signal intensity supportive of a cyst. The cystic structure is contiguous with the deep lobe of the adjacent parotid gland.

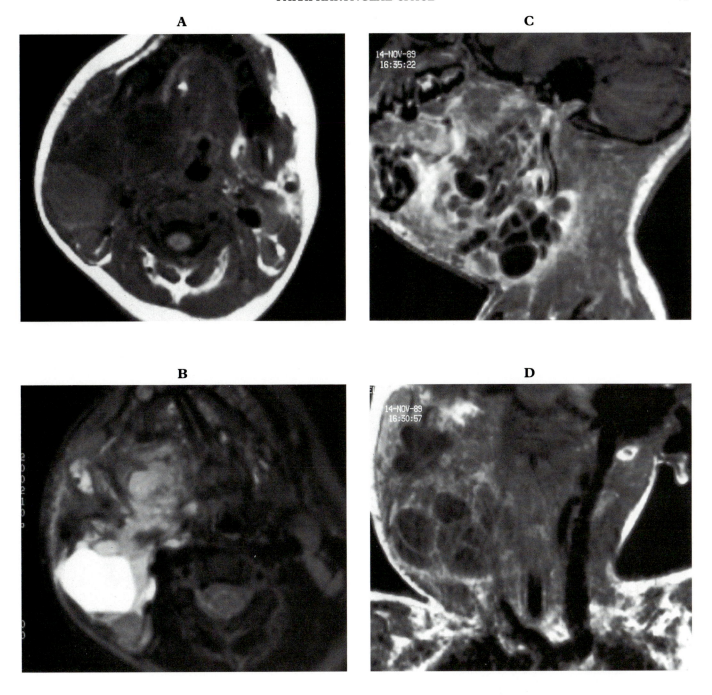

FIGURE 2.11

Large multiloculated cystic hygroma (lymphangioma) of the right posterior triangle and PPS. (**A,B**) Axial T1-weighted (TR = 600 ms, TE = 15 ms) and T2-weighted (TR = 2500 ms, TE = 90 ms) MR images. There is a large predominantly cystic right posterior triangle and PPS mass. Note the mixed signal intensity of this lesion. (**C,D**) Sagittal and coronal postgadolinium infusion T1-weighted MR images (TR = 600 ms, TE = 15 ms). This multiloculated mass demonstrates enhancement of several cyst walls, possibly the result of inflammation.

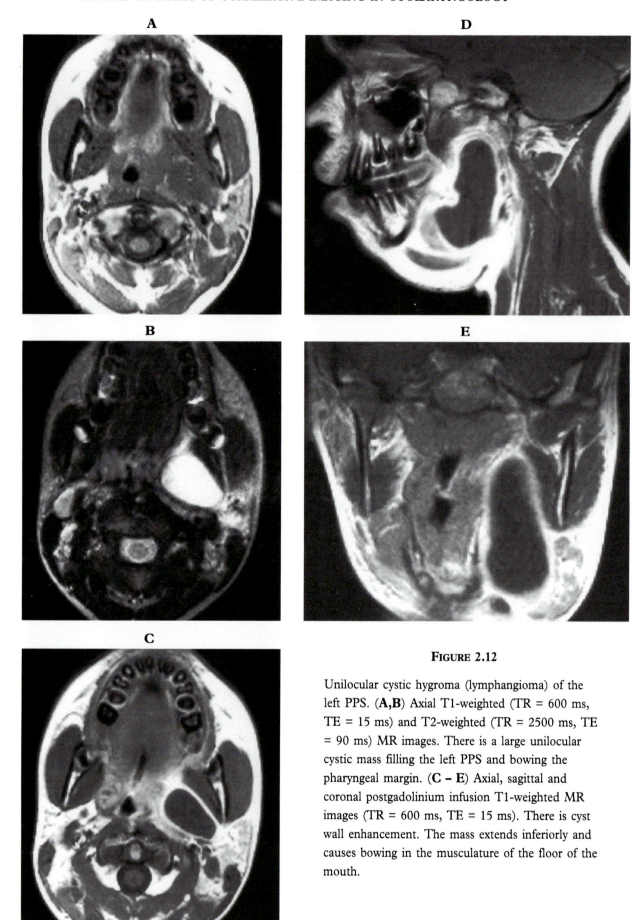

FIGURE 2.12

Unilocular cystic hygroma (lymphangioma) of the left PPS. (**A,B**) Axial T1-weighted (TR = 600 ms, TE = 15 ms) and T2-weighted (TR = 2500 ms, TE = 90 ms) MR images. There is a large unilocular cystic mass filling the left PPS and bowing the pharyngeal margin. (**C – E**) Axial, sagittal and coronal postgadolinium infusion T1-weighted MR images (TR = 600 ms, TE = 15 ms). There is cyst wall enhancement. The mass extends inferiorly and causes bowing in the musculature of the floor of the mouth.

A

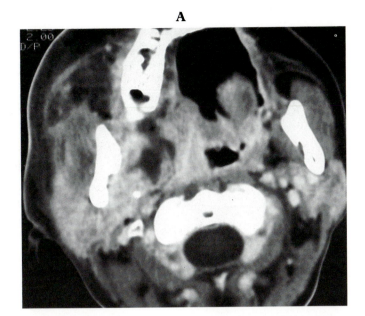

B

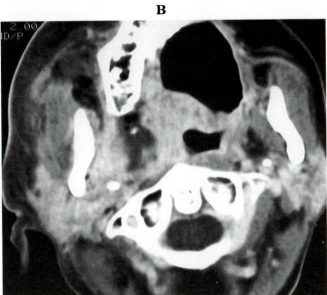

FIGURE 2.13

Abscess of the right masticator space spreading to the right PPS. (**A,B**) Contiguous axial images from a contrast-enhanced CT study. Note the low density inflammatory process involving the right masseter muscle and the right pterygoid muscles extending into the right PPS.

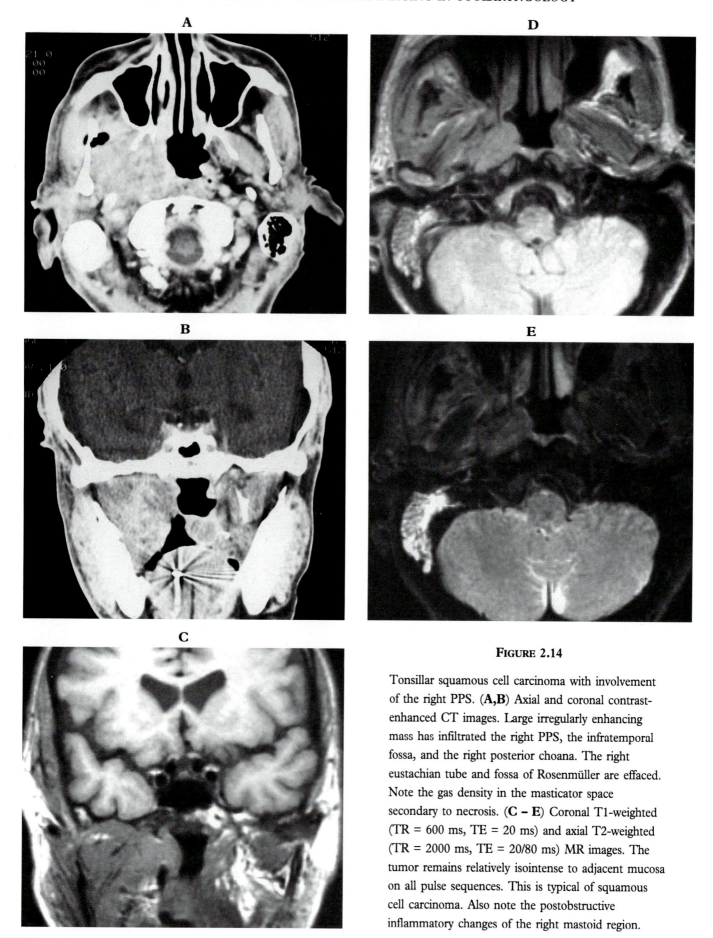

A

B

C

D

E

FIGURE 2.14

Tonsillar squamous cell carcinoma with involvement of the right PPS. (**A,B**) Axial and coronal contrast-enhanced CT images. Large irregularly enhancing mass has infiltrated the right PPS, the infratemporal fossa, and the right posterior choana. The right eustachian tube and fossa of Rosenmüller are effaced. Note the gas density in the masticator space secondary to necrosis. (**C – E**) Coronal T1-weighted (TR = 600 ms, TE = 20 ms) and axial T2-weighted (TR = 2000 ms, TE = 20/80 ms) MR images. The tumor remains relatively isointense to adjacent mucosa on all pulse sequences. This is typical of squamous cell carcinoma. Also note the postobstructive inflammatory changes of the right mastoid region.

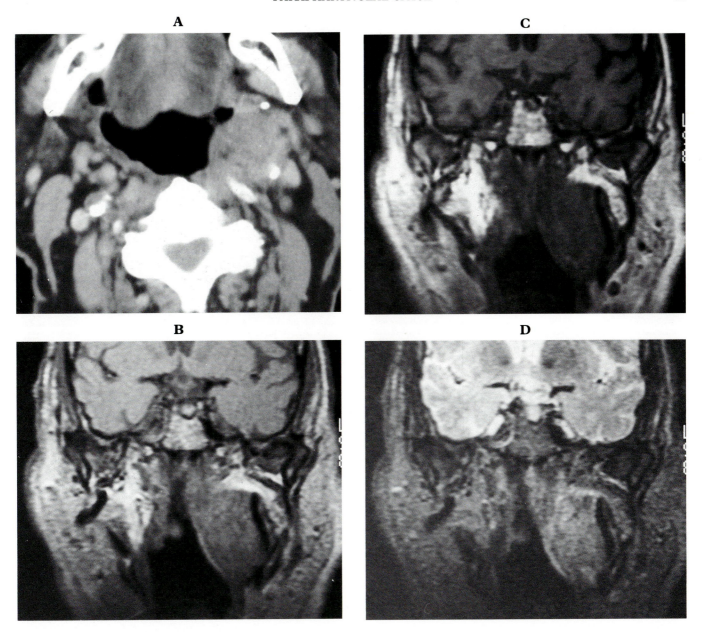

FIGURE 2.15

Squamous cell carcinoma presenting as a predominantly PPS mass. (**A**) Axial contrast-enhanced CT demonstrates a left PPS mass with associated bowing of the lateral oropharyngeal margin. (**B–D**) Coronal T1-weighted (TR = 800 ms, TE = 20 ms) and T2-weighted (TR = 2000 ms, TE = 20/80 ms) MR images. The mass is almost completely contained within the left PPS. Note the isointensity to adjacent mucosa on all the pulse sequences.

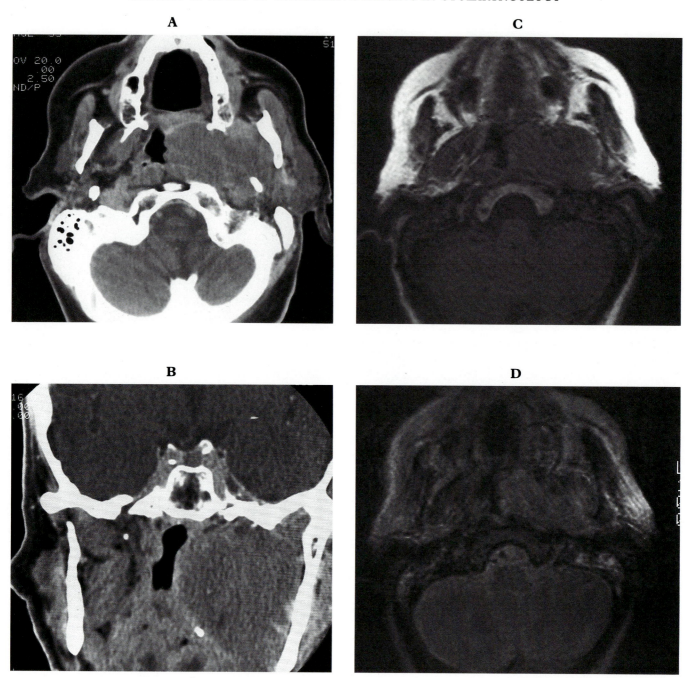

FIGURE 2.16

Lymphoma infiltrating the left PPS. (**A,B**) Axial and coronal contrast-enhanced CT images. There is a large mass infiltrating the left PPS and infratemporal fossa with superior extent to the skull base.

(**C,D**) Axial T1-weighted (TR = 600 ms, TE = 20 ms) and T2-weighted (TR = 2000 ms, TE = 80 ms) MR images. The mass has completely deformed the nasopharynx. There is only slight increase in T2 signal intensity.

continued

E

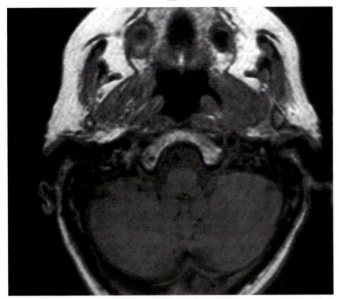

F

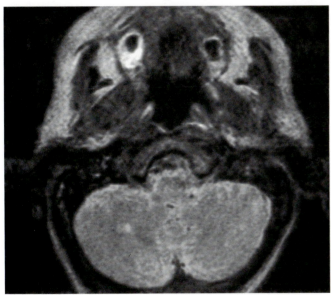

FIGURE 2.16 *(continued)*

(**E,F**) Axial T1- and T2-weighted MR images 3 months later following radiation therapy. There has been a significant interval improvement. There is only a small residual of the original mass.

CHAPTER 3

SALIVARY GLANDS

Introduction

Magnetic resonance (MR) imaging provides a noninvasive source of information in the evaluation of salivary gland neoplasms. Magnetic resonance offers superior soft tissue contrast, excellent spatial resolution, and direct multiplanar imaging. These inherent MR features aid in demonstrating: (a) intra- and extra-glandular lesions; (b) the margins of the lesion (discrete versus indistinct); (c) relationship to the facial nerve; and (d) multicentricity of the lesion.

Magnetic resonance is the examination of choice in the initial evaluation of salivary gland masses;[1] however, in many cases computed tomography (CT) is equally good. Plain films, sialography and CT remain as the principal imaging modalities in patients with a history or clinical picture of inflammatory or calculus disease.

Normal anatomy

Parotid gland

The parotid glands, which are bilaterally symmetric, are located anterior and inferior to the ear lobes. Each gland is arbitrarily divided into superficial and deep lobes by the course of the facial nerve.

The course of the facial nerve and its relationship to a parotid mass is of surgical significance. Malignant lesions in close proximity to the facial nerve may require partial excision of the facial nerve trunk and subsequent microsurgical repair. A large lesion in the deep lobe may need improved access by division and reflection of the mandibular ramus.[2]

The facial nerve exits the brainstem near the pontomedullary junction. After a short course through the cerebellopontine angle cistern, the facial nerve enters the internal auditory canal in close proximity to the eighth cranial nerve. The labyrinthine segment of the facial nerve then travels anterior to the geniculate ganglion. The tympanic portion of the nerve then runs posteriorly under the lateral semicircular canal along the medial wall of the tympanic cavity. At the level of the tympanic sinus, the nerve bends inferiorly and forms the vertical portion within the facial nerve canal. The vertical segment exits the skull base at the stylomastoid foramen (Fig. 3.1).

There is a short segment of nerve distal to the stylomastoid foramen and proximal to the parotid gland. This segment of nerve courses through the fat located between the sternocleidomastoid and the digastric muscles. This segment is routinely demonstrated on axial CT and MR scans. Magnetic resonance becomes important in the detection of perineural tumor spread.[3]

The facial nerve enters the parotid gland posteriorly and courses lateral to the external carotid artery and the retromandibular vein. Just behind the posterior border of the mandibular ramus, the facial nerve trunk divides into its two major branches, the temporofacial and cervicofacial nerves. These major branches then further ramify into the zygomatic, temporal, buccal, cervical and mandibular branches. Within the parotid gland, the facial nerve and its branches follow an arciform course within a plane that is concave superiorly and medially. This arciform plane divides the superficial and deep lobes of the parotid gland.[4,5]

Direct MR imaging of the facial nerve and its branches within the parotid gland has been described.[6] On MR, a variable yet characteristic 's-shaped' appearance is formed by the intraparotid facial nerve and its branches. Consistent MR demonstration of the intraparotid facial nerve is difficult and somewhat controversial.

Injuries to the extracranial portion of the facial nerve result in ipsilateral facial paralysis (peripheral facial nerve paralysis). The special functions of the facial nerve (lacrimation, stapedial reflex and taste in the anterior two-thirds of the tongue) are spared by injuries to the extracranial segment of the facial nerve.

Other important structures within the parotid gland include the external carotid artery, the retromandibular vein and scattered lymph nodes. The external carotid artery is located just medial to the retromandibular vein. These two vessels are readily identified on both CT and MR. The facial nerve travels immediately lateral to the retromandibular vein.

The parotid gland is the only salivary gland which contains lymph nodes. These nodes serve as a first-order drainage site for malignancies of the adjacent scalp, external auditory canal and deep face. There are approximately 20–30 lymph nodes within a normal parotid gland and the majority of these are situated lateral to the intraglandular course of the retromandibular vein.

The parotid duct (Stensen's duct) emerges from the gland anteriorly. The duct courses superficially over the masseter muscle and then curves medially to pierce the buccinator muscle near the second molar.

The extent and boundaries of the parotid space are well delineated by CT and MR (Figs 3.2 and 3.3). Along with the masticator space and its contents, the parotid space contributes to the structures of the infratemporal fossa. Superiorly the parotid space extends to the level of the external auditory canal. Inferiorly the gland extends down to the mandibular angle and often the tail of the parotid gland will dip below this level. The posterior belly of the digastric muscle and its fascia form the posteromedial border of the parotid space. The posterior belly of the digastric muscle also separates the parotid space from the posteriorly located carotid space.

Directly medial to the deep lobe of the parotid gland is the parapharyngeal space. The deep lobe of the parotid gland extends between the mandibular ramus and the styloid process (stylomandibular tunnel) into the parapharyngeal space. Lesions of the prestyloid parapharyngeal compartment are almost always of salivary gland origin, arising either from the deep lobe of the parotid gland or, on occasion, from minor salivary gland rests. The superficial lobe of the parotid gland extends subcutaneously at the anterior border of the sternocleidomastoid muscle and on the outer surface of the masseter muscles.

Accessory parotid tissue can be found in approximately 20% of the population.[7] When present, these accessory rests of tissue are found on or above the parotid duct and are bound to the masseter by extensions of the masseteric fascia. These accessory rests drain via a single major conduit into Stensen's duct. Parotid rests are histologically and functionally identical to the main gland.[8]

Submandibular gland

The paired submandibular glands are located within the submandibular spaces bilaterally (Figs 3.2 and 3.3). The larger superficial portion of the gland lies inferior to the mylohyoid muscle and is covered by the platysma. The deep portion of the gland lies just posterior and inferior to the mylohyoid muscle. Often a small portion of the gland extends superiorly over the posterior margin of the mylohyoid muscle to lie within the sublingual space. The submandibular duct runs forward through the sublingual space to its opening in the papilla in the anterior floor of the mouth.[1,9] Numerous lymph nodes are present within the submandibular space adjacent to the glandular parenchyma. There are no lymph nodes contained within the glandular capsule.

Sublingual gland

The sublingual glands are the smallest of the major salivary glands. They are contained within the sublingual space, superior to the mylohyoid muscle and lateral to the geniohyoid and genioglossus muscles. The submandibular duct, the lingual and hypoglossal nerves, the lingual artery and vein also course through the sublingual space.

Minor salivary glands

Minor salivary gland tissue is present throughout the nasal cavity, sinuses, oral cavity, pharynx and larynx. Although tumors of minor salivary origin are uncommon, the majority of these lesions are malignant.[10]

Imaging strategies

Plain films

Plain films are reserved primarily for the detection of salivary gland calculi. Approximately 80% of submandibular stones and 60% of parotid stones are radiopaque.[11] Various angled projections can be used to avoid superimposition over facial and skull base bony structures.

Sialography

Sialography today is used sparingly and only for the evaluation of various inflammatory diseases that affect ductal morphology, and in the detection of nonopaque calculi. Radiopaque contrast material is injected into the parotid or submandibular ducts and multiple images are obtained. Sialography is contraindicated in the acutely inflamed gland due to the potential of retrograde spread of infection.

Computed tomography

Computed tomography offers precise anatomic detail in the evaluation of salivary gland neoplasms. Computed tomography has few shortcomings, the most pronounced of which is image degradation by dental amalgam. Often slight gantry angle is necessary to avoid the streaking produced by dental fillings. In severe cases, MR is a valuable alternative.

Computed tomography of the salivary glands is routinely performed in the axial and coronal planes. Contiguous 5 mm sections are usually sufficient. Because the parotid gland contains fatty stroma, in contrast to most parotid lesions which are of soft tissue attenuation, unenhanced CT usually adequately demonstrates intraparotid lesions.[7,12] However, the use of iodinated contrast agents often increases the conspicuity of the lesions and more clearly demonstrates tumor margins.

The normal parotid gland contains a variable amount of fat and is consistently less dense (−25 to −10 HU) than adjacent muscle (30–60 HU). The retromandibular vein and external carotid artery within the parotid parenchyma are routinely demonstrated (Fig. 3.2). The intraparotid facial nerve and parotid duct are not demonstrated by routine CT.

The submandibular glands are usually more dense (35–60 HU) than the parotid glands and near isodense with the adjacent musculature (Fig. 3.2). Submandibular adenopathy is easily differentiated from an intraglandular lesion in patients with clinically palpable submandibular region masses.

The sublingual glands are fatty structures contained within the sublingual space bilaterally just below the lateral mucosa of the floor of the mouth. These glands are of similar attenuation to the surrounding fat and are not routinely identified.[13]

Although MR has several distinct advantages over CT, many authors believe that CT is as good as MR in the evaluation of salivary gland masses.

Calculus disease of the salivary glands may be evaluated with plain films and sialography, but CT is being increasingly utilized in the detection of calculi and evaluation of inflammatory disease. When parotid abscess is a clinical concern, CT with contrast allows identification of abscess versus cellulitis.

Magnetic resonance imaging

Magnetic resonance offers superior soft tissue contrast and direct multiplanar imaging without the use of ionizing radiation and without significant image degradation by dental amalgam. Disadvantages of MR include susceptibility to motion artifacts and the inability to demonstrate calcium and subtle bone erosion. Magnetic resonance is contraindicated in patients with pacemakers and cerebral aneurysm clips.

Routine MR of the salivary glands consists of T1- and T2-weighted images in multiple planes. The axial and coronal planes tend to be most helpful when assessing tumor margins. Gadolinium enhancement is useful in the detection of perineural tumor extent.

The normal parotid gland is hyperintense in relation to adjacent musculature on T1-, proton density, and T2-weighted images. Because of the parotid fat content, the gland is closer in signal intensity to fat. The intraparotid segments of the retromandibular vein and external carotid artery are routinely demonstrated by MR as side-by-side oval signal voids (Fig. 3.3). The intraparotid facial nerve has been described and can be demonstrated by MR.[6] The parotid duct is not normally seen.

The submandibular gland demonstrates signal intensity similar to adjacent musculature on all pulse sequences (Fig. 3.3). The duct is not normally visualized.

Magnetic resonance provides a non-invasive source of information when evaluating salivary gland masses. Magnetic resonance is superior to CT in the demonstration of intra- versus extra-glandular tumors, tumor margins, multicentricity and relationship to the facial nerve. Computed tomography becomes a valuable alternative in patients with contraindications to MR, and in demonstrating calcium and bone erosion.

Pathology

Calculus and inflammatory diseases

Salivary gland inflammation may be the result of obstructive (stone, mucous plug, or stricture) (Figs 3.4 and 3.5) or non-obstructive pathology (Sjögren's syndrome).

Inflammation of the gland itself (sialadenitis) may be categorized as autoimmune (Figs 3.6 and 3.7) or non-autoimmune (Figs 3.8–3.10). Non-autoimmune sialadenitis may be acute or chronic. Acute pyogenic parotitis (staphylococcal, streptococcal, Gram-negative or pneumococcal), which is seen in children, is initially unilateral but invariably progresses to bilateral involvement. Approximately 35% of acute pyogenic parotitis occurs in postoperative patients ('surgical parotitis'); 20% of these cases are bilateral.[14,15] Acute parotitis may also be viral (mumps, Coxsackie A or ECHO viruses). Chronic or granulomatous sialadenitis may be secondary to tuberculosis, sarcoidosis or actino-

mycosis. Of the salivary glands, sarcoidosis and tuberculosis most frequently involve the parotids. Sarcoidosis will involve the salivary glands in 6% of cases and involvement is usually bilateral. Tuberculosis of the parotids is frequently unilateral.

Autoimmune sialadenitis refers to a group of entities believed to have an autoimmune etiology and similar radiologic and histologic findings. Mikulicz disease and Sjögren's syndrome are examples of autoimmune sialadenitis. Mikulicz disease is a nonspecific entity assigned to patients with simultaneous lacrimal and parotid enlargement. Sjögren's syndrome consists of xerostomia, keratoconjunctivitis and collagen vascular disease. Rheumatoid arthritis is most commonly encountered in the syndrome; however, Sjögren's syndrome may be seen with scleroderma, lupus erythematosus and periarteritis nodosa. The 'sicca syndrome' refers to xerostomia and keratoconjunctivitis in the absence of collagen vascular disease. Complications of Sjögren's syndrome include a wide variety of lymphoreticular disorders ranging from benign lymphocytic infiltration to malignant lymphoma (Figs 3.7 and 3.27).

Cystic lesion

Branchial cleft cyst

Branchial cleft cysts represent embryologic remnants of the parapharyngeal pouch system (Figs 3.12 and 3.13). A persistent epithelial lined tract in the developmental course of a pharyngeal pouch produces the branchial cyst seen in adults. Approximately 95% of branchial cleft cysts are remnants of the second branchial cleft. Although first branchial cleft cysts are rare, a parotid region cyst is often a remnant of the first branchial cleft. In general, cysts in the parotid region are most commonly retention cysts (Fig. 3.11). Branchial cleft cysts are the second most common cyst in the parotid region.

Branchial cleft cysts may occur superficially, within, or medial to the parotid gland. The usual clinical picture is a middle-aged female with a history of recurrent parotid abscesses unresponsive to antibiotics or drainage. If the cyst is connected to the external auditory canal, otorrhea will be present. The connection is usually at the junction of the bony and cartilaginous canals.

Computed tomography will demonstrate a cystic structure. Enhancement may or may not be apparent in the cyst wall according to the degree of cyst inflammation. Typical MR features of a cyst with prolongation of T1 and T2 relaxation are usually the case. Again, wall thickness and enhancement will reflect inflammatory status.

Multicentric parotid cysts (lymphoepithelial cysts) in AIDS patients

Several recent investigators[16,17] have reported an entity in AIDS patients characterized by multicentric benign lymphoepithelial parotid cysts associated with hyperplastic cervical adenopathy (Fig. 3.14). The appearance of multiple parotid cysts and hyperplastic cervical lymphadenopathy is very characteristic of AIDS or pre-AIDS patients.[16] Intraparotid cyst and neoplasm may appear similar on MR with prolonged T1 and T2 relaxation times. Although MR identifies parotid masses more reliably than CT, CT is a better modality for differentiating solid from cystic lesion.

Ranula

The ranula is a retention phenomenon which occurs in the floor of the mouth and is the result of obstruction of the sublingual gland (Fig. 3.15). There are two types of ranulas, simple and plunging. Each has a different clinical behavior and appearance and each requires different treatment. The simple ranula is a true retention cyst contained within the sublingual space. It is epithelial lined and results from obstructed ducts. The plunging ranula extends below the floor of the mouth into the fascial planes of the upper neck. The extent is usually over the posterior edge of the mylohyoid muscle into the submandibular space or actually through a small defect in the mylohyoid following a vascular pedicle. A plunging ranula progresses with time and is the result of mucous extravasation. Simple ranulas are excised or marsupialized. Plunging ranulas require further dissection for complete removal. The sublingual gland of origin is also excised.

Posttraumatic sialocele

Posttraumatic sialocele and fistula are best demonstrated by sialography (Fig. 3.16). Computed tomography sialography is often helpful in identifying the relationship to the main duct. Fistula and sialocele are the result of direct injury to the salivary duct system.

Benign neoplasms

Pleomorphic adenoma

Pleomorphic adenoma (mixed tumor) is the most common benign tumor, comprising 70% of all benign salivary gland tumors and 70–80% of all parotid tumors (Figs 3.17–3.19). These are slow-growing tumors which usually present between the fourth and sixth decades of life. This tumor is exceedingly rare in children and there is a slight female predominance.[18] Approximately 80% of the parotid mixed tumors occur in the superficial lobe; however, they may occur in the deep lobe and also in the parapharyngeal space arising from salivary rests. Mixed tumors which arise in the deep lobe and grow anteriorly and medially to approximate the parapharyngeal space often assume a 'dumb-bell' configuration. This configuration is produced by constriction as the mass passes through the stylomandibular tunnel.

The MR appearance of a pleomorphic adenoma is a well-circumscribed mass which demonstrates low to intermediate signal on T1-weighted images and high signal intensity on the T2-weighted images. Occasionally, large tumors may demonstrate lobulated margins and foci of low signal intensity (fibrosis or dystrophic calcification). The inability to detect calcium on MR is a disadvantage since the presence of calcium within a parotid mass makes pleomorphic adenoma a likely diagnosis.

Warthin's tumor (papillary cystadenoma lymphomatosum)

Warthin's tumor is a benign slow-growing tumor of the parotid gland. There is a definite male predominance. This tumor is typically located in the tail of the parotid and is frequently multiple and bilateral (Figs 3.20 and 3.21). Intraparotid lymphadenopathy is the major differential consideration. The typical MR appearance is a well-circumscribed or partially lobulated mass which exhibits intermediate signal intensity on T1-weighted images and high signal intensity on T2-weighted images. Preoperative diagnostic specificity can be obtained on Tc-99m radionuclide scans. Warthin's tumor is characteristically 'hot' on these studies.

Hemangioma

Hemangioma is the most common parotid neoplasm in infants (Fig. 3.22). Parotid enlargement in childhood is almost always inflammatory in nature. Hemangioma is a benign tumor which demonstrates intermediate signal on T1-weighted images and high signal on T2-weighted images. Due to the vascular nature of this tumor, 'channel-voids' and the 'salt-and-pepper' appearance may be apparent.[19]

Malignant neoplasms

Mucoepidermoid carcinoma

Mucoepidermoid carcinoma comprises approximately 6% of all salivary gland tumors. The parotid gland is the most commonly involved salivary gland (Figs 3.23 and 3.24). Other than the parotid gland, the palate is the most frequent site for this tumor. Mucoepidermoid carcinoma has been reported in all ages. However, there is a peak in patients who are in the fourth and fifth decades of life, and a slight female predominance. Although cyst formation is highly unusual in the high-grade variety, the tumor may exhibit cystic components.[13]

The MR appearance of mucoepidermoid carcinoma varies with grade of aggressiveness. Low grade carcinomas may mimic benign tumors and demonstrate intermediate signal intensity on T1-weighted images and high signal intensity on T2-weighted images. High-grade malignancies tend to be highly cellular with decreased amounts of serous and mucoid material and also tend to exhibit low signal intensity on T1- and T2-weighted images.[20] Involvement of the deep lobe of the parotid gland and poor delineation of the tumor margins are additional MR findings suggestive of malignancy. Facial nerve paralysis associated with a parotid mass is almost always indicative of underlying malignancy.[21] However, peripheral facial nerve paralysis is only present in 8–33% of patients with parotid malignancies.[22] Although rapid growth and pain associated with a parotid mass are also suggestive of malignancy, a similar clinical picture can be produced by inflammatory disease.[22,23]

Adenoid cystic carcinoma

Adenoid cystic carcinoma comprises 4% of all tumors involving the major salivary glands and approximately 3% of all parotid tumors. This is the most common malignant neoplasm of the submandibular and minor salivary glands (Figs 3.25 and 3.26). Both sexes are equally affected. Of patients with this malignancy, 35% present with spontaneous facial nerve paralysis and pain.[24] Regardless of its site of origin, this neoplasm is notorious for perineural tumor spread. This proclivity accounts for the high frequency of pain and facial nerve paralysis when the neoplasm involves the parotid gland. Perineural tumor extent is almost always associated with a near hopeless prognosis.

Magnetic resonance becomes especially useful in the evaluation of perineural tumor extent. Findings supportive of facial nerve invasion include nerve enlargement, obliteration of the normal fat below the stylomastoid foramen and nerve enhancement.

Lymphoma

Primary lymphoma of the parotid gland is exceedingly rare. Systemic lymphoma with secondary parotid involvement is comparatively more common. Lymphocytic and histiocytic lymphomas account for more than half of the lymphomas with parotid involvement. There is a definite association between lymphoma and autoimmune disease. Lymphoma of the salivary glands is more common in patients with Sjogren's syndrome (Figs 3.7 and 3.27).

Magnetic resonance of parotid lymphoma demonstrates multiple and often bilateral intraglandular masses which exhibit low signal intensity on T1-weighted images and high signal intensity on T2-weighted images. Frequently there is associated cervical lymphadenopathy.

Miscellaneous primary malignancies

Acinic cell carcinoma, adenocarcinoma, squamous cell carcinoma and undifferentiated carcinoma comprise the remainder of primary salivary gland malignancies.[25] These as a group are rare.

There are a few malignant variations of benign tumors. These include malignant mixed tumor (3% of all mixed tumors), carcinoma ex pleomorphic adenoma (Fig. 3.28), and metastasizing benign mixed tumor (Fig. 3.29).[26] Malignant mixed tumor and carcinoma ex pleomorphic adenoma are much more frequent than metastasizing benign mixed tumor, which is exceedingly rare.

Parotid gland metastases

In most cases metastatic involvement of the parotid gland is of a regional nature. Primary tumors of the scalp, external ears, eyelids, external nose and lacrimal glands may metastasize to the parotid gland via lymphatic spread. Deeply invasive melanoma and poorly differentiated squamous cell carcinoma are responsible for the majority of intraparotid lymphatic metastases. Patients with regional parotid metastases frequently manifest cervical and distal metastases (Fig. 3.30).

Involvement of the salivary glands by contiguous spread of an adjacent malignancy is less common. The primary neoplasm in this instance is usually a sarcoma (Fig. 3.31).

References

1 TABOR EK, CURTIN HD, MR of the salivary glands, *Radiol Clin North Am* (1989) **27**:379–92.

2 WARD CM, Injury of the facial nerve during surgery of the parotid, *Br J Surg* (1975) **62**:401–3.

3 CURTIN HD, WOLFE P, SNYDERMAN N, The facial nerve between the stylomastoid foramen and the parotid, *Radiology* (1983) **149**:165–9.

4 CONN IG, WIESENFELD D, FERFUSON MM, The anatomy of the facial nerve in relation to CT/sialography of the parotid gland, *Br J Radiol* (1983) **56**:901–5.

5 DAVIS RA, ANSON BJ, BUDINGER JM, Surgical anatomy of the facial nerve and parotid gland based upon a study of 350 cervicofacial dissections, *Surg Gynecol Obstet* (1956) **102**:385–412.

6 TERESI LM, KOLIN E, LUFKIN RB, MR imaging of the intraparotid facial nerve; normal anatomy and pathology, *AJNR* (1987) **8**:253–8.

7 FROMMER J, The human accessory parotid gland; its incidence, nature and significance, *Oral Surg* (1977) **43**:671–3.

8 BATSAKIS JG, ed, *Tumors of the head and neck: clinical and pathological considerations*, 2nd edn (Williams and Wilkins: Baltimore 1979) 12–35.

9 BRYAN RN, MILLER RH, FERREYRO RI, Computed tomography of the major salivary glands, *Am J Radiol* (1982) **139**:547–54.

10 CURTIN HD, Assessment of salivary gland pathology, *Otolaryngol Clin North Am* (1988) **21**:547–73.

11 SOM PM, The salivary glands. In: Som P, Bergeron RT, eds, *Head and Neck Imaging* (CV Mosby: St Louis 1991) 277–348.

12 GOLDING S, Computed tomography in the diagnosis of parotid gland tumors, *Br J Radiol* (1982) **55**:182–8.

13 RABINOV K, THORNTON K, GORDON PH, CT of the salivary glands, *Radiol Clin North Am* (1984) **22**:145–59.

14 SCHWARTZ AW, DEVINE KN, BEARHS OH, Acute postoperative parotitis ('surgical-mumps'), *Plast Reconstr Surg* (1966) **25**:51–3.

15 BEARHS OH, WOOLNER LB, Surgical treatment of disease of salivary glands, *J Oral Surg* (1969) **27**:119–22.

16 SHUGAR JM, SOM PM, JACOBSEN AL, Multicentric parotid cysts and cervical adenopathy in AIDS patients. A newly recognized entity: CT and MR manifestations, *Laryngoscope* (1988) **98**:772–5.

17 HOLLIDAY RA, COHEN WA, SCHINELLA RA, Benign lymphoepithelial parotid cysts and hyperplastic cervical adenopathy in AIDS-risk patients: a new CT appearance, *Radiology* (1988) **168**:439–41.

18 DYKUN RJ, DEITEL M, BOROWY ZJ, Treatment of parotid neoplasms, *Can J Surg* (1980) **23**:14–19.

19 SOM PM, BRAUN IF, SHAPIRO MD, Tumors of the parapharyngeal space and upper neck: MR imaging characteristics, *Radiology* (1987) **164**:823–9.

20 SOM PM, BILLER HF, High-grade malignancies of the parotid gland; identification with MR imaging, *Radiology* (1989) **173**:823–6.

21 BERDAL P, GRONAS HE, MYLIUS EA, Parotid tumors; clinical and histological aspects, *Acta Otolaryngol* (1979) **263**:160–3.

22 BATSAKIS JG, ed, *Tumors of the head and neck: clinical and pathological considerations*, 2nd edn (Williams and Wilkins: Baltimore 1979) 1–75.

23 LEEGAARD T, LINDERMAN H, Salivary gland tumors: clinical picture and treatment, *Acta Otolaryngol* (1970) **263**:155–9.

24   BERDAL P, DEBESCHE A, MYLIUS E, Cylindroma of salivary glands: report of 80 cases, *Acta Otolaryngol* (1970) **263**:170–7.

25   MANCUSO AA, HANAFEE WN, *Computed tomography of the head and neck*, 2nd edn (Williams and Wilkins: Baltimore 1985) 139–60.

26   SOM PM, SHUGAR JA, SACHER M, Benign and malignant parotid pleomorphic adenomas: CT and MR studies, *J Comput Assist Tomogr* (1988) **12**:65–9.

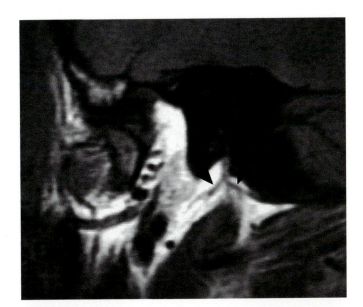

A

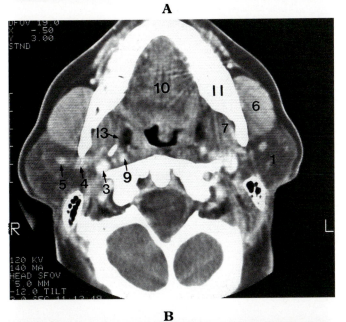

B

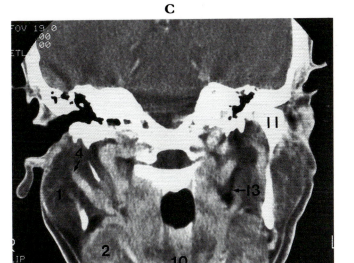

C

FIGURE 3.1

Sagittal MR image of the seventh cranial nerve. T1-weighted (TR = 700 ms, TE = 20 ms) sagittal MR image through the temporomandibular joint demonstrating the mastoid (arrows) and parotid (arrowheads) segments of the facial nerve.

FIGURE 3.2

Normal salivary gland anatomy (CT). (**A – C**) Axial and coronal contrast enhanced CT images of normal parotid and submandibular glands. Key: 1, parotid gland; 2, submandibular gland; 3, internal jugular vein; 4, external carotid artery; 5, retromandibular vein; 6, masseter muscle; 7, medial pterygoid muscle; 8, lateral pterygoid muscle; 9, internal carotid artery; 10, tongue; 11, mandible; 12, sternocleidomastoid muscle; 13, parapharyngeal space; 14, common carotid artery.

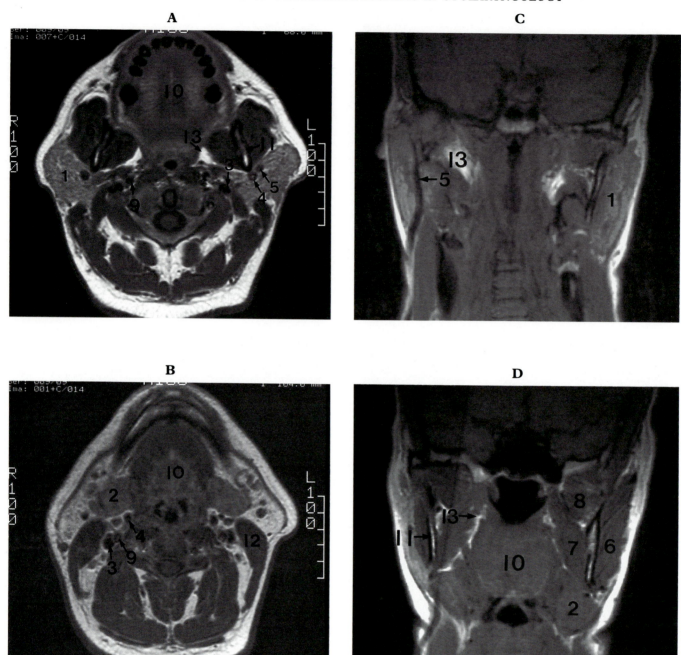

FIGURE 3.3

Normal salivary gland anatomy (MRI) (**A – D**) Axial and coronal T1-weighted (TR = 600 ms, TE = 20 ms) MR images of normal parotid and submandibular glands. See Fig. 3.2 for key.

A

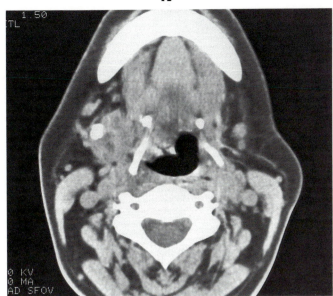

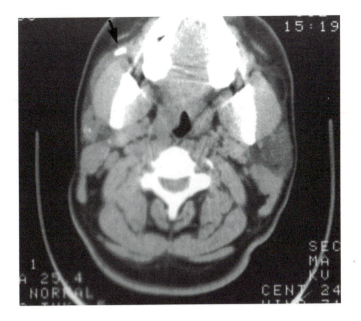

B

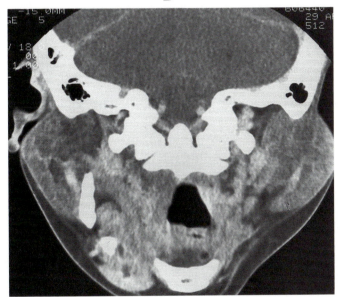

FIGURE 3.5

Calculus right parotid gland. Axial CT image demonstrates a calculus (arrow) in the distal portion of Stensen's duct.

FIGURE 3.4

Calculus right submandibular gland. (**A,B**) Axial and coronal CT images demonstrate a 1.0 cm calculus of the right submandibular gland. Note the hypodensities within the glandular parenchyma consistent with sialectasis. The left submandibular gland was removed due to calculus disease.

A

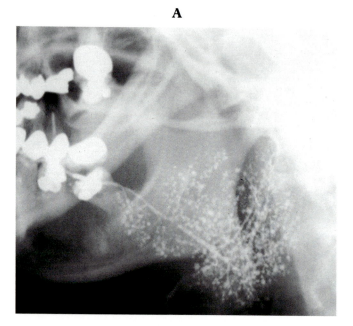

A

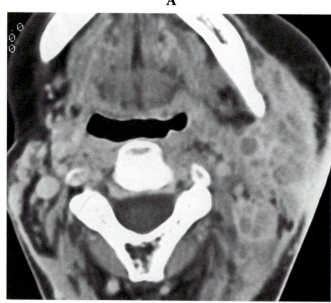

B

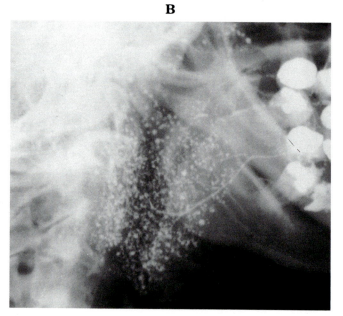

B

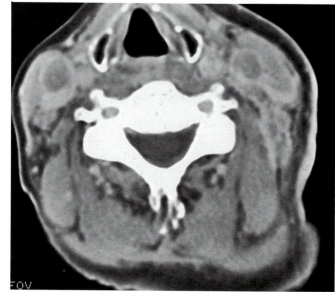

FIGURE 3.6

Autoimmune sialectasis. (**A,B**) Bilateral sialogram in a patient with Sjögren's syndrome. Note the punctate pools of contrast typical of autoimmune sialectasis.

FIGURE 3.7

Sjögren's syndrome complicated by lymphoma. (**A,B**) Axial contrast-enhanced CT images demonstrate an enlarged left parotid gland with multiple intraglandular nodes and extensive cervical adenopathy.

A

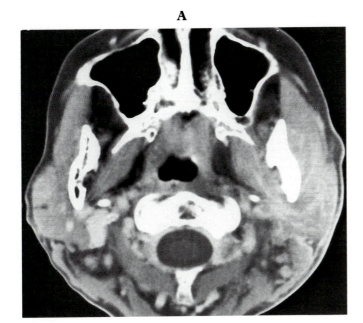

FIGURE 3.8

Acute left parotitis. (**A,B**) Axial and coronal contrast-enhanced CT images. The left parotid gland is enlarged and enhances. Also note the overlying skin thickening suggestive of inflammation.

B

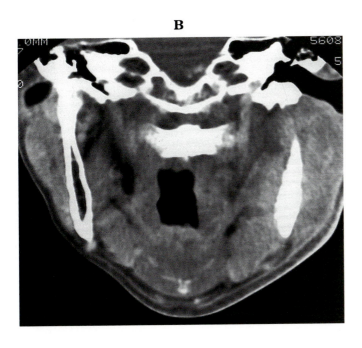

A

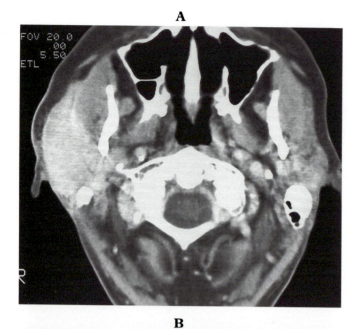

D

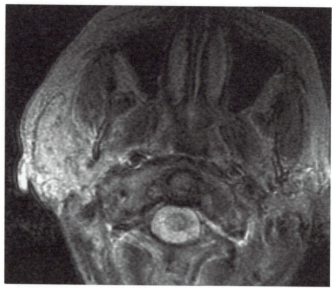

B

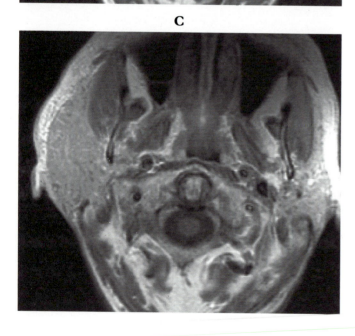

C

FIGURE 3.9

Acute right parotitis. (**A**) Contrast-enhanced CT image. The right parotid gland is diffusely enlarged and enhances uniformly. Note the overlying soft tissue induration and skin thickening. (**B,C**) Pre- and post-gadolinium enhancement T1-weighted (TR = 500 ms, TE = 15 ms) MR images. The gland is large and demonstrates moderate enhancement. (**D**) T2-weighted (TR = 2300 ms, TE = 80 ms) MR image. The gland exhibits diffuse increase in signal intensity. There is also increased signal intensity in the overlying skin and soft tissues.

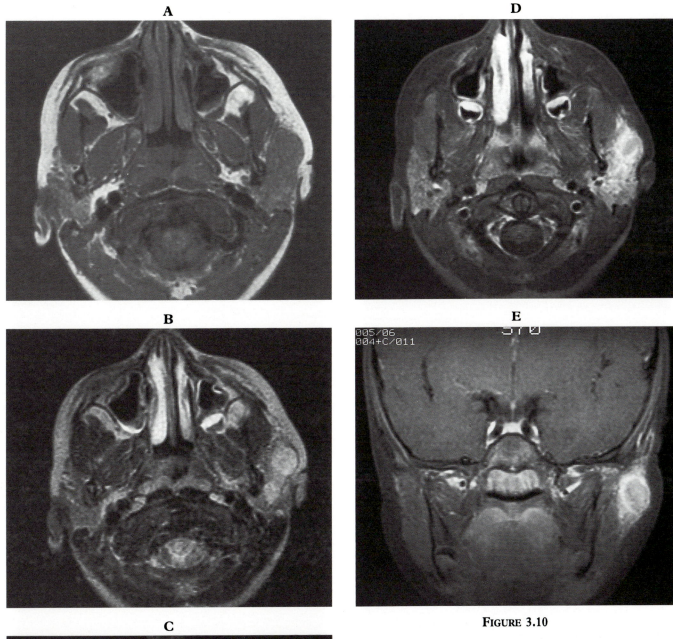

FIGURE 3.10

Parinaud's oculoglandular syndrome. This 7-year-old boy presented with left conjunctivitis and a palpable pre-auricular mass. (**A,B**) T1-weighted (TR = 750 ms, TE = 20 ms) and T2-weighted (TR = 2000 ms, TE = 80 ms) axial MR images. There is soft tissue fullness in the orbital preseptal region on the left side. The left parotid gland is enlarged with several large intraglandular nodes. (**C – E**) Axial and coronal T1-weighted (TR = 700 ms, TE = 20 ms) postgadolinium fat suppression images. There is diffuse parotid enhancement as well as enhancement in the left orbital preseptal soft tissues. Parinaud's oculoglandular syndrome refers to conjunctivitis followed by pre-auricular and or parotid adenopathy in response to a leptothrix infection.

A

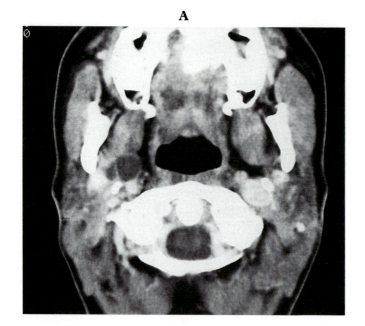

FIGURE 3.11

Retention cyst deep lobe right parotid gland. (**A**) Contrast-enhanced CT. There is a 2.0 cm low attenuation cystic structure involving the deep lobe of the right parotid gland. There is associated deformity of the parapharyngeal space. (**B**) Axial T2-weighted (TR = 2400 ms, TE = 80 ms) MR image. The cystic lesion exhibits marked increase in signal intensity.

B

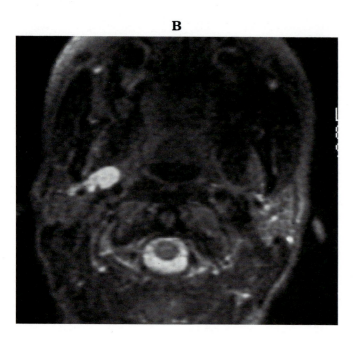

A

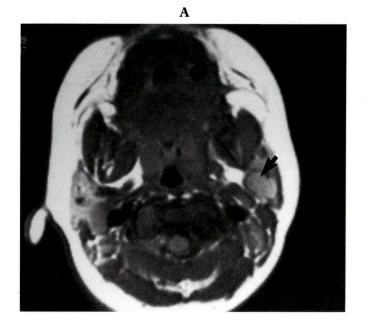

C

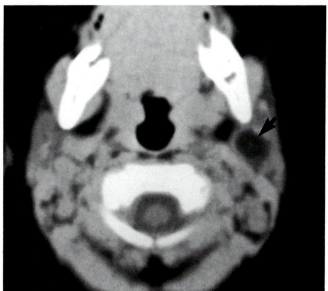

B

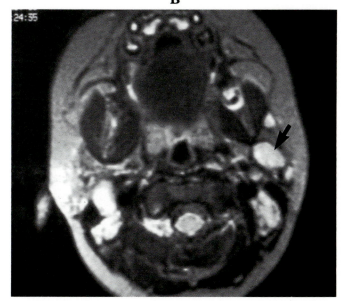

FIGURE 3.12

First branchial cleft cyst left parotid region. (**A,B**) Axial T1-weighted (TR = 700 ms, TE = 20 ms) and T2-weighted (TR = 3000 ms, TE = 90 ms) MR images in a 1-year-old. There are bilateral posterior triangle lymph nodes as well as a similar appearing structure within the left parotid gland (arrow). (**C**) Noncontrast axial CT demonstrates a low attenuation cystic structure (arrow) within the parotid gland. This case demonstrates the utility of CT in distinguishing lymph node from cyst. These may appear identical on MR images.

A

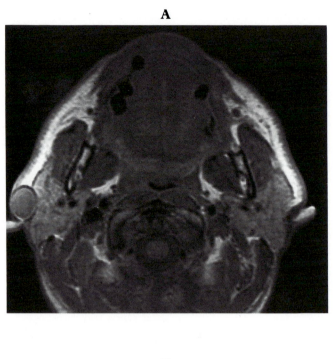

A

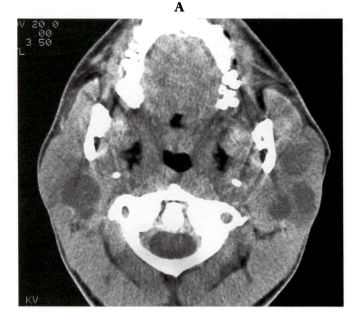

B

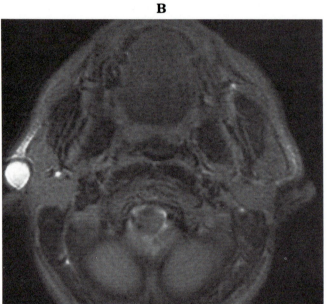

B

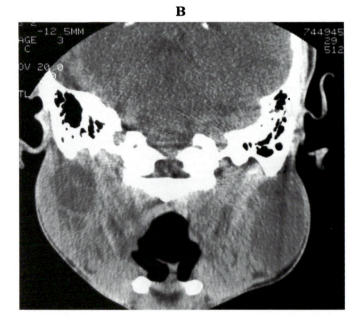

FIGURE 3.13

First branchial cleft cyst superficial to the right parotid gland. (**A,B**) T1-weighted (TR = 800 ms, TE = 20 ms) and T2-weighted (TR = 2400 ms, TE = 80 ms) axial MR images. There is a 2.0 cm cystic structure in the soft tissues overlying the right parotid gland.

FIGURE 3.14

Lymphoepithelial parotid cysts in a 37-year-old transsexual patient. (**A,B**) Axial and coronal unenhanced CT images. The parotid glands are enlarged and demonstrate multiple intraparenchymal cysts.

A

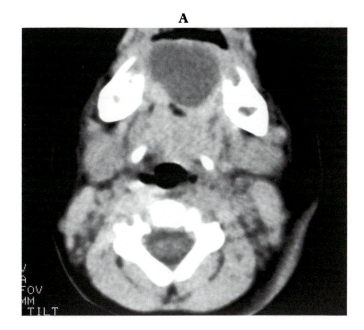

B

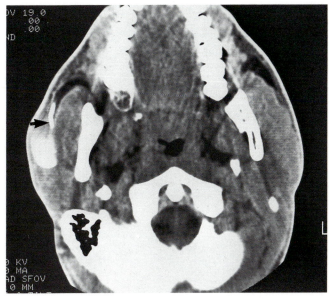

FIGURE 3.16

Post-traumatic sialocele right parotid gland. Post-sialogram CT image. There is a 2.5 cm cyst filled with contrast in the superficial lobe of the parotid gland. Stensen's duct (arrow) is opacified proximally. The patient suffered a stab wound to this region in the past.

FIGURE 3.15

Midline floor of the mouth ranula in a 3-month-old. (**A**) Noncontrast axial CT image reveals a large cystic floor of the mouth lesion. (**B**) T2-weighted (TR = 2000 ms, TE = 80 ms) coronal MR image. The cystic mass is high in signal intensity and contained within the floor of the mouth.

A   C

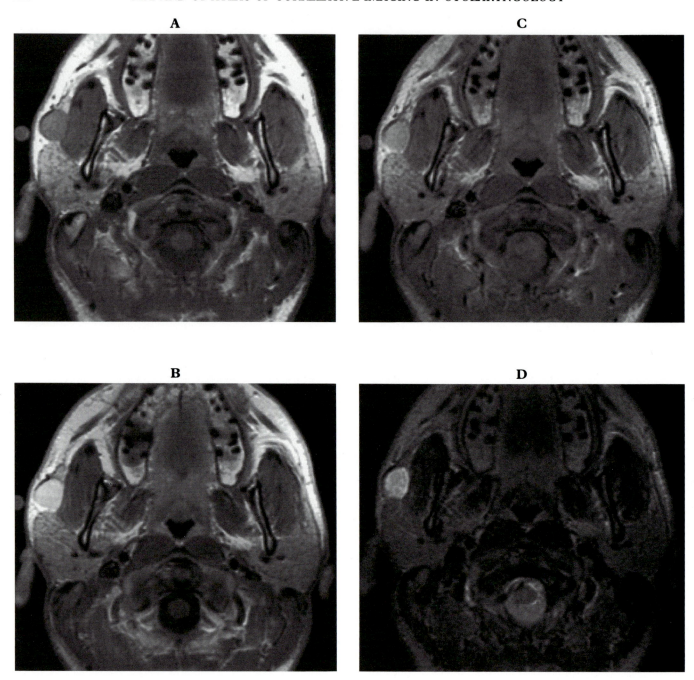

B   D

FIGURE 3.17

Pleomorphic adenoma (benign mixed tumor). (**A,B**) T1-weighted (TR = 700 ms, TE = 20 ms) axial MR images before and after intravenous gadolinium administration. There is a round sharply marginated mass which demonstrates moderate contrast enhancement. (**C,D**) T2-weighted (TR = 2600 ms, TE = 20/80 ms) axial MR images. The mass exhibits prolonged T2 relaxation times as manifested by increased signal intensity.

A

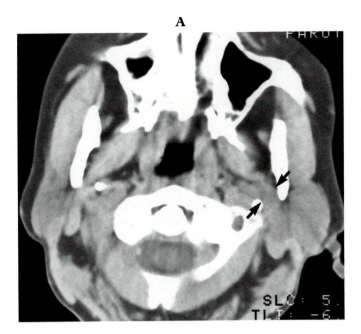

C

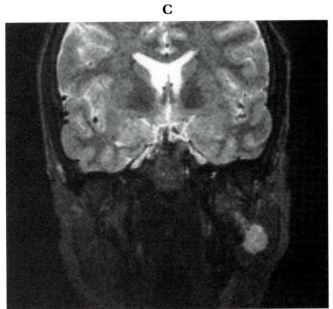

B

FIGURE 3.18

Pleomorphic adenoma of the deep lobe extending through the stylomandibular tunnel. (**A**) Non-contrast axial CT image. There is subtle widening of the stylomandibular tunnel and prominence in the deep lobe of the left parotid gland (arrows). (**B,C**) T2-weighted (TR = 2000 ms, TE = 80 ms) axial and coronal MR images. There is a hyperintense mass involving the deep lobe of the left parotid gland. The mass assumes a 'dumb-bell' configuration as it passes through the stylomandibular tunnel.

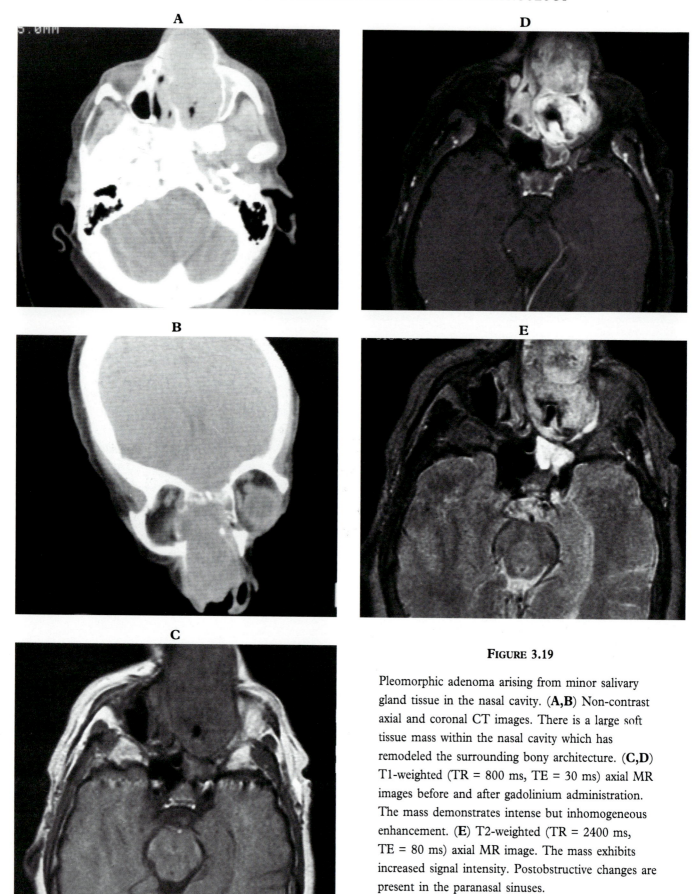

FIGURE 3.19

Pleomorphic adenoma arising from minor salivary gland tissue in the nasal cavity. (**A,B**) Non-contrast axial and coronal CT images. There is a large soft tissue mass within the nasal cavity which has remodeled the surrounding bony architecture. (**C,D**) T1-weighted (TR = 800 ms, TE = 30 ms) axial MR images before and after gadolinium administration. The mass demonstrates intense but inhomogeneous enhancement. (**E**) T2-weighted (TR = 2400 ms, TE = 80 ms) axial MR image. The mass exhibits increased signal intensity. Postobstructive changes are present in the paranasal sinuses.

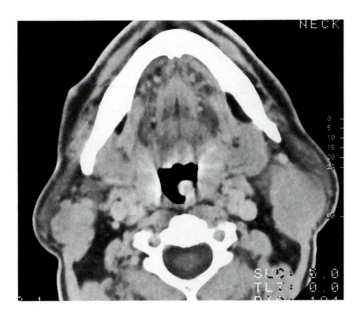

FIGURE 3.20

Bilateral Warthin's tumors (papillary cystadenoma lymphomatosum). Contrast-enhanced axial CT image reveals bilateral parotid masses. Differential considerations include Warthin's tumor, lymphoma and adenopathy.

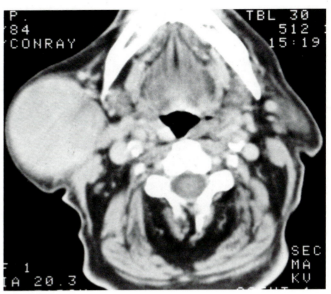

FIGURE 3.21

Large solitary Warthin's tumor. Axial contrast-enhanced CT demonstrates a large mass in the tail of the right parotid gland. The mass exhibits moderate enhancement.

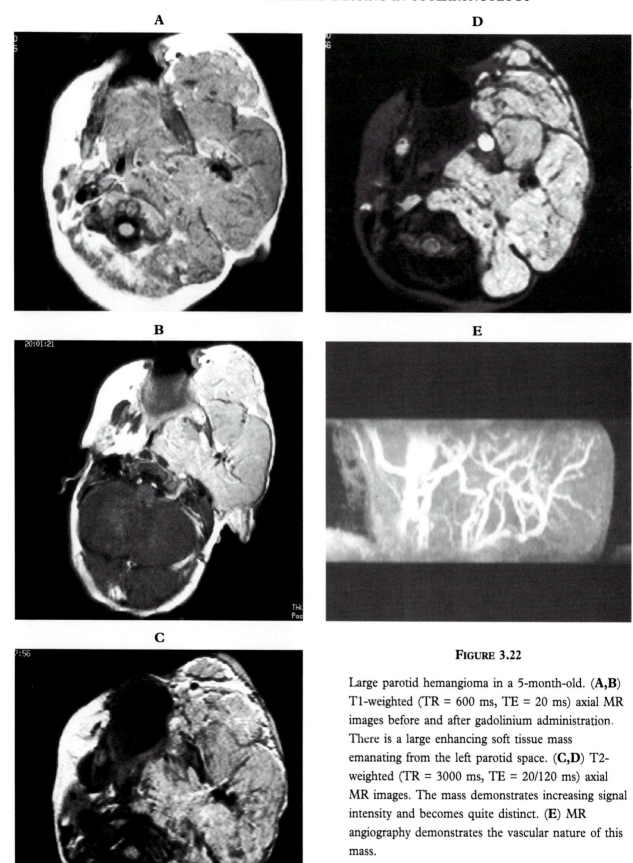

FIGURE 3.22

Large parotid hemangioma in a 5-month-old. (**A,B**) T1-weighted (TR = 600 ms, TE = 20 ms) axial MR images before and after gadolinium administration. There is a large enhancing soft tissue mass emanating from the left parotid space. (**C,D**) T2-weighted (TR = 3000 ms, TE = 20/120 ms) axial MR images. The mass demonstrates increasing signal intensity and becomes quite distinct. (**E**) MR angiography demonstrates the vascular nature of this mass.

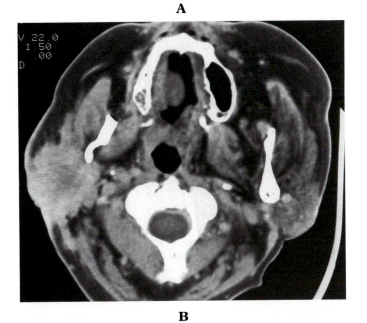

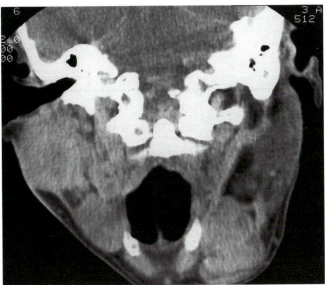

FIGURE 3.23

Mucoepidermoid carcinoma of the right parotid gland in a patient with left facial hemihypertrophy. (**A,B**) Pre- and post-contrast axial CT images. There is a large enhancing mass involving the right parotid gland which demonstrates moderate enhancement. (**C**) Coronal postcontrast CT image. The mass is well demonstrated. Also note the congenital facial hemihypertrophy.

A

D

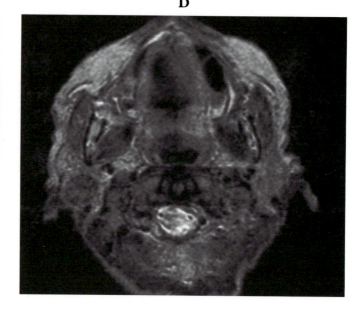

B

C

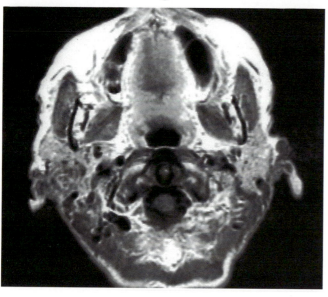

FIGURE 3.24

Mucoepidermoid carcinoma arising in a pleomorphic adenoma. (**A,B**) Enhanced axial and coronal CT images. There is an enhancing partially calcified right parotid mass. (**C**) Axial T1-weighted (TR = 800 ms, TE = 20 ms) postgadolinium MR image demonstrates an inhomogeneously enhancing mass with areas of decreased signal intensity produced by the calcifications. (**D**) Axial T2-weighted (TR = 2000 ms, TE = 80 ms) MR image. The mass is inhomogeneous and demonstrates intermediate signal intensity isointense to muscle. Salivary gland malignancies frequently do not exhibit prolonged T2 relaxation time and are often low to intermediate in signal intensity.

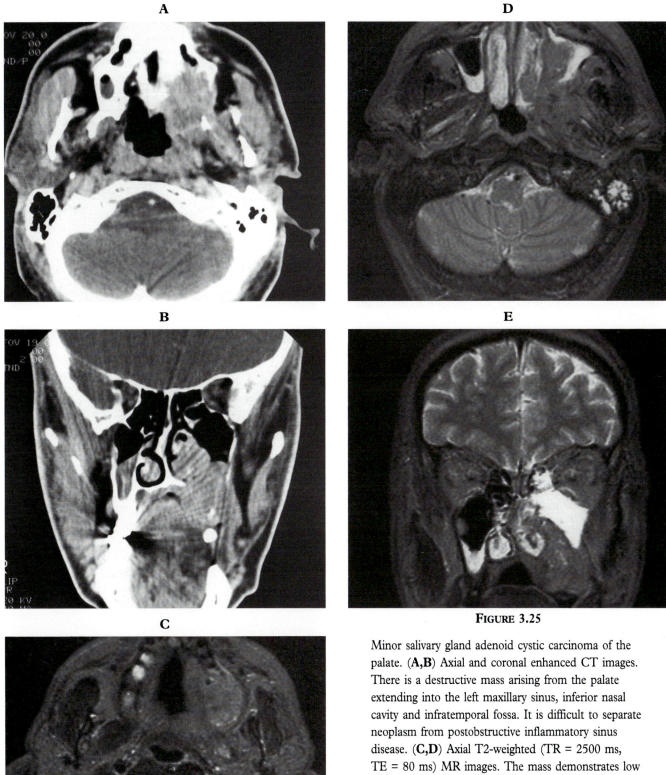

FIGURE 3.25

Minor salivary gland adenoid cystic carcinoma of the palate. (**A,B**) Axial and coronal enhanced CT images. There is a destructive mass arising from the palate extending into the left maxillary sinus, inferior nasal cavity and infratemporal fossa. It is difficult to separate neoplasm from postobstructive inflammatory sinus disease. (**C,D**) Axial T2-weighted (TR = 2500 ms, TE = 80 ms) MR images. The mass demonstrates low to intermediate signal intensity and can be clearly separated from the high signal intensity inflammatory sinus disease. Also note the retained fluid in the left mastoid air cells as the result of eustachian tube blockage. (**E**) Coronal T2-weighted (TR = 2400 ms, TE = 80 ms) MR image again demonstrates the utility of MR in distinguishing neoplasm from postobstructive sinus disease.

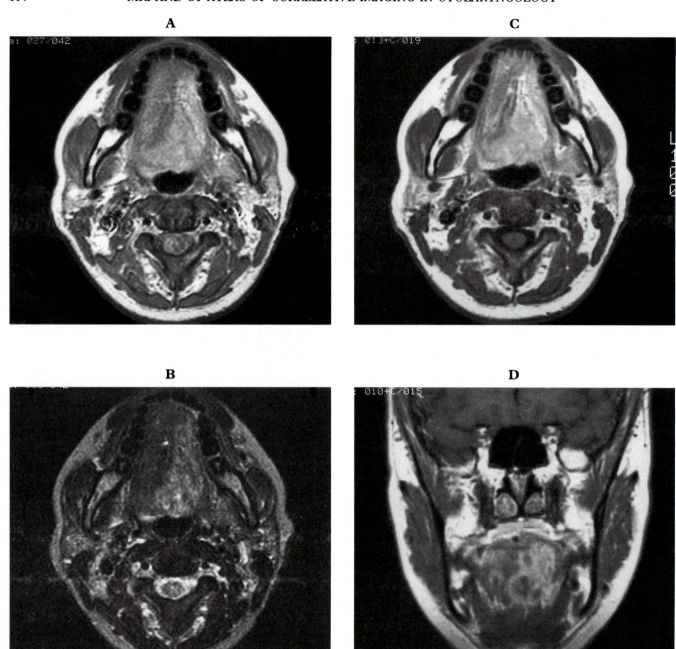

FIGURE 3.26

Adenoid cystic carcinoma of the tongue. (**A,B**) Axial T2-weighted (TR = 2400 ms, TE = 20/80 ms) MR images of the tongue. There is an infiltrating hyperintense mass of the left side of the tongue which crosses the midline near the tongue base. (**C,D**) Axial and coronal T1-weighted (TR = 800 ms, TE = 20 ms) postgadolinium MR images. The mass enhances and is well demonstrated.

A

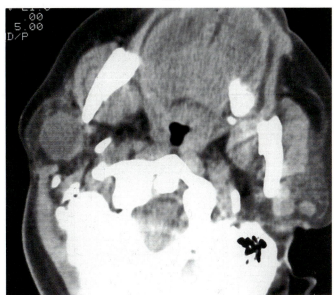

B

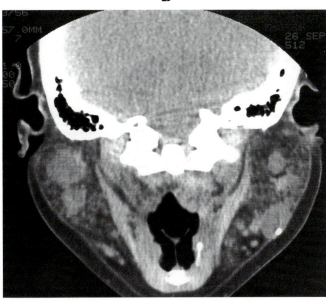

FIGURE 3.27

Lymphoma of the parotid glands in a patient with Sjogren's syndrome. Axial and coronal unenhanced CT images demonstrate bilateral intraglandular masses. Images of the lower neck revealed cervical adenopathy.

A

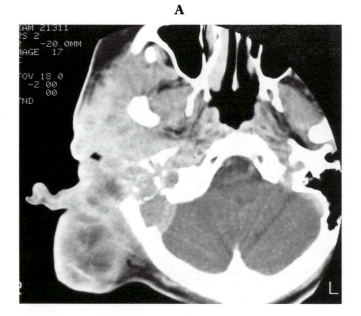

D

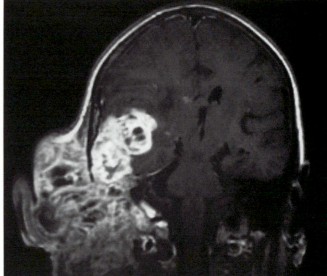

B

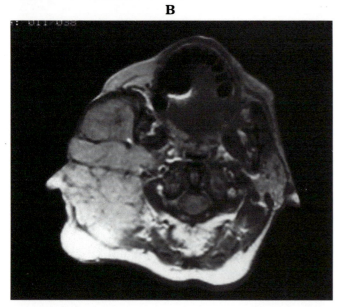

FIGURE 3.28

Carcinoma ex pleomorphic adenoma with intracranial extension. (**A**) Enhanced axial CT image shows a large enhancing right parotid mass. The mass has invaded the masticator and parapharyngeal spaces, and the intracranial compartment. (**B,C**) Axial proton density (TR = 2000 ms, TE = 30 ms) MR images. The mass demonstrates intermediate signal intensity and has grown through the calvarium. (**D**) Gadolinium-enhanced T1-weighted (TR = 600 ms, TE = 20 ms) MR image. The enhancing lesion and its extent are well demonstrated.

C

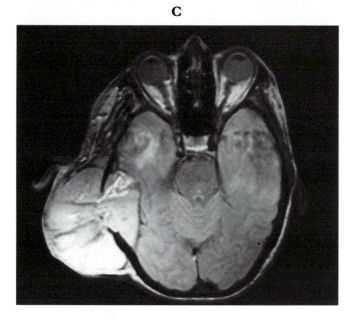

A

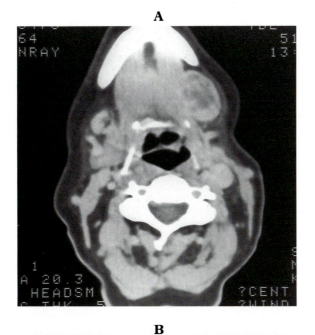

B

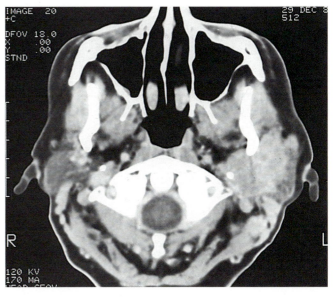

FIGURE 3.30

Breast carcinoma metastatic to the left parotid gland. Enhanced axial CT image. There is a large enhancing intraglandular mass. Additional deep jugular and posterior triangle nodes are also present in the lower neck.

FIGURE 3.29

Metastasizing benign mixed tumor. (**A**) Enhanced axial CT image in a patient who previously had a left submandibular resection. There is a 3 cm necrotic mass in the left submandibular space representing tumor recurrence. (**B**) Frontal chest radiograph reveals a large metastatic mass.

A

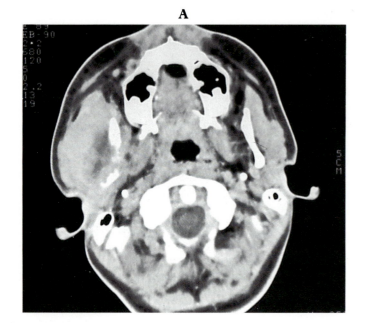

B

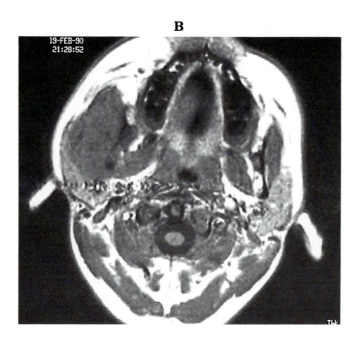

FIGURE 3.31

Mandibular sarcoma with parotid involvement. (**A**) Enhanced axial CT image. There is a large mass in the right masticator space with destruction of the mandible. The mass is inseparable from the parotid gland. The nonenhancing low attenuation central portion is suggestive of necrosis. (**B**) T1-weighted (TR = 600 ms, TE = 15 ms) axial MR image. The superficial lobe of the parotid gland is draped over this mass and the parotid gland is ill defined, suggesting invasion.

CHAPTER 4

NASOPHARYNX AND OROPHARYNX

Nasopharynx

Normal anatomy

Anatomic boundaries

The nasopharynx is a mucosal lined, tubular-shaped midline structure which constitutes the superior extent of the airway. Its cranial border is limited by the skull base (sphenoid sinus and clivus). The posterior margin of the nasopharynx extends to the prevertebral muscles and soft tissues. Anteriorly, the nasopharynx freely communicates with the nasal cavity through the posterior choanae.[1–6] At the level of the soft palate, the nasopharynx is divided from the oropharynx by a muscular sling known as Passavant's ridge.[1,6] Laterally, the nasopharynx abuts the pyramidal-shaped parapharyngeal spaces. The rigid and tough pharyngobasilar fascia provides structural support for the nasopharynx. This fascia forms a three-sided curtain which opens anteriorly towards the nasal cavity. Superiorly, the fascia is fixed to the skull base from the pterygoid plates to the carotid canal. Laterally, it is adherent to the cartilaginous portion of the eustachian tube.[1,6]

The fascia forms a closed and resistant barrier for the nasopharynx. The sinus of Morgagni is the only defect in the fascia through which the eustachian tube and levator veli palatini muscle pass. As a result of the close proximity of the foramen lacerum and foramen ovale to the sinus of Morgagni and eustachian tube there exists a potential pathway for the spread of disease to the cranial cavity.[4,7]

Internal landmarks

The most prominent superficial landmark of the mucosa is the paired torus tubariae which protrude into the nasopharynx (Figs 4.1 and 4.2). These J-shaped ridges comprise the cartilaginous portion of the eustachian tube opening.[1,3,5,6]

Posterior and superior to the tori are the paired lateral pharyngeal recesses (fossae of Rosenmuller).[1,3,4,6] These paired structures show great variability in size and shape with age and are more prominent in the elderly as the palatal musculature and lymphoid (adenoid) soft tissue regress.[3,6,8–10]

Lateral to the pharyngobasilar fascia, the nasopharynx is bounded by four spaces which are divided by three layers of deep cervical fascia. These include the masticator (infratemporal fossa), the parapharyngeal, the carotid and the parotid spaces.[11] Lateral deviation and/or infiltration of the parapharyngeal fat are sensitive indicators of the spread of nasopharyngeal disease. By contrast, tumors of the parotid space displace the fat of the parapharyngeal space medially.[7–10]

Musculature

The two palatal muscles, the levator veli palatini and tensor veli palatini, form the muscles of deglutition in the nasopharynx. Both originate lateral to the pharyngobasilar fascia, yet insert on the soft palate medial to the pharyngobasilar fascia.[3,6,7] The levator is much larger than the tensor. Originating posteriorly from the quadrate area of the petrous bone,[9] the levator traverses antero-medially and inserts into the muscular segment of the soft palate.

The tensor also originates from the skull base slightly anterior to the quadrate area from the scaphoid fossa of the sphenoid bone. It is a small slip of muscle that passes anteriorly and inferiorly, yet remains external to the pharyngobasilar fascia.[1,6] The tensor then hooks medially around the hamulus of the medial pterygoid plate, whereupon it inserts on the membranous portion of the soft palate.[4,6,9,10]

The act of swallowing initiates a coordinated contraction of the tensor and levator muscles.[6] This process effectively seals off the nasopharynx from the oropharynx during swallowing.[3,6,9,10] The tension applied by the levator and tensor muscles also acts to open the eustachian tubes, thereby equalizing the pressure in the middle ear with that of the pharynx.[1,6,10]

Lymph nodes and epithelium

Except in infants and young children, lymph nodes are not demonstrated with imaging in the retropharyngeal space. Lymph nodes are not usually visualized in the midline; however, several nodes may be present bilaterally in the high, lateral portion of the retropharyngeal space (node of Rouviere).[5,9,10]

Eighty percent of the posterior wall of the nasopharynx is covered by squamous epithelium. A transitional type of epithelium is also present in variable amounts.[1,12] The lymphatic tissue of the adenoids is located in the posterior-superior nasopharynx.

Imaging techniques

Computed tomography

Imaging evaluation of the nasopharynx is commonly performed to exclude malignancy. Computed tomography (CT) evaluation of a patient with a suspected nasopharyngeal abnormality should consist of axial images with intravenous contrast enhancement extending from the skull base to the hyoid bone. If a known malignancy exists, imaging should be extended to the level of the thoracic inlet to search for cervical adenopathy.[10] Individual three to five millimeter thick, contiguous sections through the nasopharynx in axial and coronal planes are recommended. Individual five millimeter thick axial sections of the neck are sufficient to screen for adenopathy. The images should begin anteriorly at the midpoint of the hard palate and extend (and continue) posteriorly to the cervical spine (Fig. 4.1).

Magnetic resonance imaging

Similar regions of interest should be covered with magnetic resonance imaging (MRI). Examinations can be performed in the standard head coil. To detect lower neck nodes, MRI of the neck should be performed with an anterior cervical surface coil. Magnetic resonance imaging is the preferred method of imaging nasopharyngeal disease; CT, however, still provides the best detail of osseous involvement.[1,2,5,11,13,14] The routine examination consists of images in the three conventional anatomic planes: sagittal, coronal and axial.[1,5] Midsagittal and coronal images illustrate the superior and inferior limits of disease and are most suited for defining skull base involvement and intracranial spread.[5] Axial orientation offers the best visualization of internal architecture; fossae of Rosenmuller, torus tubariae, parapharyngeal spaces and retropharyngeal nodes. As part of our routine protocol, we obtain images in the sagittal, coronal and axial planes. T1-weighted images (repetition time TR = 600–800 ms, echo delay time TE = 20 ms, 192 × 256 matrix, 1 excitation) are acquired in the sagittal plane first to plan localization of the subsequent axial and coronal images. T1-weighted images are then performed in the axial plane from the hyoid bone inferiorly to the middle cranial fossa (TR = 600–800 ms, TE = 20 ms, 192 × 256 matrix, 20 cm field-of-view, 5 mm thick, 1 mm gap, 2 excitations). The same area is studied using a T2-weighted acquisition (TR = 2000–2500 ms, TE = 20 and 80 ms, 192 × 256 matrix, 20 cm field-of-view, 5 mm thick, 1 mm gap, 1 excitation). Following gadolinium administration, the T1-weighted images are repeated in both the axial and coronal planes using a fat-suppression technique. The patient should be instructed to remain motionless during image acquisition, as even small movements of the jaw or swallowing can significantly degrade the quality of the images.

On axial T1-weighted MR images, the pharyngobasilar fascia is often seen as a low intensity band which extends from the medial pterygoid plates to the carotid foramina, reflecting medially over the pre-vertebral musculature (Fig. 4.2).[1] The mucosa and adjacent lymphoid tissue are of high signal intensity when compared to muscle on MR imaging.

The mucosal surface and superficial adenoidal tissue are poorly differentiated from the muscles of deglutition on CT, but are particularly noticeable on long TR, long TE MR sequences. On short TR, short TE (T1-weighted images), the mucosa and adenoids exhibit a moderate signal intensity similar to the surrounding muscle.[3] There is intense enhancement of the mucosa on T1-weighted MR images following administration of gadolinium-DTPA.[1] In our experience, when fat-suppression techniques are used in combination with gadolinium enhancement, there is better elaboration of tissue contrast.

Axial images show hypertrophied lymphoid tissue (adenoid) to have a lobulated configuration in younger patients.[5,9] The tissue may appear to hang down from the roof of the nasopharynx on coronal images (Fig. 4.3). When hypertrophied, the adenoids can produce nasal obstruction and hearing loss from tubal obstruction.[1] Lymphoid tissue is differentiated from invasive tumor by its discrete margins, bulk and its failure to transgress the pharyngobasilar fascia.[3,9] On MRI, the lymphoid tissue maintains a submucosal location and should not normally exist in the deeper structures of the nasopharyngeal wall.[4,11] Lymphoid tissue is normally of higher signal intensity than the musculature on T2-weighted MR images.[1,5,9,11]

The torus tubariae may be of a higher attenuation than the adjacent mucosa on CT, isointense on T1-weighted MR images, and hyperintense relative to the surrounding muscles on T2-weighted images.[4,5] The tori are virtually always recognizable on CT and MRI; slight asymmetry is considered normal.[9] The eustachian tube openings, however, should show symmetry. The eustachian tube opening appears as a small recess anterior and inferior to the torus on axial and coronal images, respectively.[1,4,6]

The levator veli palatini muscle merges with the salpingopharyngeus muscle and these are therefore seen as a single structure on axial CT as they converge on the torus tubarius. Axial MR images show the deglutitory musculature of intermediate signal intensity which flanks the airway and nasopharyngeal mucosa.[4,5] Axial images of the mid-nasopharynx show the tensor veli palatini as a thin band of tissue, slightly medial and parallel to the medial pterygoid muscle (Figs 4.1 and 4.2). The larger levator muscle is just medial to the tensor muscle, flanking the nasopharyngeal airway.[9] The eustachian tube passes between the two muscles.[1]

Administration of intravenous gadolinium-DTPA enhances tissue contrast of tumor. The ability to detect or define a nasopharyngeal tumor is not altered significantly by the administration of gadolinium, however, use of fat-suppression techniques with gadolinium may improve detection of mucosal and submucosal tumor. Specific uses for gadolinium-enhanced MR imaging include detecting perineural/perivascular invasion, providing better definition of skull base invasion and in potentially establishing criteria for malignant adenopathy.[15]

Congenital lesions

Thornwaldt's cyst

A rare, congenital lesion is the Thornwaldt's cyst. This is a remnant of the pharyngeal bursae in the nasopharynx. It is incidentally found in 4% of autopsy specimens. The cyst presents as a well-circumscribed, nonenhancing, low density mass on CT. Rim enhancement with intravenous contrast may be seen if it is infected. The Thornwaldt cyst is usually asymptomatic. However, when infected, it may give rise to pain, halitosis, nasal discharge and pre-vertebral muscle spasm. Depending on the contents of the cyst, this lesion exhibits high signal intensity on T2-weighted images and is hyper- to isointense relative to mucosa and lymphoid tissue on T1-weighted images (Fig. 4.4).[1,10] The Thornwaldt's cyst can often be differentiated from a simple mucous retention cyst by the eccentric location in the posterior nasopharynx of the latter (Fig. 4.5).

Teratoma

Teratomas and dermoids are benign polypoid masses in the nasopharynx. They are usually present at birth and are found more often in females. The lesion may be attached to an intracranial component through a skull base defect. Lesions are composed of fibroadipose tissue, cartilage, bone and muscle.[1] Those which predominate with fat have a characteristic appearance on both CT and MRI. They are relatively hypodense on CT with density similar to the subcutaneous fat. The fatty component shortens T1 relaxation time and yields a hyperintense lesion on T1-weighted images. With an increased proportion of ectodermal and mesodermal elements, a variable appearance can be seen with either modality.[12] The diagnosis is suggested by a midline mass with MR characteristics of fat and bone.[1]

Benign neoplasia

Juvenile nasopharyngeal angiofibroma

The most frequent benign tumor associated with the nasopharynx is the juvenile nasopharyngeal angiofibroma (JNA).[10] It is relatively rare, accounting for an estimated 0.5% of all head and neck neoplasms.[1] The juvenile nasopharyngeal angiofibroma characteristically occurs in teenage males. The tumor originates near the sphenopalatine foramen in the superior, postero-lateral wall of the nasal cavity or from the nasopharynx.[1,8,10] Although histologically benign, the JNA can be highly aggressive and locally invasive.[1] Sphenoid sinus invasion is present in approximately two-thirds of cases and nearly all JNA extend into the pterygopalatine fossa (Fig. 4.6). Growth into the middle cranial fossa, cavernous sinus and sella turcica has been reported.[1,10] The most common presentation is nasal congestion (60%), epistaxis (73%) or rarely, facial deformity.[1,10,12] Excellent definition of the tumor is accomplished with contrast CT and MRI. Bone destruction can be extensive. The angiofibroma reveals intermediate signal intensity on the T1-weighted images. Punctate areas of flow void are seen within the tumor mass, similar to those reported with paraganglioma.[1] Because the tumor is markedly vascular, rapid bolus contrast computed tomography reveals an intensely enhancing mass. Arteriography is useful in defining the feeding vessels and preoperative embolization of the arterial supply may decrease intraoperative blood loss and facilitate complete resection (Fig. 4.6).[10,12] Juvenile nasopharyngeal angiofibromas often recur if not completely removed (Fig. 4.7).

Nasopharyngeal malignancies

Squamous cell carcinoma

The most common type of malignant tumor in the nasopharynx is squamous cell carcinoma (80%) (Figs 4.8–4.11).[1,2,10] It constitutes up to 3% of all malignancies in the Caucasian population and up to 15% in the Chinese. The Epstein–Barr virus has been implicated in some cases.[2] In Hong Kong, nasopharyngeal carcinoma comprises 18% of all malignant neoplasms.[1] Males in the fifth decade are more commonly affected. Approximately 90% of these tumors are of the epidermoid variety. Other nasopharyngeal malignancies include lymphomas, adenocarcinomas, plasmacytomas, melanomas, sarcomas and metastatic disease from lung, breast and kidney (Figs 4.12–4.17).[1,10,12]

Symptoms of nasopharyngeal malignancy can be both subtle and severe, since malignancies may go unnoticed until disease is relatively widespread.[2] The earliest symptoms of nasopharyngeal carcinoma are those of minor irritation in the postnasal region. Atrophy of the muscles of mastication may indicate direct cranial nerve (V and X) involvement by tumor.[1,8,9] Serous otitis media is a common symptom and occurs due to blockage of the eustachian tube orifice by tumor.[1] This secondary sign of nasopharyngeal carcinoma appears as clouding of the middle ear cavity and mastoid air cells in CT. Fluid in the middle ear shows prominently as high signal intensity on T2-weighted MR images.[5,9]

Nasopharyngeal carcinomas usually arise in the postero-lateral aspect or lateral pharyngeal recess (fossa of Rosenmuller).[1–3,7] Asymmetry of this structure should prompt close scrutiny for a tissue mass.[13] A carcinoma may produce only blunting of the recess or an exophytic mass may be present (Figs 4.8 and 4.10). Submucosal spread with ulceration and fungation are relatively common.[9] Due to its greater bulk and intrapharyngeal location, the levator palatini is involved with tumor earlier and more extensively than the tensor palatini.[8–10] Although asymmetry of the torus tubariae and fossae of Rosenmuller may represent a normal anatomic variation, asymmetry of the deglutitory musculature or deep tissue planes is always abnormal.[6,8,9]

The pharyngobasilar fascia creates a natural barrier that tends to confine neoplasia to the medial compartment. The only natural opening through the fascia is the sinus of Morgagni, which offers no resistance to spread into other compartments.[7,11] A lesion which remains localized medially may only distort the local anatomy and thicken mucosal structures. Lateral extension into the parapharyngeal space is well demonstrated with CT or MRI as the parapharyngeal fat is infiltrated.[11] Magnetic resonance shows intermediate-signal tumor infiltrating the high-signal fatty planes around the eustachian tube and pharyngobasilar fascia in the nasopharynx on T1-weighted images. The tissue planes between tumor and muscle are well defined with MRI.[7,11] In practice, the T1-weighted images (short TR, short TE) offer the best anatomic information by taking advantage of the natural tissue contrasts between tumor and adjacent fat planes and marrow spaces. Soft tissue contrast may be emphasized on the long TR, long TE images due to differences in T2 relaxation between tumor (long T2) and muscle (short T2) (Fig. 4.11).[5]

Once in the parapharyngeal space, tumors have access to the floor of the middle cranial fossa through the foramen ovale and foramen lacerum by perineural or perivascular mechanisms.[2,13,14] Tumor high in the nasopharynx may sometimes gain access to the middle cranial fossa via the pterygoid canal or sphenopalatine foramen.[11] From the pterygoid canal, tumor may grow through the foramen lacerum and enter the cavernous sinus. Penetration of the sphenopalatine foramen allows extension into the pterygopalatine fossa, the inferior and superior orbital fissures, and eventually into the cavernous sinus (Figs 4.8, 4.10 and 4.11).[7,11,14]

Parapharyngeal space invasion by nasopharyngeal carcinoma (Fig. 4.9) is common, as is infratemporal fossa (masticator space) involvement.[8,11] Posterior growth or nodal metastases to the carotid space (Fig. 4.8) may produce dysfunction of the cranial nerves IX–XII.[1,7,10,11]

With direct posterior invasion of the retropharyngeal space, visible lymphadenopathy results, including the node of Rouviere.[2,8] This is shown by CT as an ill-defined mass anterior to the pre-vertebral muscles.[11] Neoplastic infiltration may only reveal mild asymmetry of the retropharyngeal tissues. Enlarged lymph nodes are more conspicuous on T2-weighted images due to their prolonged T2 relaxation time relative to that of musculature.

Skull base invasion is reported in up to 50% of nasopharyngeal carcinomas at the time of presentation (Figs 4.8, 4.10 and 4.11).[11] This occurs via two primary mechanisms: (1) intracavernous extension through the foramina lacerum and ovale affecting cranial nerves III–VI; and (2) postero-lateral spread to the carotid space and jugular fossa affecting cranial nerves IX–XII.[1,8–10] Symptoms may then consist of a cavernous sinus syndrome with multiple cranial nerve palsies and a Horner's syndrome from invasion of the sympathetic plexus. The fifth cranial nerve is most commonly affected, causing numbness and pain along its distribution.[5,8] Tumor may reach the orbit by way of the pterygopalatine fossa and inferior orbital fissure.[8,9,12]

The actual primary lesion may be so small as to remain undetected despite the presence of extensive local spread of disease (Fig. 4.11).[12] Contrast MR sometimes may be more sensitive than CT or clinical examination for detecting small lesions.[1] Nasopharyngeal carcinomas exhibit an intermediate signal intensity on T1-weighted images. The distinction between tumor, fat and muscle is sometimes more apparent on the intermediate and T2-weighted images.[1] The extent of bony destruction is often better evaluated with CT, while invasion of the marrow spaces by tumor is better assessed with MRI.[7,9,13,14] In defining an extensive nasopharyngeal lesion, CT and MRI can be complementary.

It is widely accepted that staging of nasopharyngeal carcinoma is far more accurate using CT or MRI than clinical examination alone.[2,11,13,14] Nodal metastases are present in up to 90% of patients at the time of presentation, half of which are bilateral.[2,12]

Reliable differentiation between primary malignancy and secondary (metastatic) processes are often not possible with MR or CT (Figs 4.12 and 4.13).[14] Patterns of spread of the malignancy and clinical presentation often provide important clues to origin.[7,10] Other malignancies may extend into the nasopharynx from the skull base and mimic the imaging characteristics of nasopharyngeal carcinoma (Figs 4.14–4.16).

Other malignancies

Lymphoma

Other primary nasopharyngeal malignancies include lymphoma, lymphosarcoma and chondrosarcoma.[10] In the head and neck the nasopharynx is one of the most common sites for lymphoma to originate, second only to the tonsils. Patients are usually between 50 and 90 years of age. Lymphomas appear as smoothly marginated, exophytic, submucosal masses.[1] Lymphoma in a nasopharyngeal location is detected relatively early due to symptoms related to obstruction of the eustachian tube orifice.[1]

Adenoid cystic carcinoma

Although adenoid cystic carcinomas have been reported to produce soft tissue masses in the nasopharynx, nasopharyngeal involvement is generally observed late in the clinical course of the disease (Fig. 4.16). These tumors usually show evidence of bone erosion that is disproportionate to the soft tissue component. Serous otitis media is not a common clinical finding.[8]

Rhabdomyosarcoma

Rhabdomyosarcomas are the most common soft tissue sarcomas in the pediatric age group. The peak age of incidence is between 2 and 5 years. Seventy percent become symptomatic before age ten.[1] The nasopharynx/parapharyngeal space is the second most common site of origin after the orbit. These are markedly aggressive and exhibit rapid growth, local recurrence and distant spread.[1,10] Invasion of the skull base is observed in up to 35% of patients, with encroachment upon the cavernous sinus and resultant cranial nerve palsies. Spread to regional lymph nodes occurs often (50%), and metastases to the lungs and bone are commonplace. These are bulky lesions that exhibit an intermediate signal intensity, between that of muscle and fat on the T1-weighted MR images (Fig. 4.17). As with nasopharyngeal carcinoma, skull base invasion is typical and should therefore be routinely assessed on coronal images.[1]

Chordoma

There are rare cases of chordomas presenting initially in the nasopharynx. More often, they are accompanied by a large intracranial mass. On CT, a feature of chordomas with a nasopharyngeal component is invasion of the petro-occipital fissure. Serous otitis media is not a secondary clinical finding with chordomas.[8]

Other neoplasms

Primary malignancies of the nasal cavity, oropharynx and maxillary sinuses can invade the nasopharynx secondarily.[8,9] The origin of the neoplasia can usually be inferred by the location of the bulk of the mass and pattern of bony invasion (Fig. 4.16).

Primary bone tumors such as osteochondromas and chondromas may also extend into the nasopharynx from the skull base or upper cervical spine.

Infection

Infections of the paranasal sinuses, middle ear cavities and eustachian tubes can drain to the retropharyngeal lymph nodes, causing a suppurative lymphadenitis. Inflammatory processes such as mucormycosis and necrotizing 'malignant' external otitis may also spread compartmentally and mimic a malignancy.[10] A nasopharyngeal abscess can result from direct spread of a local infectious spondylitis.

Oropharynx

Normal anatomy

Oral cavity

The perimeter of the oral cavity extends from the lips and cheeks externally to the anterior tonsillar pillars (fauces) internally. The components of the mouth include the gingivobuccal mucosa, the anterior two-thirds of the tongue, the muscular floor, the osseous roof and the mandible. The buccal and gingival mucosa consist of squamous epithelium. The gingivobuccal sulcus is the junction of these areas in the oral vestibule. The posterior aspect of the sulcus continues with the retromolar trigone which permits communication with the oral cavity proper.[15] The buccinator muscle underlies the buccal mucosa. The muscle is lateral to the maxilla and mandible and anterior to the masseter muscle. The fat-filled pterygomandibular space is limited anteriorly by the pterygomandibular raphe. This space has a posterior boundary with the deep lobe of the parotid gland; the lateral and medial margins are the mandible and the medial pterygoid muscle respectively. The pterygomandibular space contains the lingual and alveolar branches of the trigeminal nerve (Figs 4.18 and 4.19).[16]

The buccal space

The buccal space is located anterior to the mandibular ramus and lateral to the upper alveolar ridge. The space contains a fat pad just lateral to the buccinator muscle, and it is limited by the superior and inferior attachments of the buccinator muscle. The facial artery and parotid duct course through the buccal space.[16,17]

The tongue

The tongue is composed of intrinsic and extrinsic muscles. The extrinsic muscles have their origins outside the tongue. The intrinsic muscles are divided into three groups: longitudinal, vertical and transverse. Because the fibers of these muscles interdigitate, they cannot be individually distinguished. The extrinsic group includes the genioglossus, hyoglossus, styloglossus and palatoglossus muscles. Along with the geniohyoid, they form the majority of the muscles of the floor of the mouth and are all innervated by the hypoglossal nerve.[15,16,18] Several important structures course between the hyoglossus muscle medially and the mylohyoid laterally. These included lingual and hypoglossal nerves, the sublingual gland with the adjacent submandibular duct, and the lingual vein.[15,16]

The sublingual space

The entire area which is deep to the mylohyoid muscle is known as the sublingual space. The space is bounded by the mylohyoid antero-laterally, the genioglossus and geniohyoid muscles medially and the tongue and mucosa of the floor of the mouth superiorly. The superficial portion of the submandibular gland marks the confluence of the sublingual and submandibular spaces, which are the primary deep spaces related to the oral cavity.[17] The sling-shaped mylohyoid muscle and anterior belly of the digastric muscle, together with the extrinsic tongue muscles, combine to form the floor of the mouth.[16]

The oropharynx

The oropharynx includes the palatine arch complex and the oropharynx proper. The anterior pillars are formed by the palatoglossus muscles, and the posterior pillars by the palatopharyngeus muscles. The mucosal covering is squamous epithelium. Other structures which contribute to the margins of the oropharynx include the soft palate with the uvula, the base of the tongue, and the posterior and lateral pharyngeal walls. The inferior boundary is delineated from the larynx by the epiglottis and from the hypopharynx by the pharyngoepiglottic folds.[17] In the region of the palatine arch complex of the oropharynx are the faucial tonsils. The lingual tonsils underlie the mucosa at the base of the tongue. Along with the adenoids in the posterior nasopharynx, these masses of lymphoid tissue are known as Waldeyer's ring. Contiguous with the oropharynx are the parapharyngeal spaces laterally and the retropharyngeal space posteriorly. The spaces are important routes for extension of disease from the oropharynx.[17]

Imaging techniques

Computed tomography

Axial CT sections are obtained parallel to the infraorbital–meatal line. The head should be properly positioned about the cephalocaudal axis, otherwise asymmetric images may simulate pathology. A scout localizer image is obtained to document the plane of section and to avoid artifacts from dental amalgam. This preliminary scan is used to choose an optimally magnified field-of-view (14–18 cm). Contiguous axial sections of 5 mm thickness are obtained from the hard palate to the hyoid bone (Fig. 4.18). The sections from the mandibular alveolar ridge to the hyoid bone should be obtained parallel to the ramus of the mandible. This approximates the plane of attachment of the mylohyoid muscle and demonstrates the anatomic relationship of pathology to the tissue planes and spaces in the region.[16] Coronal sections are obtained from the posterior aspect of the oropharynx through the entire mandible. Coronal sections are necessary to evaluate the relationship of a pathologic process to the skull base.

To avoid motion artifact in the oral cavity and oropharynx, scans should be obtained with respiration and swallowing suspended. When detailed evaluation of the mandible is required, bone algorithms are important. The routine use of intravenous, iodinated contrast agent better determines the margins of a lesion, establishes the degree of vascularity and distinguishes normal vessels from lymph nodes. A combined bolus of 50–100 ml of 60% contrast followed by a drip infusion of 300 ml of 30% contrast is routinely recommended.[16,17]

Magnetic resonance imaging
Magnetic resonance examinations of the oral cavity and oropharynx usually may be performed with a head coil which is positioned as inferiorly as possible. An anterior neck surface coil is another preferred method.[19] The surface coil is useful, especially if the head coil cannot adequately cover the area of interest.

The examination includes several sequences. A rapid, sagittal localizer sequence is provided for cephalocaudal orientation. T1-weighted images are generated with TR = 500–1000 ms. The T2-weighted sequence is obtained with a TR ranging from 2000 to 3000 ms and a TE of 60 to 100 ms. The first echo of the T2-weighted sequence provides an image reflecting proton density. A maximum of two excitations are performed in order to maintain imaging times to a tolerable length. If the contrast agent, gadolinium-DTPA, is used, then T1-weighted images are obtained before and after its administration.[20,21] We routinely use fat suppression on all postcontrast T1-weighted sequences to increase conspicuity of pathology. When pathology involves the floor of the mouth or the lateral wall, coronal images provide the optimal view. Sagittal images are preferred for demonstrating tongue base and posterior pharyngeal wall pathology. Coronal images also provide important information for masses in the tongue base. A slice thickness of 5 mm is suggested with a 1 mm gap (Fig. 4.19).[21]

Structures which may show normal asymmetry include the tonsillar pillars, glossopalatine sulci, the pharyngoepiglottic folds and valleculae.[22] The faucial and lingual tonsils themselves can be asymmetric. The intrinsic muscles of the tongue and

the digastric muscles are usually symmetric. The parapharyngeal spaces may be asymmetric; obliteration of the space on one side is indicative of pathology. The lingual septum should always remain in the midline.[22]

Morphologic criteria for MRI studies are comparable with and based on CT criteria. However, tissue intensity signals are unique to MRI. The relative intensities of various tissues from different pulse sequences have allowed identification of patterns for normal structures relative to pathology. Contrast among tissues varies in a consistent manner. The numerous fat-to-water interfaces in soft tissues of the head and neck allow exquisite anatomic definition. Knowledge of the intrinsic tissue properties allows appropriate selection of MRI sequences for specific anatomic areas of interest.[20,23] In sites where adipose tissue is present, such as the floor of the mouth, oropharynx and hypopharynx, T1-weighted sequences are chosen to visualize fatty tissue planes and maximize contrast between fat and tumor. The images are assessed carefully for abnormal tissue bulk and deviation of tissue planes rather than for abnormal signal from the tumor. Except for the midline lingual septum, fat is sparsely distributed in the body and base of the tongue. Therefore, T2-weighted sequences that stress contrast between tumor and muscle become advantageous.[20,23,24] Differentiation between benign and malignant lesions is not feasible because there is similarity of the T1 and T2 values of such tumors.[20,23] Excessive tissue water content correlates with long T1 and T2 relaxation times noted in both neoplastic and inflammatory conditions. Cystic structures which have high water content are easily recognized. Magnetic resonance imaging may be able to discriminate complex cysts containing high protein or cellular debris from simple cysts. The complex cyst will have a shortened relaxation time which is more apparent as increased signal on T1-weighted images.[20,23] T2-weighted images alone may overestimate tumor size by incorporating surrounding tissue edema. Gadolinium allows for a more precise definition of the tumor nidus. In circumstances where natural tissue planes have been distorted by surgery and radiation, gadolinium may assist in reliably distinguishing tumor from fibrosis.[20,25]

Enhancement of normal tissues may persist for as long as six months after treatment. Use of fat-suppression techniques may augment gadolinium in producing enhancement of abnormal tissue.

Benign masses

Benign tumors may arise from the various mesenchymal cell lines which include dermoid cysts, teratomas, lipomas and hemangiomas.

Dermoid cyst

A dermoid cyst is lined with squamous epithelium. Only 7% of all dermoid cysts occur in the head and neck region, and nearly one-quarter of these arise in the floor of the mouth, submental and submandibular regions. They usually become symptomatic in the second or third decade of life. A dermoid cyst that arises in the sublingual area will raise the tongue and may interfere with deglutition. In this location a dermoid may simulate a ranula. In the submental area, a dermoid cyst presents as an external swelling above the hyoid bone.[26] Computed tomography demonstrates a hypodense mass. The presence of fat within the mass is indicative of the diagnosis (Fig. 4.20).[17,26] Magnetic resonance images typically demonstrate a hyperintense mass on T1-weighted images, confirming its fatty composition. Proton-density and T2-weighted images also reveal a homogeneous hyperintense lesion surrounded by a thin rim of low signal intensity, representing a capsule.[20]

Lipoma

A lipoma is an encapsulated, benign, subcutaneous and submucous tumor that is of little clinical significance. These tumors are unusual and constitute approximately 2% of all benign tumors of the oral cavity. The buccal mucosa, tongue, and floor of the mouth are frequent sites for occurrence.[27] Computed tomography images typically show a well-defined, homogeneous mass of fatty attenuation (Fig. 4.21). On MR images, the fat produces a homogeneous hyperintense signal on the T1-weighted sequence.

Ranula

Ranulas are acquired retention products that occur in the floor of the mouth. The etiology is obstruction of the duct of the sublingual gland. Two varieties of ranula are described: (1) the simple ranula found in the sublingual space (a true epithelial lined retention cyst) (Figs 4.22 and 4.23), and (2) the plunging type, which extends into the submandibular space via the back of the sublingual space or into the floor of the mouth and into the fascial planes of the neck (Fig. 4.24).[17] If a ranula enlarges enough, it will distort intraoral structures enough to interfere with swallowing. Computed tomography of a ranula demonstrates a hypodense mass in the sublingual or submandibular space.[16]

Hemangioma/lymphangioma

Hemangiomas are benign vascular malformations and are the most common head and neck mass in children. They may involve the oral cavity and oropharynx. They appear as a sessile, red submucosal mass usually at the base of the tongue. Histologic types include capillary, cavernous, mixed and hypertrophic.[16]

Computed tomography of hemangiomas demonstrates a well-defined mass which enhances to a variable degree. Phleboliths are diagnostic of hemangiomas when they are present.[16,20] Magnetic resonance images reveal faint increased signal intensity on T1-weighted images, while T2-weighted images show marked hyperintensity (Fig. 4.25).[20,28] Lymphangioma, on the other hand, are multiloculated masses that most commonly occur in the submandibular space. They may be difficult to distinguish from a plunging ranula or abscess radiologically (Fig. 4.26).

Thyroid rests

Embryonic rest of thyroid tissue may be located anywhere along the tract of the thyroglossal duct. The dorsal posterior third of the tongue is the most common site for this remnant of thyroid tissue. The incidence in females is far greater than in males. Such thyroid tissue may be functional, and may represent the sole source of thyroid hormones. The ectopic tissue usually is asymptomatic. However, it is subject to all forms of thyroid pathology. The tissue may enlarge to a point where the airway is compromised and there is dysphagia.[16]

Solid thyroid rests are usually discovered incidentally on CT scan. The intrinsic iodine content and the vascularity of the thyroid tissue cause it to have high attenuation in both unenhanced and enhanced scans.[16] Magnetic resonance images demonstrate a well-defined mass of intermediate signal intensity on T1-weighted sequences. The T2-weighted images show a more sharply defined lingual thyroid mass which is hyperintense.[20]

Squamous cell carcinoma

The most common malignancy of the oral cavity and oropharynx is squamous cell carcinoma which constitutes more than 90% of all oral tumors. The tumors amount to 7% of all malignancies that occur annually in the USA. The disease occurs predominantly in males, in the sixth and seventh decades and in patients with a protracted, heavy indulgence in alcohol and tobacco (Figs 4.27–4.36).[29]

Clinically, patients complain of focal pain, sore throat and poorly seated dentures. Because the external auditory canal is innervated by branches from the trigeminal, glossopharyngeal and vagus nerves, a patient may complain of otalgia. Occasionally a deeply infiltrating tumor will generate minimal symptoms, but the patient will present with a neck mass. An invasive malignancy in the tonsillar fossa may manifest itself with trismus.[16]

Tumor may gain access to other compartments by spreading along muscle bundles or fascial planes, through periosteum and perineurium or via lymphatic channels.[16,29] The loose areolar and adipose tissue that resides in the interfascial spaces surrounding the muscles of the oropharynx permit cranial and caudal extension of a malignancy. In this manner, the skull base and the upper neck become vulnerable to metastasis.[17] The periosteum usually is a formidable barrier to invasion by tumor. However, when a tumor breaches the periosteum of the mandible or the skull base it invades the bone through a neural or nutrient canal with a predilection for the marrow spaces.[16]

Early dissemination of squamous cell carcinoma in the oral cavity is to adjacent mucosal surfaces and underlying muscles and bone.[17,30] Tumors of the anterior third of the oral tongue are manifested early after minor local spread. Lesions of the middle third spread to the intrinsic muscles and the extrinsic muscles in the floor of the mouth. In the posterior third of the oral tongue, tumors behave like lesions of the tongue base. Infiltration is into the tongue musculature, the floor of the mouth and the tonsillar pillars.[17,30] Seventy-five percent of the glossal neoplasms occur in the oral portion, particularly along the lateral border of the middle third of the tongue.[29]

Lymphatic metastases from tumors of the oral cavity occur primarily in the submandibular and jugulodigastric nodes.[29,30] Clinically palpable lymph nodes reportedly have occurred on initial presentation in 10–50% of the cases (Figs 4.29, 4.31, 4.32, 4.34 and 4.36).[17,29,30] A significant percentage of lesions have contralateral nodal metastases at the time of presentation.[16,29]

In the oropharynx, the majority of the malignancies are squamous cell carcinomas (Figs 4.31–4.33).[29] The tumor most often affects the anterior faucial pillar or the faucial tonsil itself. Other regions affected by this tumor include the soft palate, oropharyngeal walls and lingual tonsils.[16,29] Squamous cell carcinoma of the anterior pillar initially will invade adjacent mucosal structures. It will extend along the palatoglossus muscle to the soft palate, to the tongue base, to the buccal mucosa and into the parapharyngeal space.

Metastases occur early, and reportedly 50% of patients with carcinoma of the tonsil will demonstrate lymph node involvement at presentation.[29,31] In a few cases, an occult tonsillar tumor is first manifested by cervical lymph node metastasis. The intrinsic aggressiveness of the tonsillar carcinoma and the paucity of symptoms account for the frequency of metastatic disease at presentation. The extensive lymphatic system in the oropharyngeal region predisposes to frequent contralateral and bilateral metastasis.

Twenty-five percent of all such carcinomas of the tongue occur in the tongue base. Diagnosis frequently is delayed because the initial mild symptoms of sore throat and otalgia are ignored. Regional extension of the tumor occurs into the oral portion of the tongue, along the glossopharyngeal sulci to the palatal arch complex and, into the valleculae and hypopharynx.[29,31] Extension of tumor into the pre-epiglottic space is recognized in both

MR and CT imaging by infiltration of the fat that separates the hyoid bone from the epiglottis.[16,17,20] With extensive primary disease, infiltration through the lingual septum may occur.

Most malignancies of the soft palate are also squamous cell carcinomas. These tumors usually affect the oral surface of the palate. The lesions tend to be well differentiated and have the best prognosis of all oropharyngeal carcinomas.[30] Extension of a palatal carcinoma occurs most commonly to the tonsillar pillars and hard palate. Lateral invasion involves the levator or tensor palatine muscles and extends into the parapharyngeal space from which it may reach the skull base.

With contrast-enhanced CT scans, the appearance of squamous cell carcinoma is that of an enhancing mass (Figs 4.27–4.34). The mass distorts normal tissue planes and infiltrates the adipose tissue within adjacent spaces. Large tumor masses and malignant nodes necrose commonly. Malignant nodes frequently demonstrate ring enhancement around a low-density necrotic core (Figs 4.29, 4.31, 4.32, 4.34 and 4.36). The probability of lymph node invasion depends on size, so that 80% of nodes greater than 2 cm and 90% of nodes greater than 3 cm will harbor metastasis.[16,17,32,33] Distinguishing between reactive and malignant adenopathy is particularly difficult in the submandibular space.

Squamous cell carcinoma demonstrates hypointense signals on T1-weighted images which makes differentiation from adjacent muscle difficult. However, the tumors on T2-weighted images exhibit varying degrees of high signal intensity, which allows for sharp demarcation from adjacent muscle. The paucity of fat and defined tissue planes within the tongue makes T2-weighted imaging essential for determining involvement of the tongue musculature (Fig. 4.30). Unilateral abnormal hyperintense signal on T1-weighted images of the tongue suggests involvement of the hypoglossal nerve with muscle atrophy and fatty infiltration (Fig. 4.33).[16] The floor of the mouth and the deep jugular and submandibular lymph nodes are assessed optimally with coronal T1- and T2-weighted images.[20,23,24] Assessment of the tongue base, epiglottis, pre-epiglottic space and intrinsic tongue muscles is best obtained with T2-weighted sagittal images. Compared with CT images, the absence of signal from cortical bone on MRI permits better visualization of adjacent soft tissues.[20,23] Assessing adenopathy on MR images relies on the size and morphologic criteria used with CT images. Magnetic resonance cannot reliably differentiate malignant from reactive lymphadenopathy.[20,23,24]

In the oropharynx, tonsillar tissue density on CT is indistinguishable from adjacent musculature in the faucial pillars (Figs 4.34–4.36).[16] On MRI, the signal from the tonsil is separated more readily from the parapharyngeal space by the hypointense signal of the tonsillar capsule and superior constrictor muscle.[20,23] On T2-weighted images, the high signal intensity of normal lymphoid tissue makes this parameter an unreliable indicator of disease in the tonsillar beds.[20,21]

Other malignancies

Lymphoma

Non-Hodgkin's lymphoma is the second most common malignancy of the oropharynx (5%). The tissue in Waldeyer's ring is second only to the lymph nodes as a source for primary lymphomas in the oropharynx. The palatine tonsils are most frequently involved with primary lymphoma and the lingual tonsils are involved the least. Lymphomas usually develop exophytically or as a submucosal mass which does not ulcerate (Fig. 4.37). Lymphomas of Waldeyer's ring produce symptoms in a delayed fashion; therefore, they usually present with a large mass. The epicenter is difficult to determine because of the usual extensive involvement upon presentation.

The density of extranodal non-Hodgkin's lymphoma on CT images is frequently indistinguishable from squamous cell carcinoma. The lymph nodes with non-Hodgkin's lymphoma on CT scans are large, multiple and bilateral. Lymphomatous nodes, despite their size may not appear necrotic on CT scans, except if treatment has been instituted previously.[16,17]

The MR signal characteristics of a tonsillar lymphoma demonstrate increased intensity compared with adjacent muscle on proton-density and T2-weighted images. The signals are similar to those obtained from a carcinoma. However, a lymphoma usually remains more sharply defined, as opposed to the infiltration typically observed with carcinomas. The MRI appearance of individual, non-necrotic nodes cannot be distinguished from metastatic nodes of squamous cell carcinoma.[20]

Adenoid cystic carcinoma

Numerous minor salivary glands are scattered throughout the oral cavity and the oropharynx. The majority of the minor salivary glands are located posterior to the level of the second molar (Figs 4.16, 4.38 and 4.39). This explains the greater incidence of minor salivary gland neoplasms in this region. Carcinomas of the minor salivary gland are uncommon and comprise 1% or less of all carcinomas of the oral cavity and oropharynx. The histologic type of neoplasms is identical to those seen in the major salivary glands. Malignant mixed cell, adenoid cystic carcinoma, mucoepidermoid carcinoma and adenocarcinoma are the most common malignant tumors.[16]

Adenoid cystic carcinoma usually arises from the soft palate, lips and buccal mucosa posterior to the second molar. The natural history demonstrates an early propensity to infiltrate along local nerves which occurs in most tumors greater than 1 cm in diameter. This behavior makes complete surgical resection problematic. Local recurrence is frequent as tumor cells usually extend beyond reasonable surgical margins.[34] Tumor can spread via the palatine canals to the pterygopalatine fossa. Metastases are typically to the regional lymph nodes and lungs.

Malignant mixed cells tumors have a predilection for women in their fourth to sixth decades. Mucoepidermoid carcinoma arises from the mucous and basal cells of the salivary gland ducts. Both low and high grade type may occur; the high grade variety is apt to recur locally and extend to regional lymph nodes. Adenocarcinoma is a rare histologic type of minor salivary gland tumor. The tumor may arise from the palate, buccal mucosa or floor of the mouth. Adenocarcinoma has a dismal prognosis compared with other neoplasms of the minor salivary glands.

In the tongue base, the imaging characteristics of minor salivary gland neoplasms obtained by CT and MRI are indistinguishable from those of a squamous cell histology (Fig. 4.39). The minor salivary gland carcinoma tends to have hypointense signals on the T1-weighted images. The tumor margins are usually well-defined when contiguous with adipose tissue; however, differentiation of the margins from adjacent muscle is difficult. On T2-weighted images, such tumors demonstrate some degree of hyperintense signal which allows a distinction from surrounding muscle. Gadolinium-DTPA may improve conspicuity of certain aspects of a lesion. Infiltrating lesions that exhibit less tumor bulk and greater bony destruction are suggestive of adenoid cystic carcinoma. The increased signal intensity of the tumor and distinction from surrounding adipose tissue may be improved with the routine use of fat-suppression techniques.[21]

Infection

Obstruction of the ducts of the sublingual and/or submandibular glands by a calculous or stenois can produce infection in the sublingual or submandibular spaces respectively (Fig. 4.40). Alternatively, periodontal infections from dental extractions can yield a peritonsillar mass that mimics a malignancy. Computed tomography well demonstrates the organized, necrotic mass (abscess) as well as the associated soft tissue cellulitis (Fig. 4.41). In most instances, the diagnosis is established by appropriate clinical history.

References

1　Braun IF, MRI of the nasopharynx, *Radiol Clin North Am* (1989) **27**:315–30.

2　Mancuso AA, Bohman L, Hanafee W et al, Computed tomography of the nasopharynx: normal and variants of normal, *Radiology* (1980) **137**:113–21.

3　Silver AJ, Mawad ME, Hilal SK et al, Computed tomography of the nasopharynx and related spaces. Part II. Pathology, *Radiology* (1983) **147**:733–8.

4　Silver AJ, Sane P, Hilal SK, CT of the nasopharyngeal region: normal and pathologic anatomy, *Radiol Clin North Am* (1984) **22**:161–76.

5 SMOKER WRK, GENTRY LR, Computed tomography of the nasopharynx and related spaces, *Semin Ultrasound CT MR* (1986) 7:107–30.

6 HOE J, CT of nasopharyngeal carcinoma: significance of widening of the preoccipital soft tissue on axial scans, *AJNR* (1989) **10**:839–44.

7 YU ZH, XU GZ, HUANG YR et al, Value of computed tomography in staging the primary lesion (t-staging) of nasopharyngeal carcinoma: an analysis of 54 patients with special reference to the parapharyngeal space, *Int J Radiat Oncol Biol Phys* (1985) **11**:2143–7.

8 WANG CC, Carcinoma of the nasopharynx. In: Wang CC, ed., *Radiation Therapy for Head and Neck Neoplasms: Indications, Techniques and Results* (John Wright and Sons, Ltd: Boston 1983) 201–12.

9 TERESI LM, LUFKIN RB, VINUELA F et al, MR imaging of the nasopharynx and floor of the middle cranial fossa. Part II. Malignant tumors, *Radiology* (1987) **164**:817–21.

10 YAMASHITA S, KONDO M, HASHIMOTO S, Conversion of T-stages of nasopharyngeal carcinoma by computed tomography, *Int J Radiat Oncol Biol Phys* (1985) **11**:1017–21.

11 SILVER AJ, MAWAD ME, HILAL SK et al, Computed tomography of the nasopharynx and related spaces. Part I. Anatomy, *Radiology* (1983) **147**:725–31.

12 CARTER BL, Nasopharynx and infratemporal fossa: anatomy and pathologic findings. In: Valvassori GE, Buckinham RA, Carter BL et al, eds, *Head and Neck Imaging* (Thieme Medical Publishers, Inc.: New York 1988) 235–50.

13 TERESI LM, LUFKIN RB, VINUELA F et al, MR imaging of the nasopharynx and floor of the middle cranial fossa. Part I. Normal anatomy, *Radiology* (1987) **164**:811–16.

14 DILLON WP, MILLS CM, KJOS B et al, Magnetic resonance imaging of the nasopharynx, *Radiology* (1984) **152**:731–8.

15 BERKOVITZ BKB, MOXHAM BJ, *A Textbook of Head and Neck Anatomy* (Year Book Medical Publishers: Chicago 1988) 272 pp.

16 DILLON WP, MANCUSO AA, The oropharynx and nasopharynx. In: Newton TH, Hasso AN, Dillon WP, eds, *Computed Tomography of the Head and Neck* (Raven Press: New York 1988) Ch. 10.

17 HARDIN CW, HARNSBERGER HR, OSBORN AG et al, CT in the evaluation of the normal and diseased oral cavity and oropharynx, *Semin Ultrasound CT MR* (1986) 7:131.

18 SMOKER WRK, HARNSBERGER R, OSBORN AG, The hypoglossal nerve, *Semin Ultrasound CT MR* (1987) **8**:301.

19 LUFKIN R, HANAFEE W, WORTHAM D et al, Magnetic resonance imaging of the larynx and hypopharynx using surface coils, *Radiology* (1986) **158**:747.

20 KASSEL EE, KELLER MA, KUCHARCZY K, MRI of the floor of the mouth tongue and orohypopharynx, *Radiol Clin North Am* (1989) **27**:331.

21 ROBINSON JD, CRAWFORD SC, TERESI LM et al, Extracranial lesions of the head and neck: preliminary experience with Gd-DTPA enhanced MR imaging, *Radiology* (1989) **172**:165–70.

22 MURAKI AS, MANCUSO AA, HARNSBERGER HR et al, CT of the oropharynx, tongue base, and floor of the mouth: normal anatomy and range of variations, and applications in staging carcinoma, *Radiology* (1983) **148**:725.

23 MAFEE MF, COMPOS M, RAJU S et al, Head and neck: high field MRI versus CT, *Otolaryngol Clin North Am* (1988) **21**:513.

24 LUFKIN RB, WORTHAM DG, DIETRICH RB et al, Tongue and oropharynx: findings on MR imaging, *Radiology* (1986) **161**:69.

25 SCHAEFER SD, MARAVILLA KR, SUSS RA et al, Magnetic resonance imaging versus computed tomography: comparison in imaging oral cavity and pharyngeal carcinoma, *Arch Otolaryngol* (1985) **111**:730.

26 BATSAKIS JG, Neoplasms of the minor and 'lesser' major salivary glands. In: Batsakis JG, ed., *Tumors of the Head and Neck: Clinical and Pathological Considerations* (Williams and Wilkins: Baltimore 1979) Ch. 10.

27 BATSAKIS JG, Soft tissue tumors of the head and neck: unusual forms. In: Batsakis JG, ed., *Tumors of the Head and Neck: Clinical and Pathological Considerations* (Williams and Wilkins: Baltimore 1979) Ch. 18.

28 COHEN EK, KRESSEL HY, PEROSIO T et al, Magnetic resonance imaging of soft tissue hemangiomas: correlations with pathologic findings, *AJR* (1988) **150**:1079–81.

29 BATSAKIS JG, Squamous cell carcinoma of the oral cavity and oropharynx. In: Batsakis JG, ed., *Tumors of the Head and Neck: Clinical and Pathological Considerations* (Williams and Wilkins: Baltimore 1979) Ch. 6.

30 WANG CC, Oral cancer. In: Wang CC, ed., *Radiation Therapy for Head and Neck: Indications, Techniques and Results* (John Wright and Sons, Ltd: Boston 1983) Ch. 8.

31 WANG CC, Carcinoma of the oropharynx. In: Wang CC, ed., *Radiation Therapy for Head and Neck: Indications, Techniques and Results* (John Wright and Sons, Ltd: Boston 1983) Ch. 9.

32 BYRD SE, SCHOEN PJ, GILL G et al, Computed tomography of palatine tonsillar carcinoma, *J Comput Assist Tomogr* (1983) 7:976.

33 ASPESTRAND F, KOLBENSTRVEDT A, BOYSEN M, Staging of carcinoma of the palatine tonsils by computed tomography, *J Comput Assist Tomogr* (1988) 12:434.

34 BATSAKIS JG, Neoplasms of the minor and 'lesser' major salivary glands. In: Batsakis JG, ed., *Tumors of the Head and Neck: Clinical and Pathological Considerations* (Williams and Wilkins: Baltimore 1979) Ch. 2.

A

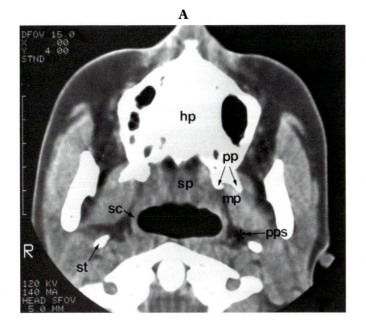

C

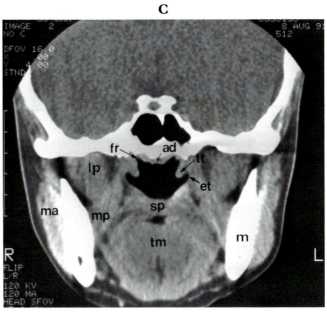

B

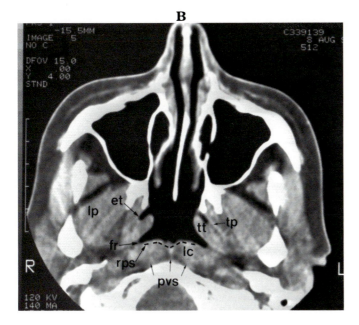

FIGURE 4.1

Normal CT anatomy of nasopharynx. (**A**) Axial image at the level of the low nasopharynx/upper oropharynx. (**B**) Axial CT image at the mid-nasopharynx level. The dotted line represents the potential retropharyngeal space. (**C**) Coronal CT image of the posterior nasopharynx.

Key: a, adenoid (lymphoid) tissue; c, carotid artery; dg, digastric muscle (posterior belly); dga, digastric muscle (anterior belly); ep, epiglottis; et, eustachian tube opening; fr, fossa of Rosenmuller; ge, genioglossus muscle; gh, geniohyoid muscle; hg, hyoglossus muscle; hp, hard palate; hy, hyoid bone; j, jugular vein; lc, longus capitus muscle; lp, lateral pterygoid muscle; ls, lingual septum; lt, lingual tonsils; lvp, levator veli palatini; m, mandible; ma, masseter muscle; my, mylohyoid muscle; mp, medial pterygoid muscle; np, nasopharynx; op, oropharynx; p, platysma muscle; pg, parotid gland; pp, pterygoid plates; pps, parapharyngeal space; pvs, prevertebral space; rps, retropharyngeal space; sc, superior constrictor muscle; sg, submandibular gland; sp, soft palate; sl, sublingual gland; st, styloid process; stg, styloglossal muscle; t, tonsil; te, temporalis muscle; tm, intrinsic tongue muscles; tp, tensor palatini muscle; tt, torus tubarius.

A

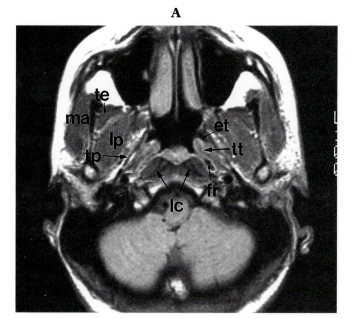

A

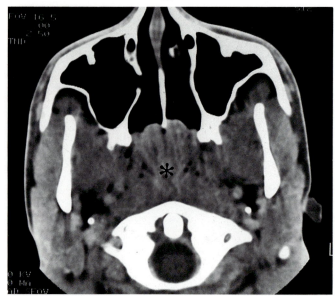

B

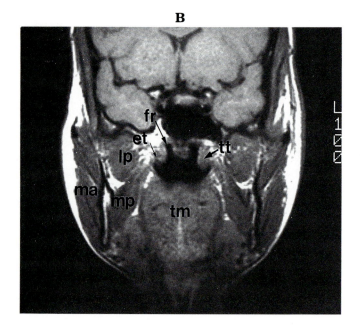

B

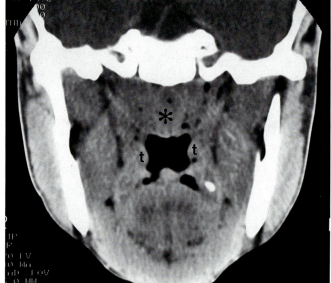

FIGURE 4.2

Normal MR anatomy of nasopharynx. (**A**) Proton-density axial MR image at the level of the mid-nasopharynx (TR = 2000 ms, TE = 20 ms). (**B**) T1-weighted coronal MR image of the nasopharynx (TR = 630 ms, TE = 20 ms).
For key, see legend to Fig. 4.1.

FIGURE 4.3

Prominent lymphoid tissue (adenoids) in a 16-year-old. (**A**) Axial CT image reveals a large, lobulated, soft tissue mass arising from the posterior–superior nasopharynx (*), extending into the posterior nasal cavity. Note that the mass conforms to the shape of the nasopharynx and does not displace or distort the adjacent mucosa or musculature. Pockets of air fill small interstices (crypts) within the lymphoid tissue. (**B**) Coronal image shows that the lymphoid tissue (*) arises well above the paired torus tubariae (t).

A

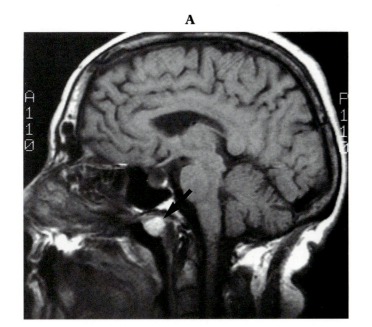

B

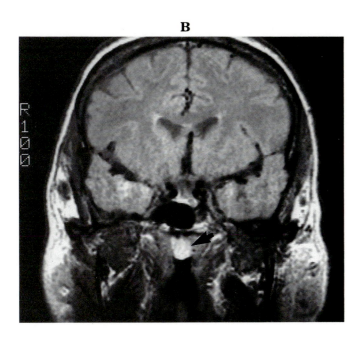

FIGURE 4.4

Thornwaldt's cyst. (**A**) Sagittal T1-weighted image of the brain (TR = 600 ms, TE = 20 ms) reveals a well-defined hyperintense mass attached to the posterior wall of the nasopharynx at the midline (arrow). The short T1 characteristics are probably due to high protein content of the cyst. (**B**) The cyst remains hyperintense (arrow) on a proton-density image (TR = 2000 ms, TE = 20 ms) in the coronal plane, and it is midline in location, without distortion or infiltration of adjacent structures.

A   **C**

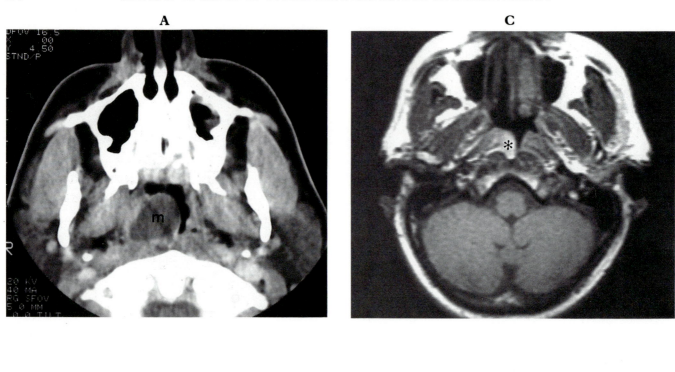

B   **D**

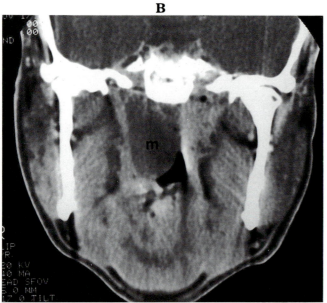   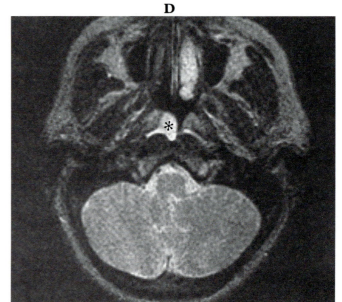

FIGURE 4.5

Mucous retention cyst. (**A**) Axial CT image in the nasopharynx shows a large ovoid mass of low density extending from the right lateral recess of the nasopharynx (m). Note that there is no evidence of invasion into adjacent tissue planes. In contrast to the Thornwaldt's cyst, which looks similar, the mucous retention cyst often arises laterally. (**B**) Coronal CT image on the same patient. Note that the cyst extends low into the oral cavity (m). (**C**) Axial MR image (TR = 700 ms, TE = 30 ms) on a different patient shows that the proteinaceous components of the cyst (*) yield a hyperintense signal on T1-weighted images. (**D**) The cyst (*) remains hyperintense on the axial T2-weighted image (TR = 2000 ms, TE = 80 ms).

A

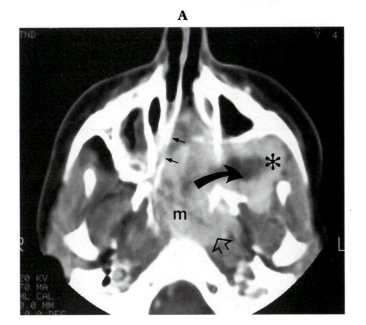

C

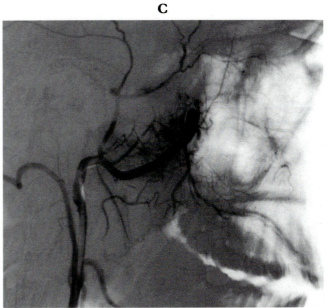

B

FIGURE 4.6

Juvenile angiofibroma in a 12-year-old male. (**A**) Postcontrast axial CT image demonstrates an enhancing mass lesion in the posterior nasal cavity and nasopharynx (m). The mass protrudes anteriorly and deviates the nasal septum to the right (small arrows). The mass extends into the left infratemporal fossa (*) through the eroded pterygoid plates and pterygopalatine fossa (curved arrow). Invasion of the left parapharyngeal space is also noted (open arrow). (**B**) The tumor has grown directly into the sphenoid sinus (arrow) as well as invaded the left sphenoid bone and skull base (*). The marked enlargement of the cavernous sinus on the left suggests that tumor has breached the skull base and has entered the cavernous sinus (open arrow). (**C**) Lateral view from a pre-embolization left external carotid arteriogram shows the marked hypervascularity of this tumor.

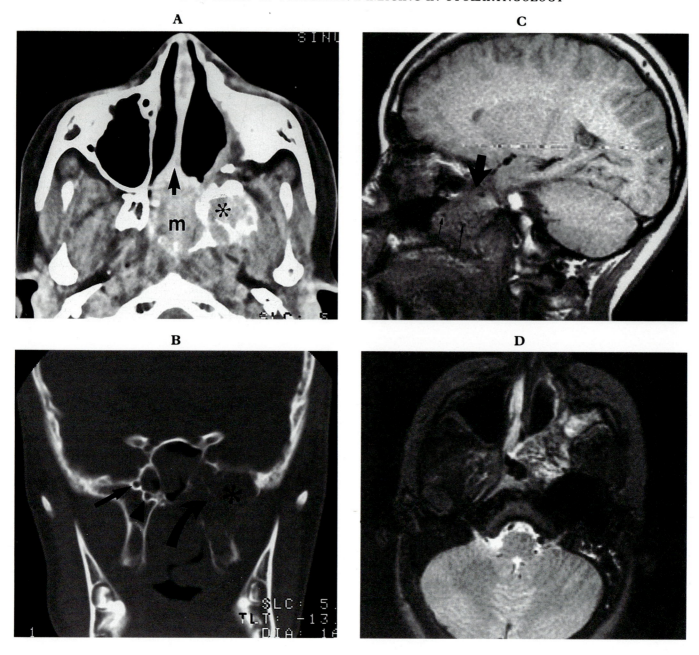

FIGURE 4.7

Recurrent juvenile angiofibroma in an 11-year-old male. (**A**) Postoperative changes are present in the left maxillary sinus on this axial CT image. Residual/recurrent tumor is present in the posterior nasal cavity (m) which has eroded the nasal septum (arrow). Erosion of the left pterygopalatine fossa and pterygoid plates (*) is also present. (**B**) A coronal CT image utilizing bone detail well illustrates the peripheral margins of the tumor. There is invasion superiorly with destruction of the sphenoid bone and skull base (*), and there is outgrowth of tumor into the left infratemporal fossa via transgression of the pterygoid plates on the left (curved arrow). This process has destroyed foramina leading to the pterygopalatine fossa (normal foramen rotundum) (arrow) and vidian canal (arrowhead) on the right. (**C**) A parasagittal T1-weighted MR image (TR = 600 ms, TE = 20 ms) shows the mass to be isointense to muscle and containing multiple linear flow voids suggestive of enlarged vascular channels (long arrows). The superior extent of the tumor and transgression of the skull base is well delineated (thick arrow). (**D**) The tumor is mildly hyperintense on the T2-weighted axial image (TR = 2600 ms, TE = 80 ms). Intratumoral linear flow voids persist on this pulse sequence, further suggesting hypervascularity.

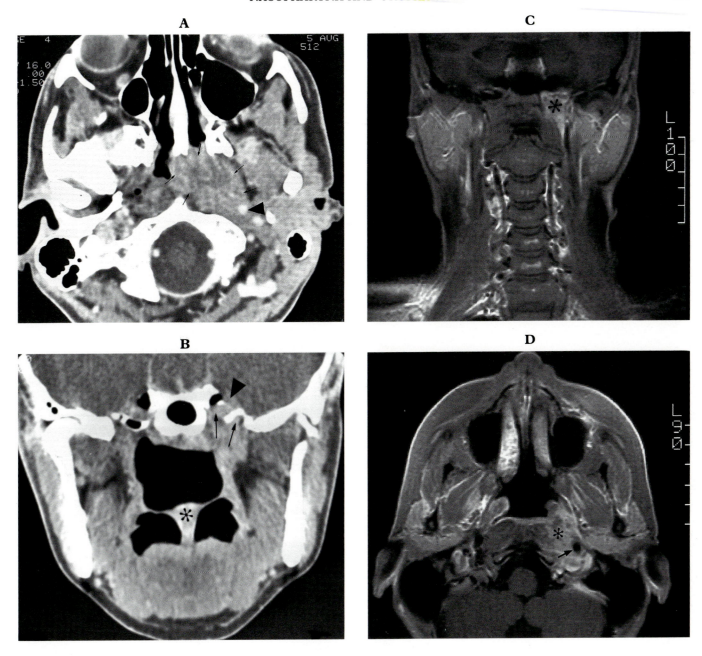

FIGURE 4.8

Nasopharyngeal carcinoma with skull base invasion. (**A**) Axial CT image with contrast material shows a bulky soft tissue mass (arrows) in the left nasopharynx, extending from the posterior nasal cavity anteriorly, to the retropharyngeal/pre-vertebral spaces posteriorly. Tumor encroaches upon the carotid space on the left (arrowhead). (**B**) The coronal CT images show the skull base invasion on the left (arrows) and extension into the left posterior cavernous sinus (arrowhead). Normal uvula (*).

(**C**) The use of fat-suppression techniques on this gadolinium-enhanced coronal T1-weighted MR image (TR = 450 ms, TE = 11 ms) creates sharp contrast between the tumor in the skull base (*) and the surrounding structures. (**D**) In axial orientation the tumor (*) is well delineated. Skull base invasion is confirmed as is posterior extension of the mass into the pre-vertebral and carotid spaces. Note the flow void in the left carotid artery (arrow) which is engulfed by tumor.

continued

E

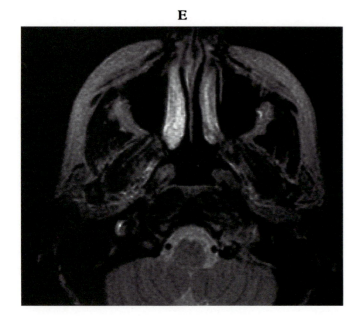

FIGURE 4.8 *(continued)*

(**E**) The tumor is difficult to visualize on a T2-weighted axial image (TR = 2150 ms, TE = 90 ms) obtained at the same location as (**D**).

A

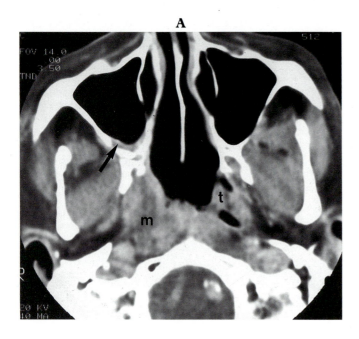

B

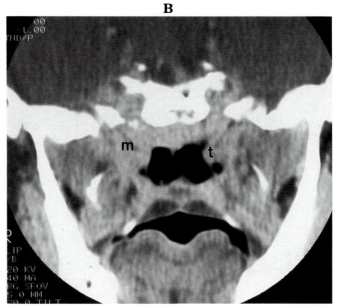

FIGURE 4.9

Nasopharyngeal carcinoma with maxillary sinus involvement. (**A**) Axial CT image reveals a mass of low attenuation (m) originating in the right nasopharynx, obliterating the right torus tubarius, eustachian tube opening and fossa of Rosenmuller. (Note the normal torus (t) on the left.) Tumor transgresses the lateral nasopharyngeal wall and pharyngobasilar fascia, effacing the parapharyngeal fat on the right. There is continuation of the mass anteriorly via the pterygopalatine fossa, with the erosion of the posterior wall of the maxillary sinus and invasion of the underlying mucosa (arrow). (**B**) Contrast-enhanced, coronal CT image shows slight enhancement of the mass (m) which abuts the skull base. There is no gross invasion of the skull base or cavernous sinus. t, normal torus.

A

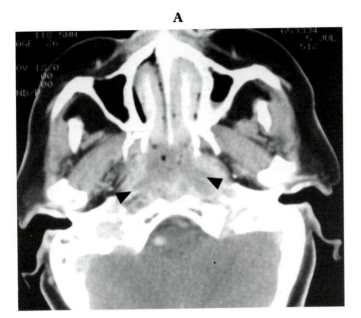

C

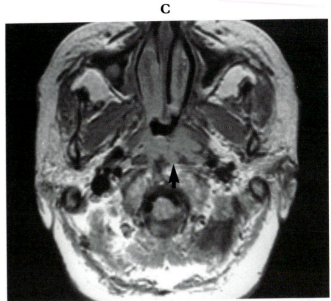

B

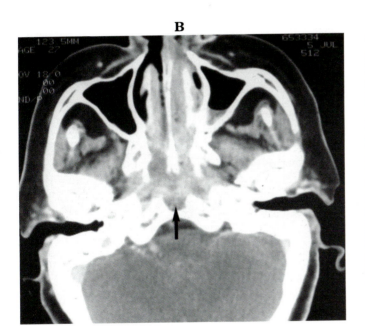

D

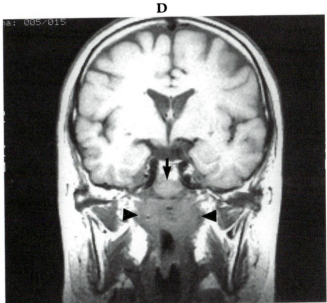

FIGURE 4.10

Nasopharyngeal carcinoma with skull base invasion. (A) Axial CT images of the nasopharynx demonstrate extensive soft tissue thickening of the nasopharyngeal mucosa and obliteration of the normal landmarks (arrowheads). (B) Axial CT image of the lower skull base shows transgression of the pharyngobasilar fascia by tumor with infiltration of the pre-vertebral fascia and invasion of the clivus (arrow). (C) Axial spin-echo MR image (TR = 2000 ms, TE = 20 ms) at the level of the lower nasopharynx shows relative containment of tumor by the lateral walls, without direct invasion of the parapharyngeal spaces. Definition of the posterior wall is less distinct and is suggestive of invasion in the pre-vertebral space (arrow). (D) Coronal spin-echo image (TR = 650 ms, TE = 20 ms) shows the bulky tumor mass of intermediate signal intensity bulging the walls of the nasopharynx laterally (arrowheads) with direct invasion of the clival marrow (arrow).   *continued*

E

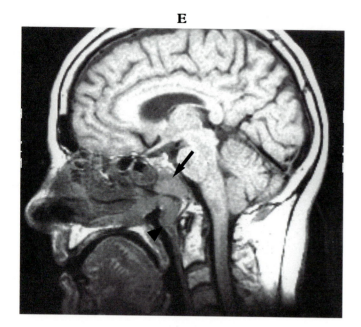

FIGURE 4.10 *(continued)*

(**E**) Sagittal spin-echo MR image (TR = 600 ms, TE = 20 ms) shows both components of the tumor well; the nasopharyngeal mass (arrowhead) and the associated skull base invasion (arrow).

A

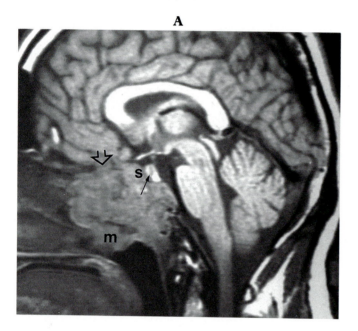

B

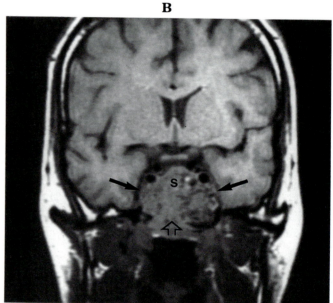

FIGURE 4.11

Nasopharyngeal carcinoma with skull base and cavernous sinus invasion. (**A**) A large lobulated mass is present in the posterior nasal cavity (m) and nasopharynx. This T1-weighted sagittal image (TR = 600 ms, TE = 20 ms) demonstrates the boundaries of this lesion. Tumor has completely replaced the clivus, sphenoid bone and sella turcica (s). The pituitary gland has been displaced posteriorly (arrow). Tumor invasion extends into the anterior cranial fossa (open arrow). Although this tumor is of nasopharyngeal origin, the bulk of tissue is in the nasal cavity and the cranial compartment.

(**B**) Coronal MR image (TR = 800 ms, TE = 25 ms) at the level of the cavernous sinus shows the result of direct invasion by tumor. Note the bulging of the lateral dural margin of the cavernous sinus bilaterally (arrows). There is complete replacement of the cavernous sinus and sella turcica (s) by tumor. Observe the large bony defect in the clivus through which tumor has gained access to the intracranial compartment (open arrow).

continued

C

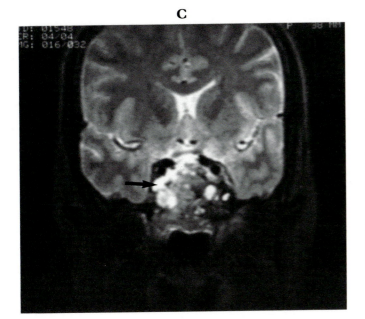

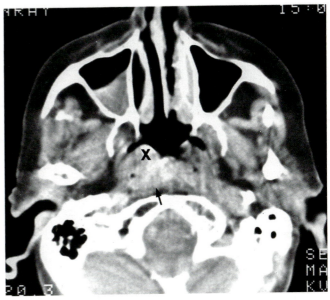

FIGURE 4.11 *(continued)*

(**C**) The tumor is of mixed signal intensity on this coronal T2-weighted MR image (TR = 2000 ms, TE = 80 ms) Tumor which has breached the cavernous sinus on the right is markedly hyperintense relative to the remainder of visualized tumor (arrow).

FIGURE 4.12

Lymphoepithelioma. Axial CT image at mid-nasopharyngeal level shows bulbous enlargement of the right torus tubarius (x) and obliteration of the ipsilateral fossa of Rosenmuller. The mass appears to cross the midline and effaces the pre-vertebral fat planes on the right (arrow) secondary to compression or direct invasion. The parapharyngeal fat is preserved. This lesion cannot be readily distinguished from a carcinoma.

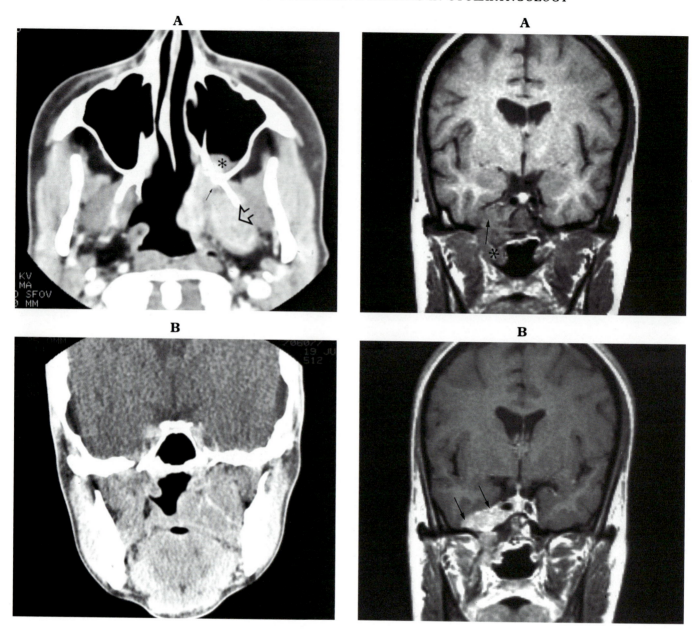

FIGURE 4.13

FIGURE 4.14

Melanoma metastases to nasopharynx and pterygoid musculature. (**A**) Axial CT image at the level of the torus tubarius reveals a lobulated, enhancing soft tissue mass which thickens the mucosa of the left lateral nasopharynx, infiltrates the adjacent fat planes and obliterates the left eustachian tube opening. The enlarged left pterygoid musculature is involved with tumor (open arrow) and there is erosion of the medial pterygoid plate (small arrow). Tissue in the posterior aspect of the left maxillary sinus suggests extension of tumor into this region (*). (**B**) Coronal CT image shows medial displacement of the pharyngobasilar fascia, distortion of the nasopharyngeal airway and collapse of the eustachian tube opening.

Meningiosarcoma simulating a nasopharyngeal malignancy. (**A**) A coronal T1-weighted image (TR = 600 ms, TE = 20 ms) shows thickening of the right torus tubarius (*) and infiltration of the infratemporal fossa with transgression of the skull base (arrow). The cavernous sinus is enlarged on the right and is occupied by tumor. The patient presented with a cavernous sinus syndrome. (**B**) Following infusion of intravenous gadolinium, there is marked enhancement of the tumor. The extent of intracranial involvement (arrows) is much more apparent in the middle cranial

continued

C

E

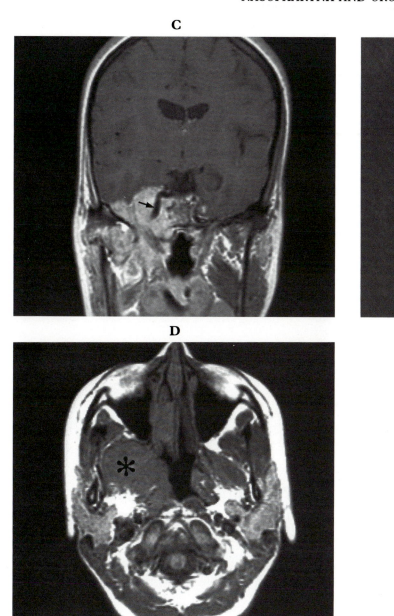

D

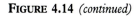

FIGURE 4.14 *(continued)*

fossa. Note that contrast enhancement tends to diminish the conspicuity of tumor extracranially as it blends in with the surrounding fat. Use of fat suppression with gadolinium counteracts this effect. (**C**) 6 weeks later, a repeat MR examination with contrast reveals marked progression in growth of the mass, both intracranially and extracranially. There is circumferential encasement of the cavernous internal carotid artery (arrow). (**D**) The tumor (*) is isointense to muscle on this noncontrast axial T1-weighted image (TR = 700 ms, TE = 20 ms)

obtained below the skull base. The tumor occupies a large portion of the infratemporal fossa and extends into the masticator space. The pterygoid musculature is infiltrated by tumor. (**E**) The mass is hyperintense on a T2-weighted sequence (TR = 2100 ms, TE = 80 ms). Clues to diagnosis in this case include age (25 years), lack of associated risk factors for nasopharyngeal carcinoma, extremely rapid growth and the observation that the bulk of disease initially presented intracranially.

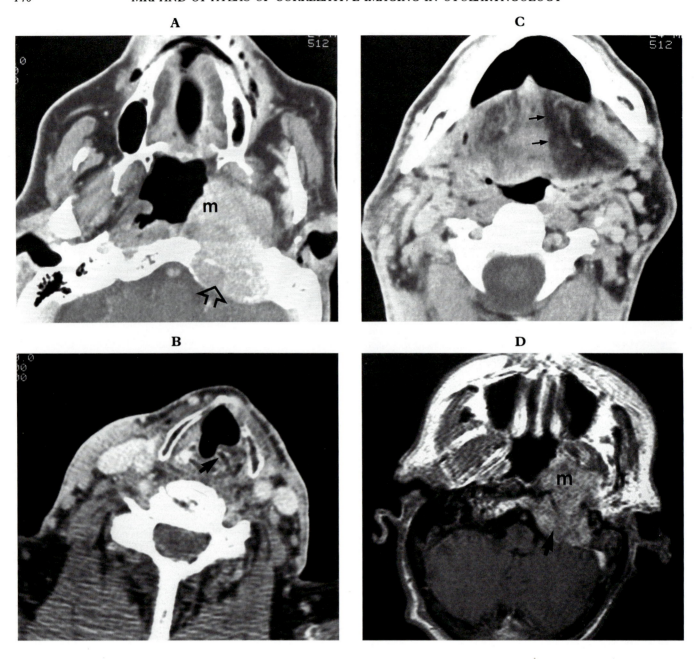

FIGURE 4.15

(A) Amyloidoma simulating a nasopharyngeal carcinoma. (**A**) A 79-year-old male with multiple cranial nerve palsies on the left. There is a large enhancing mass (m) originating in the left nasopharynx extending into the parapharyngeal space with extensive erosion of the temporal bone and occipital condyle (open arrow). (**B**) There is paralysis of the left vocal cord with medial rotation of the arytenoid cartilage (arrow) indicative of dysfunction of cranial nerve X.

(**C**) Denervation atrophy of the left tongue is present with fatty replacement of the intrinsic tongue musculature (arrows) indicative of dysfunction of cranial nerve XII. (**D**) The mass (m) enhances with gadolinium on this T1-weighted axial image (TR = 750 ms, TE = 20 ms). The tumor protrudes into the cerebellar pontine angle cistern (arrow) and contributes to the cranial nerve VII and VIII palsies.

continued

E

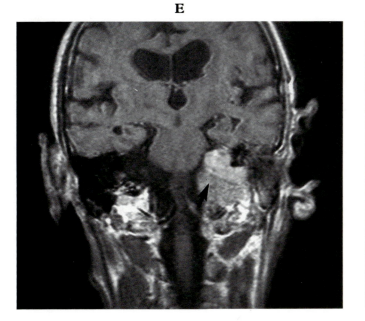

A

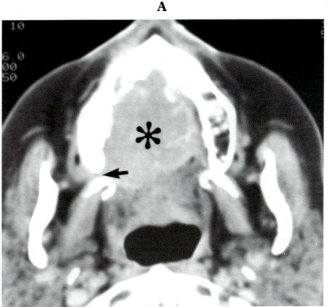

FIGURE 4.15 *(continued)*

(E) The coronal T1-weighted image shows the superior/inferior extent of the lesion to best advantage. Tumor has transgressed the skull base at the level of the jugular foramen (arrow), accounting for many of the cranial nerve deficits.

B

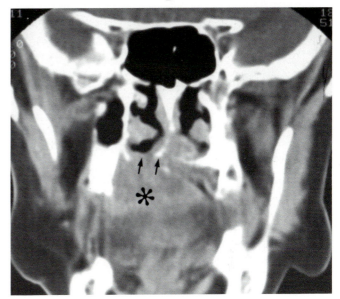

FIGURE 4.16

Adenoid cystic carcinoma of the hard palate. (A) A postcontrast axial CT image at the level of the palate shows an enhancing soft tissue mass which has destroyed the entire hard palate (*). Postero-lateral growth of tumor extends into the pterygoid plate region on the right (arrow). (B) A coronal CT image through the hard palate confirms extensive destruction of this structure with replacement by a tissue mass (*). Tumor has eroded into the nasal cavity on the right (small arrows). While this tumor extends into the posterior nasal cavity, it neither takes origin from nor involves the nasopharyngeal mucosa.

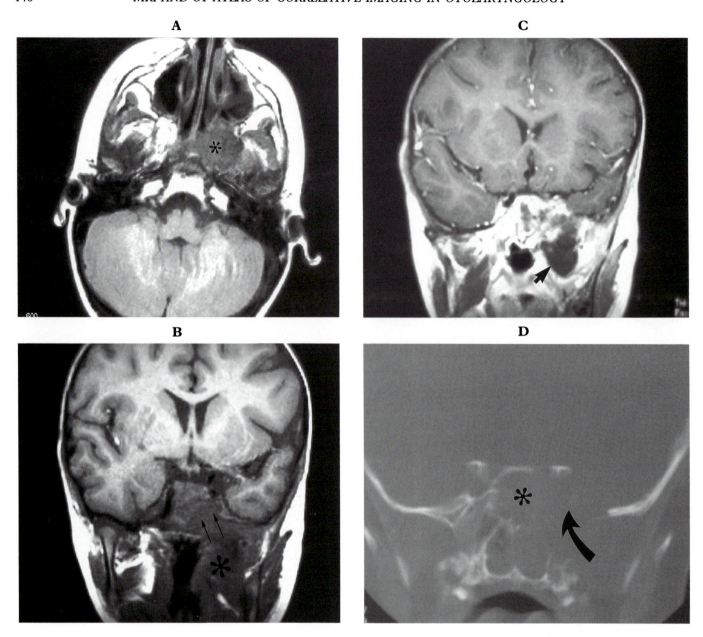

FIGURE 4.17

Nasopharyngeal rhabdomyosarcoma in a 5-year-old female. (**A**) T1-weighted axial image (TR = 600 ms, TE = 15 ms) shows that there is a tissue mass of low signal intensity within the left infratemporal fossa and posterior nasal cavity (*). (**B**) The fat/tissue planes are obliterated in the left parapharyngeal space by this large tumor (*) which has violated the boundaries of the skull base and entered the left cavernous sinus (arrows). (**C**) After infusion of gadolinium-DTPA the majority of the tumor enhances markedly, exhibiting isointensity with the surrounding fat with the exception of an area of central necrosis (arrow). (**D**) The extent of bony destruction of the skull base is most apparent in the coronal CT image. The floor of the middle cranial fossa is destroyed and tumor has direct access to the intracranial compartment (curved arrow). Tumor and/or inspissated secretions fill the sphenoid sinus and nasal cavity (*).

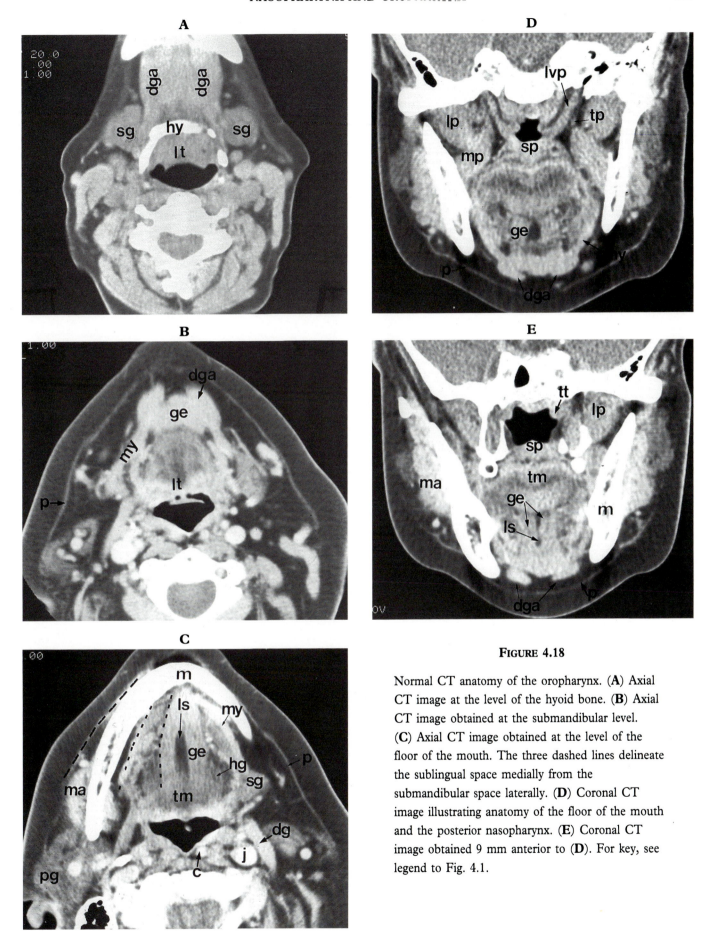

FIGURE 4.18

Normal CT anatomy of the oropharynx. (**A**) Axial CT image at the level of the hyoid bone. (**B**) Axial CT image obtained at the submandibular level. (**C**) Axial CT image obtained at the level of the floor of the mouth. The three dashed lines delineate the sublingual space medially from the submandibular space laterally. (**D**) Coronal CT image illustrating anatomy of the floor of the mouth and the posterior nasopharynx. (**E**) Coronal CT image obtained 9 mm anterior to (**D**). For key, see legend to Fig. 4.1.

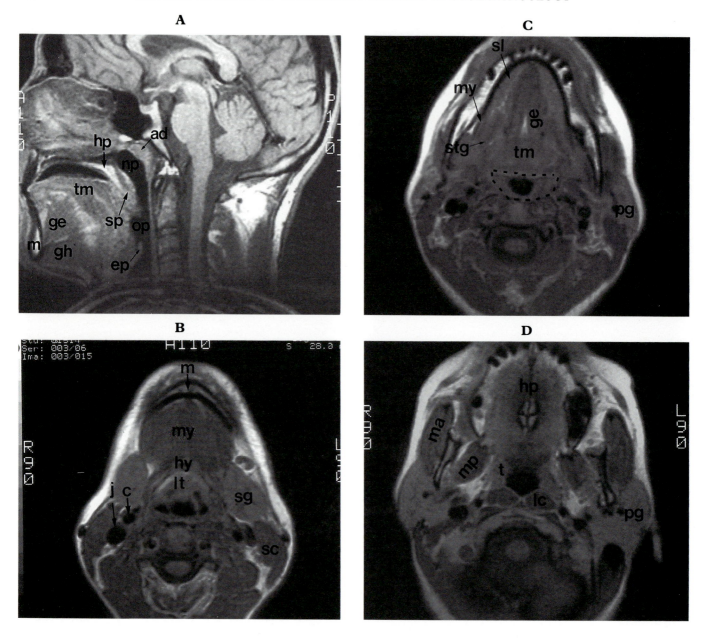

FIGURE 4.19

Normal MRI anatomy of the oropharynx. (**A**) Sagittal T1-weighted MR image (TR = 600 ms, TE = 20 ms) shows the anatomic relationships of the oropharynx to the nasopharynx. (**B**) Axial T1-weighted image (TR = 650 ms, TE = 15 ms) obtained at the level of the mental symphysis.

(**C**) Axial T1-weighted image (TR = 650 ms, TE = 15 ms) obtained at the level of the floor of the mouth. The dotted line demarcates the palatine tonsils. (**D**) Axial T1-weighted image (TR = 650 ms, TE = 15 ms) obtained at the level of the hard palate. For key, see legend to Fig. 4.1.

A

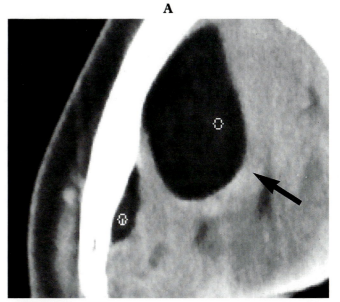

B

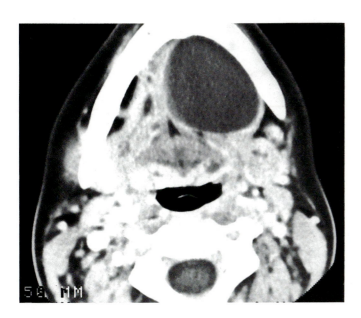

FIGURE 4.20

Dermoid cyst. 15-year-old female with progressive
swelling in the floor of the mouth for approximately
1 year. Contrast enhanced axial CT image of the
floor of the mouth reveals a large cystic mass in the
left sublingual space with the intrinsic musculature
displaced around it. This lesion cannot be
differentiated from a simple ranula.

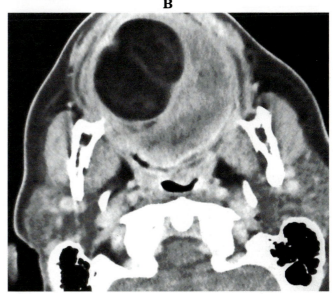

FIGURE 4.21

Lipoma of the tongue. (**A**) A magnified, axial CT
image obtained at the level of the floor of the mouth
reveals a well circumscribed ovoid mass of fat
density, insinuated within the sublingual space. The
mass is displacing the genioglossus muscle (arrow).
(**B**) Axial CT image of the tongue shows the upper
limit of extension of the lipoma which is
incorporated into the intrinsic musculature of the
tongue, resulting in generalized enlargement of that
structure.

A

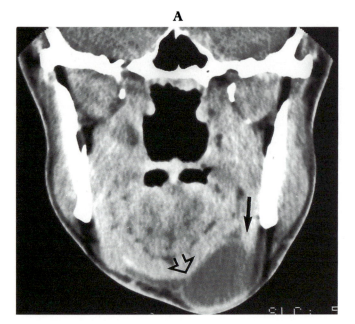

A

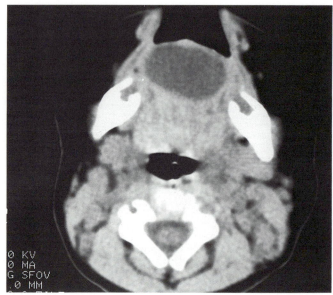

B

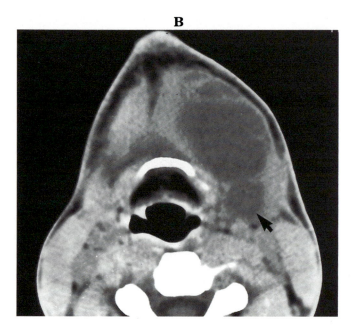

B

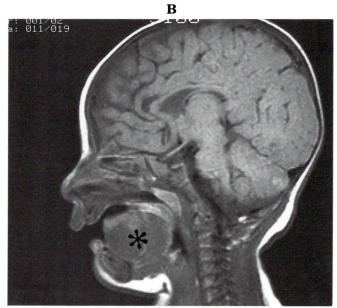

FIGURE 4.22

Simple ranula. (**A**) Coronal CT image shows a well demarcated, oval-shaped mass within the left sublingual space. The mass is homogeneous and of fluid density. Note that the ranula insinuates itself between the mylohyoid muscle laterally (arrow) and the digastric muscle medially (open arrow). (**B**) On an axial CT image, the mass is noted to be multiloculated (arrow) and extends far posteriorly.

FIGURE 4.23

Simple ranula. (**A**) 3-month-old male with a history of sublingual swelling since birth. An axial CT image shows a large and well-defined cystic lesion in the floor of the mouth. (**B**) The sagittal MR image (TR = 800 ms, TE = 20 ms) shows that the mass is relatively low in signal intensity on this T1-weighted sequence (*) and there is poor differentiation from the intrinsic musculature of the tongue and floor of

continued

C

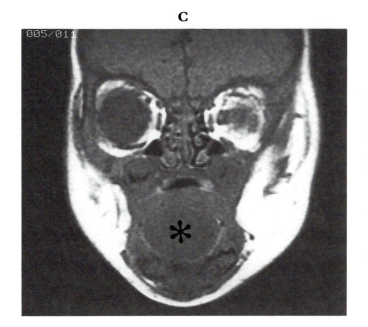

A

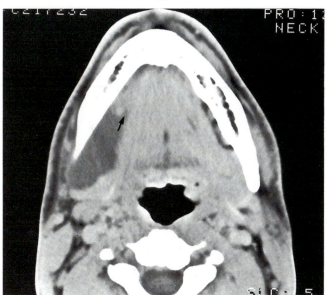

D

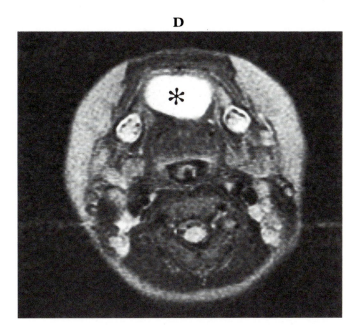

B

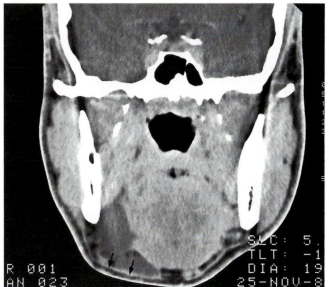

FIGURE 4.23 *(continued)*

the mouth. (**C**) A coronal MR image (TR = 600 ms, TE = 20 ms) also shows that there is poor contrast between the mass (∗) and adjacent tissues with T1 weighting. (**D**) A T2-weighted axial image (TR = 2000 ms, TE = 80 ms) confirms the cystic character of this lesion which is homogeneously hyperintense (∗).

FIGURE 4.24

Plunging ranula. (**A**) Axial CT image with contrast reveals a low attenuation (cystic) lesion in the right submandibular space. It has dissected postero-inferiorly around a slip of mylohyoid muscle (small arrow). (**B**) Coronal CT image with contrast confirms the submandibular location of the lesion. Note that the ranula abuts the platysma muscle (arrows).

A

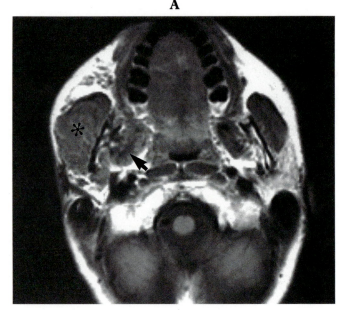

C

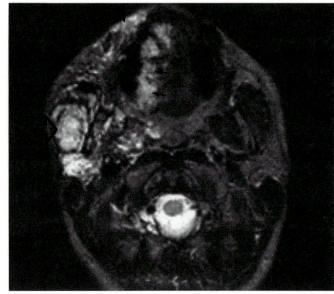

B

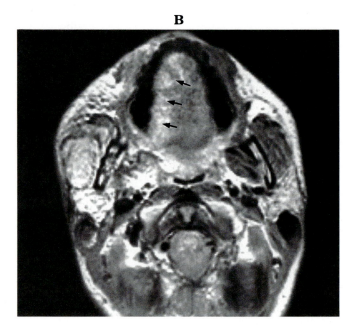

FIGURE 4.25

Hemangioma of oral cavity and face. (**A**) There is enlargement of the masseter muscle (∗) on the right as shown on this axial T1-weighted MR image (TR = 600 ms, TE = 20 ms). There is also some asymmetry of the ipsilateral pterygoid muscles (arrow). (**B**) The areas of abnormality convert to high signal intensity on the proton-density image (TR = 2000 ms, TE = 20 ms). Also note the signal abnormality adjacent to the superior alveolar ridge on the right (arrows). (**C**) Hyperintensity of tumor persists on the T2-weighted image (TR = 2000 ms, TE = 80 ms). This hemangioma is rather extensive, involving the tissues of the lip (arrowhead), the oral mucosa adjacent to the hard palate (arrows), as well as the muscles of mastication (open arrow).

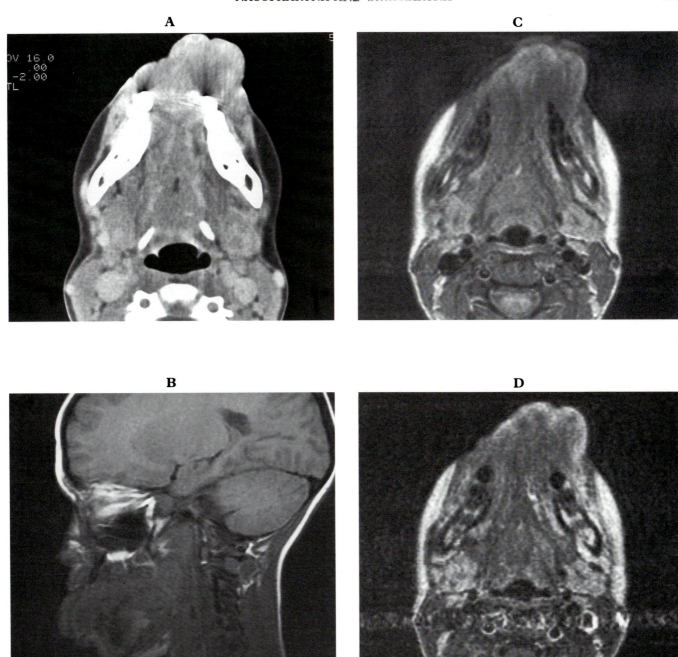

FIGURE 4.26

Lymphangioma of the tongue in a 9-year-old female. (**A**) A lobulated soft tissue mass protrudes from the oral cavity on this axial CT image taken at the level of the floor of the mouth. (**B**) T1-weighted sagittal MR image shows the mass to be isointense with the tissues of the tongue. (**C**) The mass is relatively homogeneous in appearance and has no cystic characteristics on this axial spin-echo MR image (TR = 2400 ms, TE = 20 ms). (**D**) Axial T1-weighted image with gadolinium (TR = 700 ms, TE = 20 ms) reveals minimal enhancement of the mass. The neoplasm cannot be readily differentiated from the tongue or the muscles of the floor of the mouth. The imaging characteristics of this tumor are non-specific.

A

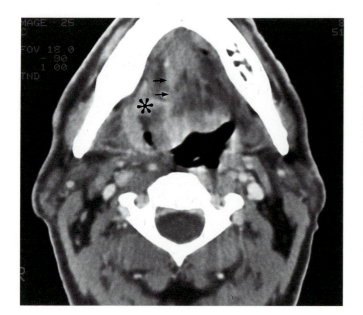
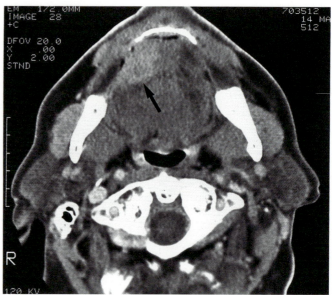

FIGURE 4.27

Squamous cell carcinoma of the tongue. Axial CT image reveals an enhancing, ulcerated mass (*) in the right sublingual space deviating the genioglossus muscle (arrows).

B

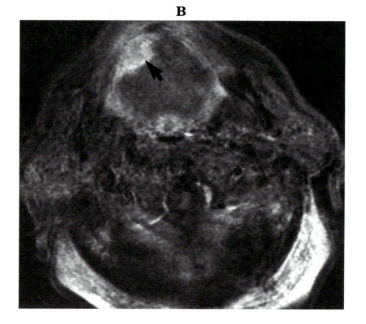

FIGURE 4.28

Carcinoma of the tongue. (**A**) Axial CT image of the oral cavity reveals an enhancing mass originating in the right anterior aspect of the tongue (arrow). (**B**) Gadolinium enhancement of this tumor (arrow) is intensified by the use of fat suppression in this T1-weighted axial image (TR = 900 ms, TE = 20 ms).

A

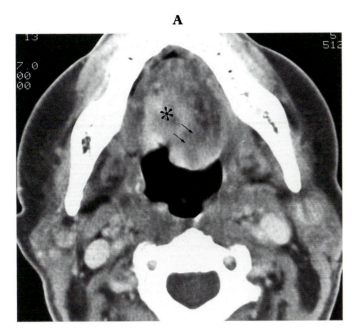

C

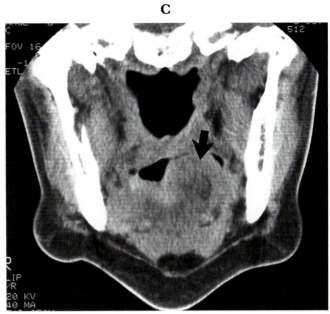

B

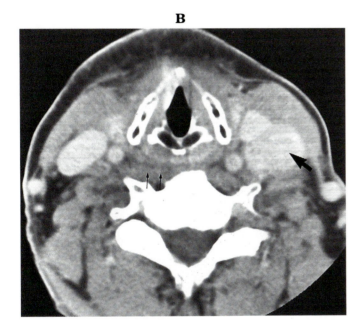

FIGURE 4.29

Squamous cell carcinoma of the tongue. (**A**) Axial CT image shows an inhomogeneous mass (*) protruding from the posterior aspect of the tongue on the left (arrows). (**B**) Lymphadenopathy of the left midjugular chain is demonstrated (arrow). There is infiltration of the retrolaryngeal space (small arrows) and reticulation of the subcutaneous soft tissues secondary to radiation changes. (**C**) The coronal CT image shows the superior exophytic component of the mass (arrow). Note that there is poor delineation of tissue planes between the mass and the intrinsic muscles of the tongue.

A   C

B   D

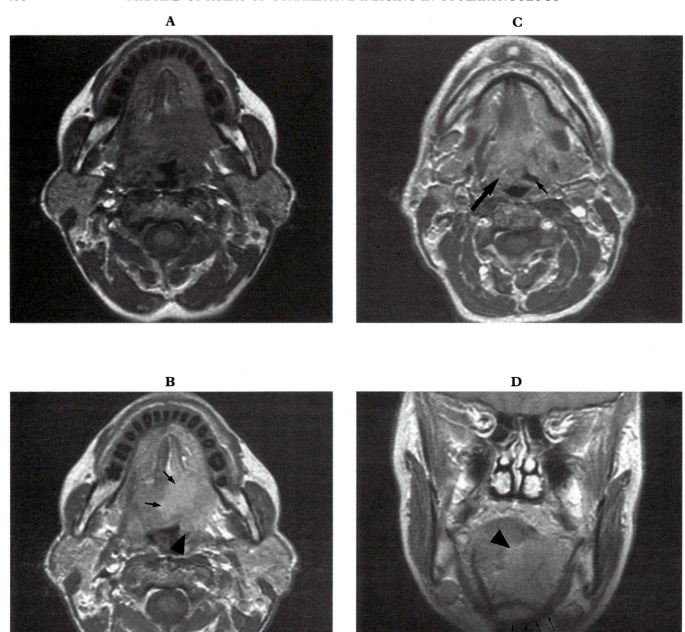

FIGURE 4.30

Squamous cell carcinoma of the tongue. (**A**) Axial
MR image (TR = 800 ms, TE = 30 ms) of the
oropharynx reveals a soft tissue mass on the left
which is isointense with the adjacent musculature.
(**B**) Following administration of intravenous
gadolinium-DTPA, there is uniform enhancement of
the tumor (arrows), allowing for better definition of
the tumor. Also note that the tumor bulges partially
into the oral cavity (arrowhead).

(**C**) A contrast-enhanced T1-weighted image (TR =
800 ms, TE = 30 ms) obtained several centimeters
caudal to figure (**B**), at the level of the hypopharynx
demonstrates extension of tumor postero-inferior to
the right with effacement of the right valleculae
(arrow) compared to normal valleculae on left (small
arrow). (**D**) A contrast-enhanced T1-weighted image
(TR = 800 ms, TE = 30 ms) in the coronal plane also
demonstrates the enhancing tumor in the left tongue
base (arrowhead). Note that tumor is contained by the
mylohyoid sling (small arrows).   *continued*

E

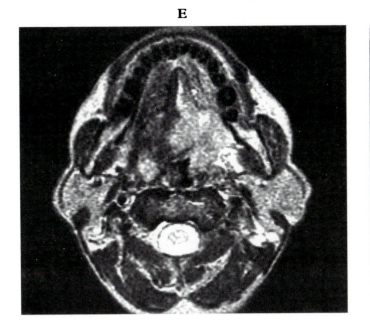

G

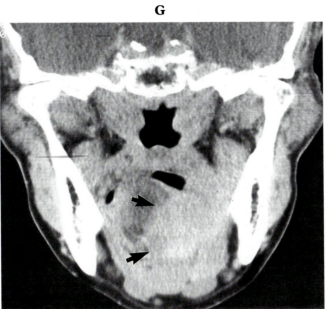

F

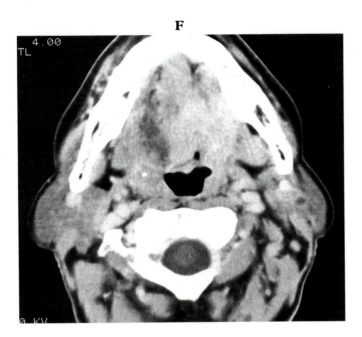

FIGURE 4.30 *(continued)*

(**E**) T2-weighted spin-echo axial image (TR = 2000 ms, TE = 80 ms) demonstrates well the hyperintense tumor contrasted against the hypointense musculature. (**F**) The tumor is well outlined on a contrast enhanced axial CT image. (**G**) Coronal CT image of the carcinoma of the left tongue (arrows).

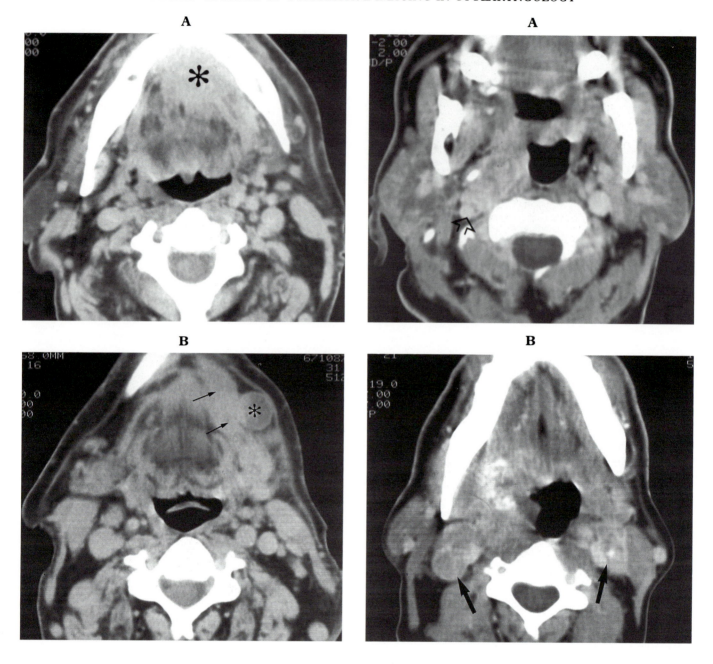

FIGURE 4.31

FIGURE 4.32

Squamous cell carcinoma of floor of the mouth. (**A**) A contrast-enhanced axial CT image demonstrates a homogeneously enhancing mass in the floor of the mouth anteriorly, extending both to the left and right of midline (∗). The mass reaches the inferior alveolar margin and most likely is within the submandibular space. (**B**) An axial CT image obtained approximately 20 mm caudal to (**A**) reveals a large, necrotic, submandibular lymph node (∗) and presumed infiltration of the mylohyoid muscle by tumor (arrows).

Squamous cell carcinoma of the oropharynx. (**A**) A contrast-enhanced axial CT image shows an enhancing lobulated soft tissue mass originating in the right oropharynx with extension into the tonsillar fossa and right carotid space (open arrow). (**B**) Axial CT image 25 mm below (**A**) reveals extensive lymphadenopathy in the deep jugular chains with bilateral necrotic nodes (arrows).

A

B

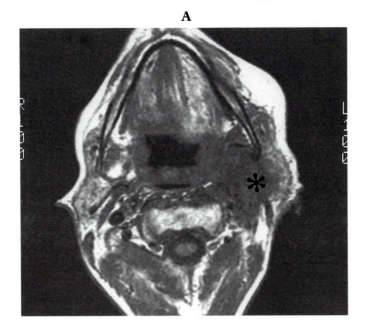
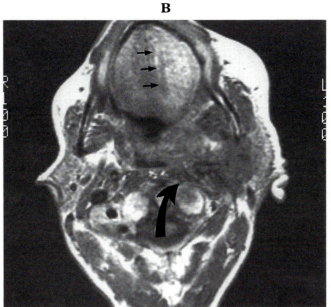

FIGURE 4.33

Oropharyngeal carcinoma with invasion of multiple compartments. 69-year-old male with a peripheral seventh nerve palsy on the left. (**A**) Axial T1-weighted MR image (TR = 600 ms, TE = 20 ms) shows a large mass of low signal intensity in the left parapharyngeal space with extension into the left parotid gland (*). The tumor also infiltrates the left carotid space, the retrostyloid region, the pre- vertebral area and anteriorly to the tongue base. (**B**) Axial T1-weighted MR image through the tongue (TR = 600 ms, TE = 20 ms) reveals denervation atrophy with fatty replacement of the intrinsic tongue muscles on the left side (small arrows), presumably secondary to direct invasion of the left hypoglossal nerve. Also note that tumor reaches the pre-vertebral space on the left (curved arrow).

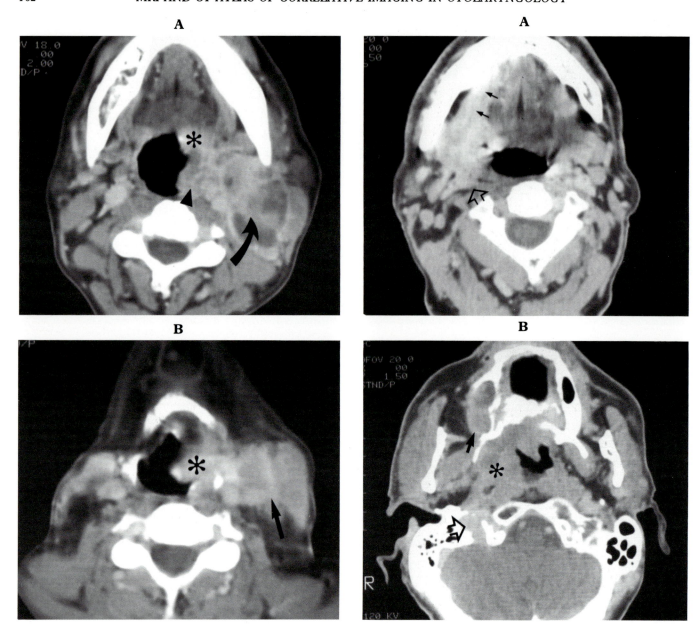

FIGURE 4.34

Tonsillar carcinoma in a 51-year-old female. (**A**) A large exophytic mass is present in the left tonsillar fossa (arrowhead) on this contrast-enhanced axial CT scan. It extends anteriorly to involve the floor of the mouth and lingual tonsils (*). Extensive lymphadenopathy is also present with multiple necrotic lymph nodes in the deep jugular chain (curved arrow). (**B**) Another image obtained at the level of the hyoid bone shows that the tumor extends inferiorly to involve the epiglottis, left aryepiglottic fold and the left false cord (*). Lymphadenopathy persists at this level as well (arrow).

FIGURE 4.35

Tonsillar carcinoma with skull base invasion. (**A**) An enhancing tissue mass occupies the right tonsillar fossa (open arrow) and extends anteriorly in the submandibular space producing thickening, infiltration and enhancement of the mylohyoid muscle (small arrows). (**B**) Another CT image taken at the level of the skull base shows the tumor has infiltrated and thickened the pharyngeal musculature on the right (*) with encroachment on the parapharyngeal space and obliteration of tissue planes around the pterygoid musculature. The right maxillary sinus is opacified, presumably from direct invasion by tumor (arrow). Tumor also extends posteriorly to abut and erode the skull base (open arrow).

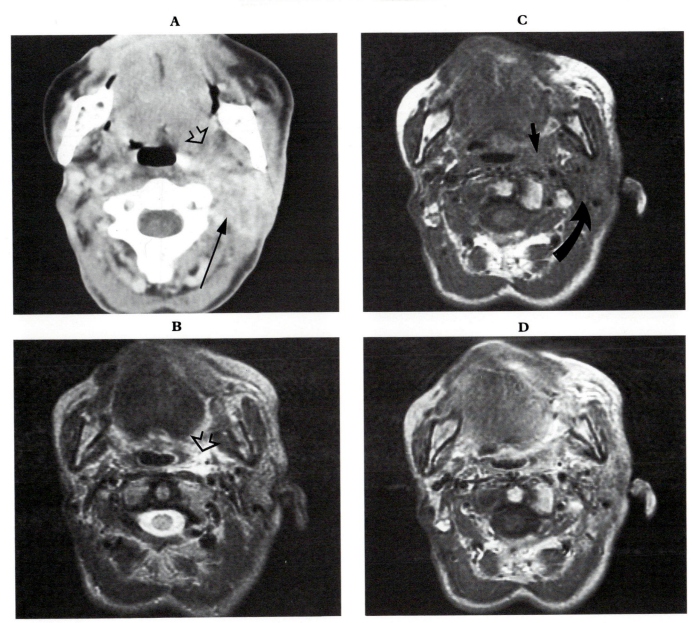

FIGURE 4.36

Carcinoma of the left tonsillar fossa. (**A**) A postcontrast axial CT image shows an irregularly enhancing mass in the region of the left tonsillar fossa with extension into the parapharyngeal space (open arrow). Note the loss of definition of the fat/fascial planes and the extensive adenopathy in the left posterior triangle (long arrow). (**B**) Axial MR image (TR = 2000 ms, TE = 80 ms) shows the hyperintense tumor from the tonsillar fossa obliterating the parapharyngeal space (open arrow). (**C**) The axial T1-weighted MR image (TR = 800 ms, TE = 20 ms) best defines the tissue planes with the isointense tumor contrasted against the hyperintense parapharyngeal fat (short arrow). The associated lymphadenopathy in the left posterior triangle (curved arrow) is also isointense with muscle. (**D**) The enhancement of tumor on the postcontrast axial MR image (TR = 800 ms, TE = 20 ms) actually results in diminished conspicuity of the lesion due to reduction of contrast between the tumor and the adjacent hyperintense fat. Fat-suppression techniques can be used to improve definition of the enhancing tumor.

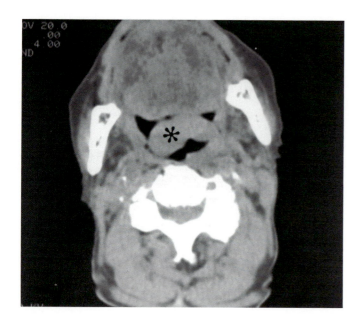

FIGURE 4.37

Lymphoma of soft palate. 79-year-old female with history of extranodal lymphoma and dysphagia. A noncontrast axial CT image demonstrates marked thickening of the soft palate (∗) secondary to infiltration by lymphoma.

A

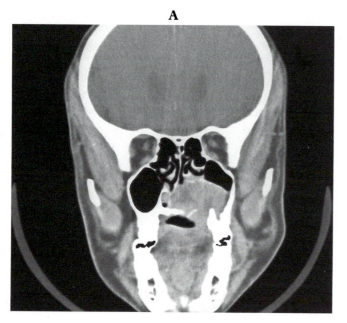

B

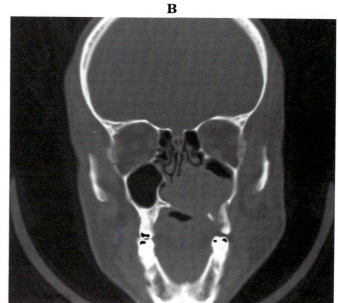

FIGURE 4.38

Adenoid cystic carcinoma of the hard palate. (**A**) Coronal CT image demonstrates a large soft tissue mass extending into the left maxillary sinus and nasal cavity associated with destruction of the hard palate and erosion of the turbinates and medial wall of the maxillary sinus. (**B**) Bone window coronal CT image immediately anterior to (**A**) shows the extensive destruction of the hard palate.

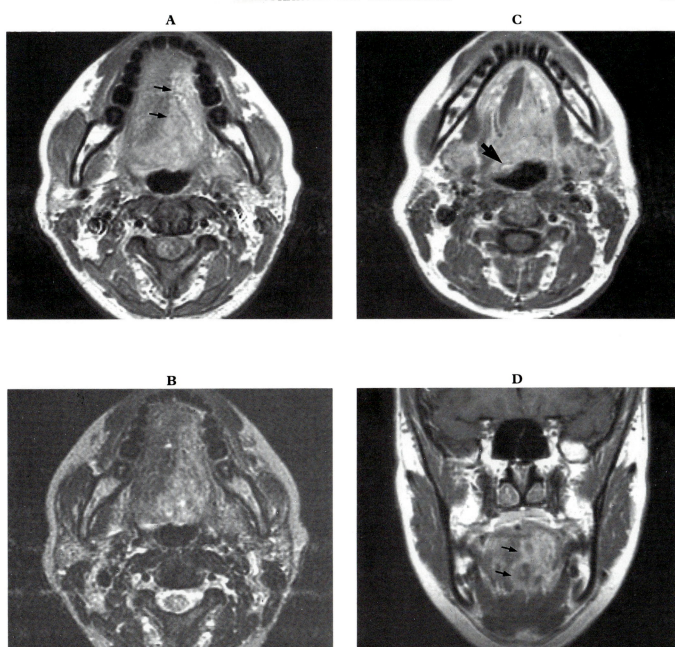

FIGURE 4.39

Adenoid cystic carcinoma of the tongue. (**A**) Axial proton-density MR image of the tongue (TR = 2400 ms, TE = 20 ms) shows an infiltrating hyperintense mass occupying the entire left side of the tongue as well as the tongue base (arrows). (**B**) T2-weighted image (TR = 2400 ms, TE = 80 ms) at the same location as (**A**). (**C**) Contrast-enhanced axial T1-weighted image (TR = 800 ms, TE = 20 ms) at the level of the tongue base shows invasion of tumor into the sublingual space and extension beyond the right of midline with encroachment on the right valleculae (arrow). (**D**) Contrast-enhanced coronal T1-weighted image (TR = 650 ms, TE = 20 ms) shows the local extent of the enhancing tumor (arrows) in the left aspect of the tongue. Note that the mylohyoid muscle is not involved with tumor.

A

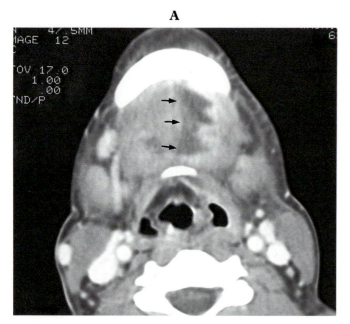

A

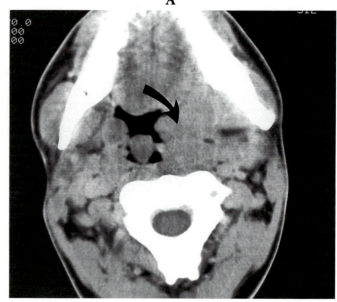

B

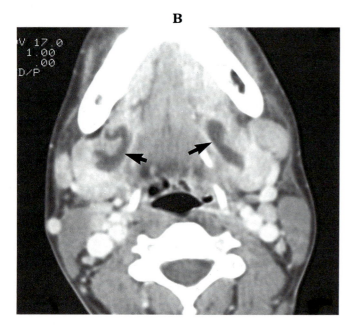

B

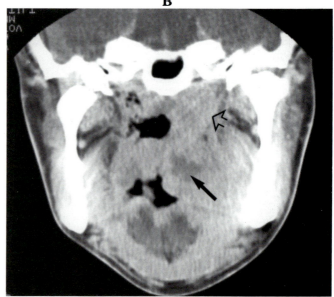

FIGURE 4.40

Submandibular abscess following removal of left third molar. (**A**) Postcontrast axial CT image at the level of the mental symphysis shows a poorly demarcated, low attenuation mass with peripheral enhancement located in the left submandibular space (arrows). Note the reticulation of the subcutaneous fat secondary to edema. (**B**) Axial image obtained at the level of the submandibular glands shows marked dilatation of Wharton's duct bilaterally (arrows).

FIGURE 4.41

Left tonsillar fossa abscess. (**A**) Postcontrast axial CT image at the level of the tonsillar pillars shows an irregularly shaped mass which protrudes into the oropharynx (curved arrow) and obscures the fascial planes of the adjacent parapharyngeal space. (**B**) A coronal CT image obtained in the middle of the mass reveals a central area of necrosis (arrow). Also note that the inflammatory process shows significant extension towards the nasopharynx (open arrow).

CHAPTER 5

INFRAHYOID NECK AND LARYNGOPHARYNX

Introduction

Advances in imaging technology during the past decade have made a dramatic impact on the detection, diagnosis and management of neck lesions. Ultrasound (US), computed tomography (CT) and magnetic resonance imaging (MRI) permit accurate localization of masses, delineate extent of lesions, and allow differentiation of solid and cystic masses. Accuracy of nodal pathology as demonstrated by CT has made a significant impact on the staging of malignant tumors.

This chapter is divided into four sections: (1) soft tissues of the neck; (2) cervical nodes; (3) larynx and hypopharynx, and (4) thyroid and parathyroid glands.

Each section briefly reviews the anatomy, addresses the imaging strategies and discusses the associated pathology.

Soft tissues of the neck

Normal anatomy

The gross anatomical neck spans from the mandible inferiorly. Using the hyoid bone as a landmark, this can be further divided into suprahyoid and infrahyoid subgroups. This chapter will focus on the infrahyoid neck.

Traditionally, the neck has been divided into anterior and posterior triangles using the sterno-cleidomastoid muscle as a dividing landmark. The anterior triangle is further subdivided into sub-mental and submandibular triangles in the suprahyoid region and the carotid and muscular triangles in the infrahyoid region (Fig. 5.1). The posterior triangle is divided into the occipital and the sub-clavian triangles.[1]

More recently, the radiologic literature has emphasized division of the neck by fascial spaces created by the three layers of the deep cervical fascia.[2,3] These include (a) the superficial (investing) layer, (b) the middle (visceral) layer and (c) the deep (pre-vertebral) layer.[4] Such an anatomic approach is better suited for cross-sectional imaging by CT and MR and facilitates an understanding of the spread of disease.

The superficial or investing layer envelopes the entire extracranial head and neck region and extends from the skull base to the clavicles. In the suprahyoid neck it defines the parotid space, masticator space, and submandibular space. Further description and discussion of these spaces are covered elsewhere in this book.

The middle or the visceral fascia extends from the central skull base to the mediastinum and encircles the aerodigestive tract. The deep or pre-vertebral layer surrounds the vertebral column, paravertebral muscles, scalene muscles, vertebral artery and vein, trunks of the branchial plexus, and the phrenic nerve. The anterior margin of the deep fascia splits into the alar layer and the pre-vertebral layer. The alar fascia contributes to the carotid sheath and also forms the lateral aspect of the retropharyngeal space. Superiorly, the pre-vertebral layer attaches to the skull base and inferiorly it continues down to the coccyx.

These fascial planes define the following spaces in the infrahyoid neck (Fig. 5.2). When the origin or center of a lesion can be assigned a space, the differential diagnosis can be further narrowed.

Visceral space

The visceral space, circumscribed by the middle layer of the deep cervical fascia, contains the thyroid gland, parathyroid glands, larynx, trachea, esophagus, recurrent laryngeal nerve and lymph nodes.

Carotid space

The carotid sheath is formed by all three layers of the deep cervical fascia and encloses the carotid space surrounding the carotid artery and jugular vein.[5] This carotid space in the suprahyoid neck is also referred to as the poststyloid space or posterior parapharyngeal space. Other contents of this space include a portion of the glossopharyngeal, spinal accessory and hypoglossal nerves. The cervical sympathetic trunk lies posterior and medial to the vessels and is often embedded within the fascia of the carotid sheath.

Posterior cervical space

The posterior cervical space is a fat-filled space located behind the carotid space. This space lies between the layers of deep cervical fascia and corresponds to the posterior triangle of the neck. It is consistently visualized as a fatty space which contains spinal accessory and dorsal scapular nerves, the spinal accessory chain of lymph nodes, and the preaxillary branchial plexus.

Retropharyngeal space

As the name indicates, the retropharyngeal space is located behind the pharynx, bordered in front by the visceral fascia and posteriorly by the deep fascia and its alar layer. It contains fat and retropharyngeal nodes at the suprahyoid level only. This space spans from the skull base to the third thoracic vertebral body. The potential danger space lies between the retropharyngeal space and the pre-vertebral space. This space extends down to the diaphragm, beyond the retropharyngeal space and provides a conduit for spread of disease. From an imaging point of view, however, the danger space cannot be differentiated from the retropharyngeal space.

Pre-vertebral space

The pre-vertebral space is enclosed by the deep layer of the deep cervical fascia. It contains the pre-vertebral muscles, longus colli muscle, scalene muscles, proximal portion of the brachial plexus, phrenic nerve, vertebral artery and vein, vertebrae up to T3 and paraspinal muscles down to the coccyx.

Imaging strategies

Computed tomography

Axial computed tomographic sections are performed in the supine position with the patient's chin slightly extended. Individual 4–5 mm thick contiguous sections are obtained parallel to the hyoid bone, extending from the angle of mandible to the clavicles (Fig. 5.3). Routine scanning is performed during quiet breathing. All examinations of the neck are obtained with administration of intravenous contrast medium. A bolus of 50 ml of 60% iodinated contrast medium is administered, followed by rapid drip infusion of 300 ml of 30% iodinated contrast medium.

Magnetic resonance imaging

With the rapid advancements in technology, MRI has shown great promise in the imaging of neck lesions. Surface coils are used as the receiver coils to increase the signal-to-noise ratio. As a rule, 5 mm-thick sections with 1 mm gap are sufficient. T1-weighted images are obtained utilizing a repetition time (TR) of 600–800 ms and echo time (TE) of 12–25 ms with a 256 × 192 acquisition matrix (Fig. 5.4). T2-weighted images utilize a TR of 2000–3000 ms with a TE of 20 ms for proton density and second echo of 80–100 ms for T2-weighted images. Additional images may be obtained following intravenous administration of gadolinium-DTPA. Postcontrast T1-weighted images may be obtained with fat suppression.

Pathology

Congenital lesions

Thyroglossal duct cyst

Thyroglossal duct cysts arise as a result of failure of a portion of the thyroglossal duct to involute. The duct originates at the foramen cecum and defines the path of extension of the thyroid gland down to its normal expected position in the lower neck. The duct descends through the tongue musculature, floor of the mouth and loops around the inferior margin of the hyoid bone followed by a slight turn upwards, either up through the hyoid bone itself or into the thin cavity along its posterior surface and finally ends at the level of the thyroid isthmus.[6,7] The thyroglossal duct cysts are classified into suprahyoid (20%), hyoid (15%) and infrahyoid (65%). The majority of the thyroglossal duct cysts occur in the midline, although a small number can be seen laterally. Fistulas are uncommon, but can occur secondary to infection, ruptured cyst or a postoperative complication. Coexisting carcinoma in a thyroglossal duct cyst is extremely rare. The reported incidence of ectopic thyroid tissue along the thyroglossal duct varies from 1% to 30%.[6]

Computed tomography reveals a low density mass with thin peripheral rim which may show enhancement with contrast. The mass is typically in the midline and embedded within the strap muscles adjacent to the thyroid cartilage. By MRI, these lesions show a low to intermediate signal intensity on T1-weighted images and intermediate to high signal intensity on T2-weighted images (Fig. 5.5).

Branchial cleft cysts

During embryogenesis the neck and facial structures develop from the branchial apparatus which includes the first several branchial arches, their interposed ectodermal clefts, primitive foregut and the corresponding endodermal pouches.

Most branchial cleft anomalies arise from the second branchial cleft apparatus. These anomalies include development of cysts, sinuses or fistulae.[8,9] The second branchial arch grows over the second, third and fourth branchial clefts and merges with the lateral branchial wall, thereby forming an ectoderm-lined cavity, the cervical sinus. It is believed that incomplete involution of the cervical sinus is responsible for the development of branchial cleft anomalies.[10]

The branchial cleft cysts most commonly present clinically in the second and third decades. Cysts are more common than sinuses and fistulae. The second or type II branchial cleft cysts are located most commonly anterior to the sternocleidomastoid muscle at the angle of the mandible, and wedged between the submandibular space and the carotid space (Fig. 5.6).[11] Less frequently, these masses can occur anywhere along the anterior border of sterno-cleidomastoid muscle. The classic second branchial cleft cyst extends beyond the internal and external carotid arteries.[11] The tract can usually be traced superiorly extending into the region of the posterior tonsillar pillar. When these lesions get large, they can extend into the posterior cervical space.

First branchial cleft abnormalities account for less than 10% of all branchial cleft anomalies. These masses generally occur near the external canal and parotid gland. Associated anomalies of the ear may exist. Persistent pre-aural discharge without middle ear disease or recurrent parotid abscesses should raise suspicion of the first branchial cleft anomalies.

Third and fourth branchial cleft anomalies are rare.

Computed tomography reveals well-defined low density masses which do not enhance. The thin surrounding rim may reveal slight enhancement (Figs 5.6 and 5.7). If the lesion is complicated by hemorrhage or infection, the density of the content may increase. Thickening and irregularity of the margins and reticulation of the surrounding fat indicate associated infection (Figs 5.8 and 5.9).

Magnetic resonance imaging reveals low to intermediate signal intensity on T1-weighted images and high signal intensity on T2-weighted images (Fig. 5.6). Rim enhancement occurs with gadolinium administration.

Cystic hygroma

Cystic hygromas are comprised of multiple dilated lymphatic channels that vary from a few millimeters to several centimeters in diameter, lined by a single layer of flattened endothelium. These masses develop from sequestered portions of primitive lymph sacs during embryogenesis.

Cystic hygromas are often detected at birth. Although most are clinically manifested during the first few years of life, they have been reported in adults. Cystic hygromas most commonly occur in the posterior cervical space. These masses can be rather large and extend superiorly into the cheek, inferiorly into the mediastinum, and laterally into the axilla. Anteriorly, they may occur in the floor of the mouth and submandibular space. Cystic hygroma, cavernous lymphangioma and lymphangioma simplex are part of the same spectrum.

Antenatal diagnosis by ultrasound may be made.[12] Ultrasound reveals a septated mass with anechoic collections. Hemorrhage into the cysts may increase the echogenicity. The margins of the mass are better defined by CT or MRI.

Computed tomography reveals a low density mass, which is often septated.[13,14] Magnetic resonance imaging demonstrates low signal or intermediate signal on T1-weighted images and high signal on T2-weighted images. Presence of hemorrhage can provide variable signals depending on the age of the hemorrhagic products (Fig. 5.10).[15]

Dermoid cysts, epidermoid cysts and teratoid cysts

Dermoid cysts, teratoid cysts and epidermal cysts are all congenital anomalies which involve pluri potent embryonal cells.[10] A dermoid cyst is lined by epithelium and contains ectodermal and mesodermal elements. A teratoid cyst or teratoma is comprised of all three germ layers. It is epithelial lined with a fibrous capsule and contains skin appendages and connective tissue derivatives. An epidermal cyst is lined with epithelium, has a fibrous capsule but does not contain skin appendages. Dermoid or epidermoid cysts occur in the midline at the floor of the mouth. Computed tomography reveals a well-circumscribed, low density, nonenhancing mass. Detection of lipid usually confirms the diagnosis.[16] Magnetic resonance imaging demonstrates low to intermediate signal intensity on the T1-weighted images, or high signal intensity if there is a lipid component. The signal intensity is intermediate or high on T2-weighted images.

Hemangioma

Whether hemangiomas are true tumors or represent vascular malformations has been debated in the literature. In any case, these are classified according to histologic appearance into capillary, cavernous and mixed, or proliferative types. Hemangiomas of the face are primarily capillary and cavernous. Hemangiomas occurring in the deep fascial planes and muscles are often poorly circumscribed and infiltrative. These are so-called 'invasive' hemangiomas and are fairly characteristic of intramuscular lesions.

Computed tomography reveals the mass to be isodense with muscle demonstrating miminal to no

enhancement. Phleboliths, if present, can aid in the diagnosis. Hemangiomas are seen as echogenic masses by ultrasound.[17] Magnetic resonance imaging is superior in delineating the extent of the hemangiomas because of better soft tissue contrast compared to CT.[18] Hemangiomas reveal low signal intensity on T1-weighted images and very high signal intensity on T2-weighted images (Fig. 5.11). Signal void channels representing vessels may be seen in capillary hemangiomas.

Inflammatory lesions

Computed tomography, and more recently magnetic resonance imaging provide a valuable means of evaluating cervical infections, the extent of such infections usually being difficult to determine clinically. Computed tomography is particularly useful in differentiating cellulitis from abscess. Soft tissue swelling with streaking of subcutaneous fat and loss of fat planes indicates cellulitis; the presence of well-defined or ill-defined collections of low attenuation within soft tissue indicates abscess formation (Figs 5.12 and 5.13). Complications of cervical infections, which include airway encroachment, osteomyelitis, and intracranial or orbital extension, are also easily assessed with cross-sectional imaging (CT and MRI).

Infection of the neck, particularly in the deep neck spaces, can be potentially life threatening. Sources of infection include extension from suppurative adenitis secondary to dental disease, salivary gland infections, pharyngeal and tonsillar infections, intravenous drug abuse, hematogenous spread from infective endocarditis, and direct extension from osteomyelitis. The deep neck infections may be dominant in one fascial compartment with extension to other compartments, depending on the source of infection.[19] Knowledge of fascial anatomy as discussed at the beginning is essential in analyzing the extent of pathology.[19,20] Skin and fascial thickening with linear streaking of subcutaneous fat similar to cellulitis may also be seen in irradiated necks.

Vascular lesions

Asymmetry of the internal jugular veins is more a rule than the exception. Usually the right internal jugular vein is larger than the left and should not be mistaken for an enhancing mass. An ectatic common carotid artery, especially near the bifurcation, may mimic carotid body tumor. Venous thrombosis in the neck occurs as a complication of intravenous catheterization and drug abuse. Computed tomography reveals central lucency surrounded by contrast-enhanced blood. The blood vessel wall may enhance as a result of flow through the vasa vasorum. In the presence of thrombophlebitis, abnormal density in the adjacent soft tissues may be seen (Figs 5.14 and 5.15).

Venous thrombosis can be easily diagnosed by ultrasound and MRI in addition to CT.[21–23] Ultrasound reveals the thrombosed vessel to be enlarged with internal echoes. Real-time scanning reveals lack of compressibility and absence of venous pulsations. Doppler ultrasound is useful in cases of acute thrombosis where the clot may be soft and less echogenic.

Magnetic resonance imaging has great potential in vascular imaging. The blood flow can be imaged as 'black blood' (signal void) or 'white blood' (high signal), depending on the pulse sequences utilized. Thrombus, slow flow and flow-related enhancement, all showing high signal in the vessel, can be distinguished by using gradient-echo imaging or using phase shift properties of the signal.[24]

Neoplasms

In this section, only non-nodal acquired lesions are addressed.

Neural tumors

The most common tumor of neural origin is the schwannoma, which arises from the nerve sheath of the peripheral nerves or sympathetic chain.[25] Schwannomas are usually solitary masses and can occur at any age. Multiple schwannomas may occur in patients with vonRecklinghausen's disease. By histopathology, schwannomas reveal a cellular component and a myxoid component; neurofibromas show swirls of neuronal elements.[10] Only about 10% of patients with neurofibromas have vonRecklinghausen's disease. Computed tomography reveals the neural tumors to be of variable density, but low density is more characteristic. These tumors may be homogeneous or inhomogeneous. Contrast enhancement is also variable.[26] Neuromas can enhance intensely, mimicking paragangliomas. Neural tumors

are hypointense or isointense to muscle on the MRI T1-weighted images and hyperintense on T2-weighted images (Fig. 5.16). Signal void areas are not seen with neural tumors on MRI. Angiography reveals these tumors to be hypovascular.

Paragangliomas

The most common paraganglioma seen in the neck is the carotid body tumor.[27] The glomus vagale arises along the nodose ganglion of the vagus nerve in the parapharyngeal space and can extend inferiorly into the neck.

Carotid body tumor presents as a painless, pulsatile mass below the angle of the mandible. Although there is a slight female predominance, it can occur at any age. These tumors arise from the paraganglionic cells in the vicinity of carotid bifurcation. The lesions are usually unilateral but may be bilateral and familial. Computed tomography reveals lesions that are isodense with the surrounding muscles and enhance intensely with contrast administration. Carotid body tumors are characteristically located at the bifurcation of the common carotid artery, with splaying of the internal and external carotid arteries (Fig. 5.17). Dynamic CT can more reliably differentiate paragangliomas from neurofibromas.[28] Magnetic resonance imaging reveals a mass that is hypointense or isointense with muscle on T1-weighted images and hyperintense on T2-weighted images. Signal voids within the tumors on MRI are characteristic of vascular tumors and help in differentiating paragangliomas from neuromas.[29] However, lack of signal void does not exclude paraganglioma because the vessels may be very small or thrombosed. Angiography reveals an intense blush because of the vascular nature of the tumor.

Lipomas

Lipomas are benign, encapsulated lesions that may involve the lateral and posterior neck. Lipomas are more common in obese people and are more frequent in women over 40 years of age.[30]

Lipomas are easily diagnosed by CT or MRI (Figs 5.18 and 5.19). These lesions have the same density as subcutaneous fat, are homogeneous and do not show enhancement with intravenous contrast.[31,32] Lipomas often compress and displace adjacent structures without invasion. On MRI, lipomas show high signal intensity on T1-weighted images similar to subcutaneous fat and intermediate signal intensity on T2-weighted images. Nodularity or soft tissue density within a primarily lipomatous matrix should suggest the possibility of liposarcoma (Fig. 5.20). Hemorrhage can also occur within a benign lipoma, making differentiation from liposarcoma difficult.

Neuroblastoma

Neuroblastoma is a solid tumor of the sympathetic nervous system. Most of the neuroblastomas are of adrenal origin. Less than 5% arise from the cervical sympathetic chain and present as a neck mass.[10] On US examination, neuroblastoma is seen as an echogenic mass. Computed tomography demonstrates an isodense mass which shows variable patchy enhancement. Magnetic resonance imaging reveals the neuroblastomas to be isointense with muscles on T1-weighted images and usually hyperintense on T2-weighted images.

Rhabdomyosarcoma

Rhabdomyosarcoma is the most common soft tissue sarcoma in children. Forty percent of all rhabdomyosarcomas arise in the head and neck region. These most commonly occur in the orbit, nasopharynx, paranasal sinuses and neck. Computed tomography reveals poorly marginated soft tissue masses with bone destruction. Rim enhancement may be seen with contrast.[33] Magnetic resonance imaging reveals intermediate signal intensity on both T1- and T2-weighted images.

Cervical nodes

Anatomic considerations

One-third of the entire body's lymph nodes are located in the neck. In the suprahyoid neck, well-defined groups of nodes form a pericervical collar and are classified into the following groups.[34–37]

    Occipital
    Mastoid
    Parotid
    Submandibular
    Facial

    Submental
    Sublingual
    Retropharyngeal

In the infrahyoid neck, two longitudinal chains of cervical nodes are present, the anterior cervical chain and the lateral cervical chain.

Adenopathy involving occipital, mastoid, facial and sublingual groups are uncommon. The submandibular and submental groups of nodes lie in the suprahyoid neck and primarily drain the anterior portion of the tongue and floor of the mouth, submandibular and sublingual glands. The efferent lymph drains into the lateral deep cervical chain. The parotid group of nodes can be intraparotid or periparotid in location. Skin lesions along the temporal and frontal regions typically drain into the parotid nodes. Parotid adenopathy can also be seen as a part of a more generalized process such as lymphoma or sarcoidosis.

Retropharyngeal nodes are the dominant nodes for drainage of nasopharyngeal carcinomas and are located in the retrovisceral space. Since these nodes are not amenable to clinical examination, imaging has contributed significantly to the detection of retropharyngeal adenopathy.

Infrahyoid nodes

The anterior cervical chain runs along the anterior jugular veins and includes the juxtavisceral group of nodes, as well as pre-laryngeal, pre-tracheal, pre-thyroid and para-tracheal nodes. The lateral cervical chain is further divided into deep and superficial groups. The superficial nodes are located along the external jugular vein. The deep nodes are subdivided into three components: the internal jugular chain, the spinal accessory chain and the transverse cervical chain.

All head and neck carcinomas ultimately drain into the deep group of lymph nodes. The internal jugular chain follows the course of the internal jugular vein and lies within or adjacent to the carotid sheath. The internal jugular chain is further subdivided into high (suprahyoid), mid (hyoid to cricoid level), and low (infracricoid) jugular nodes. The highest node in the internal jugular chain is also known as the jugular digastric node, which is located at the level of the posterior belly of the digastric along the inferior-medial surface of the parotid gland. This node is particularly important because it forms the primary station drainage node for all head and neck carcinomas. The spinal accessory group of lymph nodes courses obliquely through the posterior neck and along the spinal accessory nerve. The transverse cervical chain bridges the lower limbs of the internal jugular and spinal accessory chain along the course of the transverse cervical artery and vein. These nodes which are clinically within the supraclavicular chain, also drain any neoplasms present in the chest and abdomen (Fig. 5.21).

Imaging strategies

Most imagers prefer CT over MRI in detection of nodal disease in the neck. The CT criteria for pathologic nodes are well established. The experience with MRI evaluation of adenopathy is still somewhat scant. While nodal necrosis is easily determined by CT, the sensitivity of MR is debatable. However, the use of gadolinium may increase the sensitivity of the diagnosis.

Pathology

The following are the well-accepted criteria used to determine abnormal nodes by CT.[35–39]

Size. Nodes greater than 1.5 cm in the upper neck (submental, submandibular and high internal jugular chain) and 1 cm in the lower neck should be considered abnormal. This discrepancy in size is due to recurrent upper respiratory tract infections resulting in reactive hyperplasia of the upper neck nodes.

Density. Central lucency (excluding fatty replacement) within any size node is abnormal. Fatty replacement can be seen in postinflammatory or postradiated nodes, is usually peripheral in location, and should not be confused with nodal necrosis.

Extranodal extension. When an abnormal node demonstrates ill-defined margins and poor demarcation from the adjacent soft tissues, this should suggest extranodal spread of tumor. Previous surgery and radiation can also lead to loss of fascial planes and should not be confused with extranodal spread of disease. In addition, inflammatory disease with changes in the skin and subcutaneous tissues may mimic metastatic nodal disease with extracapsular extension.

Fixation. In the presence of extranodal spread of disease and loss of fascial planes between the node and adjacent structures, the node should be considered as being adherent to those structures. This becomes particularly important when the node is adjacent to the carotid sheath. True invasion of the carotid may be difficult to assess by any of the imaging modalities—CT, MR or US.

Metastatic neck adenopathy

The presence of nodal metastasis is associated with significant reduction in the cure rate of squamous cell carcinomas of the aerodigestive tract.[39] Therefore, accurate staging is of the utmost importance in determining clinical management. Adenopathy usually occurs along the expected drainage route of the site of squamous cell carcinoma.

Knowledge of patterns of nodal spread from the various primary neoplastic sites is useful in diagnostic imaging. Retropharyngeal adenopathy is typically noted with nasopharyngeal carcinoma followed by the internal jugular chain. Presence of an enlarged Delphian node (anterior node along the cricothyroid membrane) signifies the presence of subglottic disease. Jugulodigastric node involvement is typically seen with oral cavity, oropharynx and hypopharyngeal lesions (Figs 5.22–5.24). Presence of lower cervical adenopathy without associated upper neck adenopathy is more suggestive of a primary neoplasm below the diaphragm.

The radiologist performing neck imaging for nodal staging should be familiar with the following classifications by the American Joint Committee on Cancer:[40]

N0: No regional lymph node metastasis

N1: Metastasis in a single ipsilateral lymph node, 3 cm or less in greater dimension

N2a: Metastasis in a single ipsilateral lymph node, more than 3 cm but not more than 6 cm in greatest dimension

N2b: Metastasis in multiple ipsilateral lymph nodes, none more than 6 cm in greatest dimension

N2c: Metastasis in bilateral or contralateral lymph nodes, none more than 6 cm in greatest dimension

N3: Metastasis in a lymph node, more than 6 cm in greatest dimension

Extranodal spread of tumor reduces the long-term survival by 50%. Accuracy of nodal staging by CT is in the range of 90–95% compared to 70–80% clinical accuracy. Not enough data are presently available with MRI to determine its accuracy.

Lymphoma

Hodgkin's and non-Hodgkin's lymphoma may present with cervical adenopathy.[41,42] In the head and neck regions, non-Hodgkin's lymphoma is more common and may involve extranodal lymphatic sites such as the Waldeyer's ring or even extranodal extralymphatic sites which include the nasal cavity, paranasal sinuses, orbits, etc. Lymphomatous adenopathy is more often bilateral than unilateral and is commonly found in the middle and lower jugular nodes (Figs 5.25–5.27). Isolated involvement of the upper jugular nodes is rare with lymphoma in contrast to metastatic squamous cell carcinoma. Usually homogeneous in density, the lymphomatous nodes are variable in size, ranging from 0.5 cm to greater than 1 cm. Calcification may occasionally be seen with Hodgkin's disease, particularly with the nodular sclerosing form. Extranodal lymphatic lymphoma in the Waldeyer's ring is difficult to differentiate from nasopharyngeal carcinoma. Lack of bone erosion at the skull base favors a diagnosis of lymphoma. Masses secondary to lymphoma in the extranodal, extralymphatic sites may also mimic carcinomas. Multiple extralymphatic masses are more suggestive of lymphoma than of synchronous sites of carcinoma.

Inflammatory

Tuberculous adenitis (scrofula)

Tuberculous adenitis accounts for approximately 5% of cervical adenopathy.[36] Tuberculous adenitis secondary to mycobacterium tuberculosis is a manifestation of systemic disease. Bilateral diffuse adenopathy involving the lateral deep cervical chain is usually seen. Associated pulmonary tuberculosis may be present. Computed tomography reveals a variable appearance with or without peripheral rim enhancement, central necrosis and calcifications (Fig. 5.28).[43] Most frequently, multiple nodes with thick rims of peripheral enhancement are noted.[43] Coalescence and breakdown may develop into a 'cold abscess'.

Atypical mycobacterium have also been implicated in cervical adenitis. This occurs more frequently in children. Involvement of the upper cervical nodes and Waldeyer's tonsillar ring predominate. The CT appearance of adenitis is similar to that described above.

AIDS/ARC adenopathy

Diffuse cervical adenopathy in association with parotid lymphoepithelial cysts is described in patients with acquired immunodeficiency syndrome or acquired immune related complex.[44] The adenopathy may be secondary to inflammation, neoplasm or benign hyperplasia (Fig. 5.29). Infections may be bacterial and related to atypical mycobacterium, particularly *Mycobacterium avium–intracellulare*.

Sarcoidosis

Diffuse adenopathy may occur in patients with sarcoidosis, which is a multisystemic granulomatous disease. The enlarged nodes reveal smooth margins and are homogeneous in appearance by CT.[45] There may also be an associated abnormality in the Waldeyer's ring.

Larynx and hypopharynx

Anatomic considerations

The larynx is supported by a cartilaginous framework consisting of the cricoid, thyroid, paired arytenoid and corniculate cartilages.[46–49] Because it is a complete ring, the cricoid cartilage can be considered the foundation. The paired arytenoid cartilages are perched on top of the cricoid and provide attachment for the false vocal cords and the true vocal cords. The thyroid cartilage encloses the larynx anteriorly and laterally. The true vocal cords are composed of the mucosa covering the thyroarytenoideus muscle, the medial-most portion of which is referred to as the vocalis muscle. The medial margin of the true vocal cord is formed by the vocal ligament. The paired vocal ligaments attach to the vocal process of the arytenoid and also to the thyroid cartilage near the midline at the region of the anterior commissure. The soft tissue thickness at this level should not exceed 1 mm on CT. The posterior commissure refers to the mucosa over the cricoid between the posterior margin of the true vocal ligaments.

The paraglottic space, filled with fat and muscle, lies between the laryngeal mucosa and the skeletal framework. It is continuous anteriorly with the pre-epiglottic space. The laryngeal ventricle is the small space between the true and false vocal cords. The false vocal cords are the under surface of the aryepiglottic folds, which run from the broad lateral surfaces of the epiglottis to the arytenoid cartilages. The epiglottis is a broad leaf-like structure which narrows at its tip (the petiole) and attaches to the thyroid cartilage by the thyroepiglottic ligament just above the anterior commissure. The aryepiglottic folds separate the larynx from the hypopharyngeal pyriform sinuses. The epiglottis, pharyngo-epiglottic folds, and glossoepiglottic fold separate the superior extent of the larynx from the oropharynx.

The larynx is divided into the three parts: (1) the glottic region, which consists of the true cords, the anterior and posterior commissures; (2) the supra-glottic region, which incorporates the laryngeal ventricle, the false cords, the aryepiglottic folds, the epiglottis and the laryngeal vestibule; and (3) the infraglottic region, which is the region from the under surface of the true cords to the lower margin of the cricoid cartilage.

The hypopharynx is the caudal continuation of the pharynx and is subdivided into pyriform sinuses, the postcricoid region and the posterior hypopharyngeal wall. The paired pyriform sinuses are the lateral recesses of the hypopharynx and are separated from the endolarynx by the aryepiglottic folds. Posteriorly, the mucosa of the pyriform sinus is contiguous with the mucosa of the posterior hypopharyngeal wall. The postcricoid region extends from the level of the arytenoid cartilages and the connecting folds to the inferior border of the cricoid cartilage.

Imaging strategies

Computed tomography or MR may be used to image the larynx and hypopharynx.[46–61] The choice of imaging modality depends upon the availability and the personal preference of the radiologist. Although the mucosal surfaces are best evaluated by endoscopy, deep extension of tumor is better defined by imaging studies. The advantages of CT are the speed of the examination and thin section capability. The multiplanar capability of MR, coupled with superior soft tissue contrast, offers distinct advantages over CT. However, longer scanning time allows for image degradation by motion. Magnetic resonance is better in evaluating cartilage involvement and subglottic extension of disease. Computed tomography scans are obtained during quiet breathing. Contiguous sections 1.5 mm or 3 mm thick are obtained parallel to the laryngeal ventricle. It is of the utmost importance that the patient be coached to limit swallowing during the scanning. Magnetic resonance scans are performed using the anterior neck surface coil as the receiver coil. T1- and T2-weighted images are obtained in the axial and coronal planes, using 3 mm or 5 mm thick slices with 1 mm gap. Peripheral gating and/or flow compensation may be utilized to decrease artifact from vascular flow.

Pathology

Malignant neoplasm

Approximately 95% of all laryngeal and hypopharyngeal malignant tumors are squamous cell carcinomas.[56,57] Other carcinomas include adenocarcinoma, verrucous carcinoma, and anaplastic carcinomas. The laryngeal carcinoma can be divided into: supraglottic, glottic, and subglottic lesions (Figs 5.30–5.32). Supraglottic tumors account for 30% of all laryngeal carcinomas and can be further classified into three subgroups: (1) anterior lesions involving the epiglottis, (2) marginal lesions involving the aryepiglottic fold and (3) lesions involving the false cords and laryngeal ventricle.[56] The epiglottic carcinomas tend to grow circumferentially and extend into the pre-epiglottic fatty space. Marginal tumors spread along the aryepiglottic fold to the epiglottis or to the arytenoid and cricoarytenoid articulation. False cord and laryngeal ventricle tumors tend to grow submucosally into the paraglottic space. As a result of the rich lymphatic supply of supraglottic larynx and late clinical presentation, approximately 50% of these patients have adenopathy at the time of initial diagnosis.

The glottic carcinomas, which are the most common, account for 60–65% of all laryngeal tumors. The glottic carcinomas arise from the true cords, the anterior commissure or the posterior commissure. Glottic carcinomas clinically manifest early due to hoarseness and carry the best prognosis.

The subglottic carcinomas are rare and account for only 5% of all laryngeal carcinomas. The subglottic region is more commonly involved by direct extension from the glottic or supraglottic carcinoma.

Cord mobility plays a major role in classification of laryngeal tumors. Classification, as defined by the American Joint Committee on Cancer,[40] includes the following:

Supraglottis

T1: Tumor confined to the site of origin with normal cord mobility

T2: Tumor invades an adjacent supraglottic site(s) or glottis with normal cord mobility

T3: Tumor limited to the larynx with fixation or extension to postcricoid area, medial wall of pyriform sinus or pre-epiglottic space

T4: Massive tumor with extension beyond the larynx or erosion of thyroid cartilage.

Glottis

T1: Tumor confined to vocal cords with normal cord mobility

T2: Tumor with extension to supraglottis or subglottis with normal or impaired vocal cord mobility

T3: Tumor confined to larynx with cord fixation

T4: Tumor with extension beyond the larynx or thyroid cartilage erosion

Subglottis

T1: Tumor limited to subglottis

T2: Tumor extension to vocal cords with normal or impaired mobility

T3: Tumor limited to larynx with vocal cord fixation

T4: Tumor extension beyond larynx or thyroid/cricoid cartilage erosion.

Speech conservation surgery includes supraglottic laryngectomy for supraglottic tumor and vertical hemilaryngectomy for vocal cord tumors.[46] Cartilage involvement leads to total laryngectomy and should be carefully sought on imaging studies. The thyroid cartilage calcifies irregularly and involvement is definite only if tumor is demonstrated beyond the cartilage in the soft tissues. Thyroid cartilage involvement is rare without involvement of the anterior commissure and the ventricle.[46] Magnetic resonance imaging may be more sensitive than CT in demonstrating cartilage involvement.[54,58] The fatty marrow in the ossified cartilage reveals high signal intensity on T1-weighted images. Tumor infiltration into the cartilage results in decreased signal intensity of the marrow. If the cartilage is non-ossified, T2-weighted images are more helpful because the tumor is usually hyperintense relative to the non-ossified cartilage.

Extension of tumor beyond the ventricle in supraglottic tumors and into the subglottis from glottic tumors is equally important in patient management. Since CT is performed only in the axial plane, detection of extension across these horizontal planes can be difficult. Magnetic resonance imaging has an advantage because it can be performed in the coronal plane. Tumors usually cross the laryngeal ventricle along the lateral aspect of the paraglottic space.

Carcinoma of the hypopharynx is most common in the pyriform sinus (60%), followed by the postcricoid region (25%) and posterior pharyngeal wall (15%) (Figs 5.33–5.35). Like the supraglottic tumors, hypopharyngeal tumors present late, and 50% of the patients reveal cervical adenopathy at the initial presentation.[59] Hypopharyngeal carcinoma is more common in men, and is associated with smoking and drinking. In women, an association with Plummer–Vinson syndrome is described.[39] Pyriform sinus carcinomas can be seen as extending between the thyroid and arytenoid cartilages through the thyroarytenoid gap. Lesions arising from the anterior wall of the pyriform sinuses tend to invade into the paraglottic space at the level of the false cords. Postcricoid carcinomas are difficult to assess because the soft tissue thickness of the pre-vertebral and the pharyngeal muscles at the pharyngo-esophageal junction is variable. Among the hypopharyngeal carcinomas, postcricoid carcinoma results in the poorest prognosis. Posterior hypopharyngeal carcinoma can arise anywhere along the posterior pharyngeal region, extending from the level of vallecula to that of cricoarytenoid joints. These tumors generally spread superiorly and inferiorly along the posterior margin into the nasopharynx and oropharynx. Retropharyngeal adenopathy is often associated.

Non-epithelial malignant tumors

Lymphoma involving the larynx is uncommon and accounts for less than 1% of all laryngeal neoplasms. The majority of lymphomas present as smooth, supraglottic masses, usually of the epiglottis or the aryepiglottic folds. Mesenchymal tumors such as malignant fibrous histiocytomas, liposarcomas, chondrosarcomas are also rarely encountered (Figs 5.36–5.38).

Benign tumors

Papillomas are benign, wart-like lesions that are common in children. These lesions are usually multiple and involve the larynx and trachea. The larynx may be the origin of any of the mesenchymal tumors such as lipoma, neurofibroma, hemangioma, etc. (Figs 5.39 and 5.40).

Laryngocele

A laryngocele usually results from dilatation of the laryngeal saccule either due to increased intraglottic pressure secondary to playing wind instruments, blowing glass, etc. or less commonly, due to obstruction of the saccule due to inflammatory disease or tumor. The laryngocele may be air-filled or fluid-filled. These are classified as internal, external or mixed. An internal laryngocele is confined within the larynx. The external laryngocele extends through the thyrohyoid membrane and may present as a neck mass. The mixed type has an internal and external component. Air-filled laryngoceles are easily detected by CT and MRI. Fluid-filled laryngoceles are also known as saccular cysts and mimic a soft tissue mass in the supraglottic region (Figs 5.41 and 5.42).

Miscellaneous

Teflon implant

In patients with unilateral cord paralysis where the vocal cord is in the intermediate or paramedian position, incomplete glottic closure results in a soft breathy voice, cough and recurrent aspiration. The injection of synthetic substances such as Teflon paste into the paralyzed cord is a well recognized therapeutic procedure to lessen the clinical manifestations of cord paralysis. Teflon paste is detected on CT as a high density collection (Fig. 5.43).

Cervical osteophytes

Significant compression on the posterior pharyngeal margin may occur with large osteophytes, leading to dysphagia. This is easily demonstrated by CT or MRI (Fig. 5.44).

Carotid position

The internal carotid artery may be positioned rather medially and create a bulge along the posterior pharyngeal margin. Such variation should be considered before biopsy of these pseudomasses. This is equally well demonstrated by CT and MRI (Fig. 5.45).

Thyroid and parathyroid

Anatomic considerations

The thyroid gland originates at the level of foramen cecum at the tongue base. It then descends as a bilobed structure along the thyroglossal duct to its permanent position in the neck below the thyroid cartilage. The two thyroid lobes are connected by the thyroid isthmus, which is anterior to the trachea. This embryologic development and migration are completed by about 7 weeks of gestation. The thyroglossal duct involutes by 8–10 weeks of gestation. Most people have four parathyroid glands. They are paired glands located behind the superior and inferior poles of the thyroid gland. Variable migration of the lower parathyroid glands may result in ectopic location at the cervicothoracic junction or in the upper mediastinum.

Imaging strategies

Radionuclide scanning, ultrasound, CT and more recently MR are all utilized in thyroid imaging. Scintigraphy with radioactive iodine has traditionally been the primary imaging modality in evaluation of thyroid abnormalities. Scintigraphy assesses the function of the thyroid gland and determines if the palpable nodule is 'cold' or a functioning nodule. It is also useful in demonstrating extrathyroidal metastatic disease from thyroid carcinoma. Spatial resolution, however, is poor. Ultrasound using a 7.5 MHz transducer is useful in differentiating cystic from solid masses. Computed tomography scanning of the thyroid gland is satisfactorily performed by using 5 mm-thick contiguous sections in the axial plane. The thyroid gland, by virtue of its high iodine content, is fairly dense on CT without intravenous contrast. Use of iodinated contrast for CT precludes radionuclide scanning at least for 6 weeks because of the iodine overload. The CT characteristics are not useful in differentiating benign from malignant thyroid masses.

Magnetic resonance imaging appears promising in thyroid imaging. Magnetic resonance imaging may be performed in the body coil or with the use of surface coils as the receiver coils. Five-millimeter-thick sections with MR are obtained using a field-of-view of 20 cm, 256 × 256 matrix and two excitations. Pulse sequences include T1-weighted images using TR of 600 ms and TE of 20 ms and T2-weighted images using TR of 2500 ms and TE of 20/80 ms. Sagittal and coronal planes are complementary to the standard axial plane.

The normal parathyroid glands cannot be visualized by any imaging technique. Ultrasound, CT and MRI as described above are all utilized in parathyroid evaluation. In addition, a radionuclide scan utilizing thallium-201/technetium-99m pertechnetate subtraction technique is successful in 65–80% of patients for parathyroid localization.

Pathology

Malignant tumors

Carcinoma

Histologically, thyroid carcinoma may be divided into papillary, follicular, medullary, anaplastic and Hurthle cell types in descending order of frequency. Papillary carcinoma carries the best prognosis, spreading locally by lymphatics; nodal metastases are often cystic and may mimic a branchial cleft cyst. Computed tomography and MRI are useful in defining the extent of the tumor (Figs 5.46–5.48).[62–64] The margins of the lesion are ill-defined. Magnetic resonance imaging shows penetration of the pseudocapsule by tumor and high signal intensity on T2-weighted images.[63] Calcification by CT may be seen on 30–35% of patients.

Recurrent thyroid carcinoma may potentially be differentiated from postoperative scarring by MRI.[65] Local recurrence reveals low signal on T1-weighted images and high signal on T2-weighted images. Scarring in the postoperative bed shows low signal intensity on both T1- and T2-weighted images.[65] Postoperative edema, infection or hemorrhage, however, can give high signal on T2-weighted images and simulate recurrent tumor.

Lymphoma

Primary thyroid lymphoma is rare and accounts for about 4% of all thyroid malignancies. A strong association between thyroid lymphoma and Hashimoto's thyroiditis is described.[64,66] Primary thyroid lymphoma is more commonly seen in elderly women. With the use of CT imaging characteristics and clinical findings, a diagnosis of thyroid lymphoma can be predicted in about 87% of the cases.[67] Computed tomography may reveal single or multiple nodules and occasionally, a diffuse goiter. Compression, or less commonly infiltration, of surrounding structures is noted. Calcification and necrosis are uncommon (7%). Computed tomography is considered superior to US in the evaluation of thyroid lymphoma (Fig. 5.49).[66] Experience with MR is limited at the time of writing.

Benign lesions

Colloid cyst

A colloid cyst usually manifests as a single cystic mass within the thyroid gland and may be difficult to differentiate from goiter or carcinoma with cystic degeneration. Computed tomography reveals well-marginated low-density masses. Ultrasound confirms the cystic nature and fluid can be aspirated under US guidance. Magnetic resonance imaging shows high signal intensity on both T1- and T2-weighted images because of the high protein content (Fig. 5.50).[64] Hemorrhagic cysts also reveal high signal on T1- and T2-weighted images because of the paramagnetic effect of blood products.

Follicular adenoma

Adenomas are seen as solitary thyroid masses ranging from 1 to 4 cm in size which are inhomogeneous in appearance. Computed tomography may reveal calcifications. Magnetic resonance imaging reveals an intact pseudocapsule.[63] Because of hemorrhagic degeneration, this mass is often inhomogeneous. Microscopic foci of carcinoma within an adenoma are not detected by MR imaging.[64]

Multinodular goiter

Multinodular goiter refers to a diffusely enlarged nodular thyroid gland which occurs on a familial basis due to iodine deficiency. Both lobes of the thyroid gland reveal multiple, well-circumscribed masses. Radionuclide scanning identifies patchy areas of increased and decreased uptake. Computed tomography shows enlargement of both lobes with areas of low and high attenuation. Calcification is common. The enlarged gland shows well-defined margins and causes compression of the adjacent structures (Fig. 5.51). Magnetic resonance imaging delineates heterogeneous foci of high and low signal intensity on T1- and T2-weighted images (Fig. 5.52).[64]

Diffuse thyroid disease

Patients with Graves' disease show diffuse glandular enlargement which is relatively homogeneous. Magnetic resonance imaging detects multiple signal voids due to intense vascularity. A moderate to marked diffuse increase in signal intensity with T1- and T2-weighted MRI is reported in patients with Graves' disease.[68] Furthermore, a linear relationship between the thyroid gland to muscle signal intensity contrast ratio and the serum thyronine (T4) level in Graves' disease is described.[68] Patients with Hashimoto's thyroiditis also show diffuse enlargement which is heterogeneous. There is a high association between primary thyroid lymphoma and Hashimoto's thyroiditis.

Parathyroid adenoma

The most common cause of primary hyperparathyroidism is a single parathyroid adenoma (80%) followed by glandular hyperplasia (12%), multiple adenomas (4%) and parathyroid carcinoma (1%).[69] Secondary hyperparathyroidism occurs with renal disease and malabsorption. There are reports in the literature of comparable success rates in parathyroid adenoma localization by US and CT in the range of 61–80%.[70–75] The sensitivity of combined thallium-201 and technetium-99m pertechnetate scintigraphy ranges from 65 to 80%.[76] Hyperplastic glands are usually smaller than adenomas and thus more difficult to detect.[76] Ultrasound shows a mass between the longus colli muscles and the thyroid gland anteriorly. Computed tomography reveals an enhancing lesion in the tracheo-esophageal groove. The double isotope subtraction technique utilizes both thallium 201 chloride and technetium-99m pertechnetate. The thallium is accumulated by both the thyroid and the parathyroid glands, but the technetium-99m pertechnetate is selectively concentrated by the thyroid gland only. Subtraction of the technetium image from the thallium image by computer provides imaging of the parathyroid glands. Ultrasound has difficulty depicting adenomas in the mediastinum because of acoustic shadowing by the sternum and by the air column. Computed tomography suffers from the artifact of streaking at the cervico-thoracic inlet. Scintigraphy also is limited in the mediastinum because of the low energy and penetration of photons and narrow beam. Magnetic resonance imaging is particularly useful in detecting parathyroid abnormality in patients with prior surgery and ectopic parathyroid adenomas.[69,77] The adenomas usually demonstrate low signal intensity on T1-weighted and high signal intensity on T2-weighted images.[69] On MRI, a periadenomal vessel is described as a marker for localizing parathyroid adenoma.[78] Adenomas cannot be differentiated from carcinomas and hyperplasia with MRI. An accuracy of up to 90% with MRI in detecting parathyroid abnormality is reported (Figs 5.53–5.55).[79]

References

1 REEDE DL, WHELAN MA, BERGERON RT, CT of the soft tissue structures of the neck, *Rad Clin North Am* (1984) **22**:239–50.

2 SMOKER WRK, HARNSBERGER HR, REEDE DL et al, The neck. In: Som P, Bergeron RT, eds, *Head and Neck Imaging*, 2nd edn (Mosby/Year Book: St Louis 1991) 497–530.

3 HARNSBERGER HR, *Head and Neck Imaging*, Handbooks in Radiology (Year Book Medical Publishers: Chicago 1990) 138–223.

4 HOLLINSHEAD WH, Anatomy for surgeons. In: *The Head and Neck*, 2nd edn, Vol. 1 (Harper and Row: New York 1968) 306–30.

5 SILVER AJ, MAWAD ME, HILAL SK et al, Computed tomography of the carotid and related cervical spaces. I: Anatomy, *Radiology* (1984) **150**:723–8.

6 REEDE DL, BERGERON RT, SOM PM, CT of thyroglossal duct cysts, *Radiology* (1985) **157**:121–5.

7 REEDE DL, BERGERON RT, The CT evaluation of the normal and diseased neck, *Semin Ultrasound, CT, MR* (1986) **7**:181–201.

8 MORAN AG, BUCHANAN PR, Branchial cysts, sinuses and fistulae, *Clin Otolaryngol* (1978) **3**:77–92.

9 LISTON SL, SIEGEL LG, Branchial cyst, sinuses and fistulas, *Ear Nose Throat J* (1979) **58**:504–9.

10 BATSAKIS JG, Cysts, sinuses and 'coeles'. In: *Tumors of the Head and Neck. Clinical and Pathological Considerations* (Williams and Wilkins: Baltimore 1979) 514–30.

11 HARNSBERGER HR, MANCUSO AA, MURAKI AS et al, Branchial cleft anomalies and their mimics: computed tomographic evaluation, *Radiology* (1984) **152**:739–48.

12 PHILLIPS HE, MCGAHAN JP, Intrauterine fetal cystic hygromas: sonographic detection, *AJR* (1981) **136**:799–802.

13 SILVERMAN PM, KOROBKIN M, MOORE AV, CT diagnosis of cystic hygroma of the neck, *J Comput Assist Tomogr* (1983) **7**:519–20.

14 PILLA TJ, WOLVERSON MK, SUNDARAM M et al, CT evaluation of cystic lymphangiomas of the mediastinum, *Radiology* (1982) **144**:841–2.

15 MANCUSO AA, DILLON WP, The neck, *Radiol Clin North Am* (1989) **27**:407–34.

16 HUNTER TB, PAPLANUS SH, CHERNIN MM et al, Dermoid cyst of the floor of the mouth: CT appearance, *AJR* (1983) **141**:1239–40.

17 KRAUS R, HAN BK, BABCOCK DS et al, Sonography of neck masses in children, *AJR* (1986) **146**:609–13.

18 ITOH K, NISHIMURA K, TOGASHI K, MR imaging of cavernous hemangioma of the face and neck, *J Comput Assist Tomogr* (1986) **10**:831–5.

19 NYBERG DA, JEFFREY RB, BRANT-ZAWADZKI M et al, Computed tomography of cervical infections, *J Comput Assist Tomogr* (1985) **9**:288–96.

20 HOLT GR, MCMANUS K, NEWMAN RK et al, Computerized tomography in the diagnosis of deep neck infections, *Arch Otolaryngol Head Neck Surg* (1982) **108**:693–6.

21 FISHMAN EK, PAKTER RL, GAYLER BW et al, Jugular venous thrombosis: diagnosis by computed tomography, *J Comput Assist Tomogr* (1984) **8**:963–8.

22 WING V, SCHEIBLE W, Sonography of jugular vein thrombosis, *AJR* (1983) **140**:333–6.

23 BRAUN IF, HOFFMAN JC JR, MALKO JA et al, Jugular venous thrombosis MR imaging, *Radiology* (1985) **157**:357–60.

24 DINSMORE RE, WEEDEN VJ, ROSEN B et al, Phase-offset techniques to distinguish slow blood flow and thrombus on MR images, *AJR* (1987) **418**:634–6.

25 SILVER AJ, MAWAD ME, HILAL SK, Computed tomography of the carotid space and related cervical spaces. II. Neurogenic tumors, *Radiology* (1984) **150**:729–35.

26 REEDE DL, WHELAN MA, BERGERON RT, Computed tomography of the infrahyoid neck. II, *Radiology* (1982) **145**:397–402.

27 SWARTZ JD, KORSVIK H, High resolution computed tomography of paragangliomas of the head and neck, *J Comput Tomograph. CT* (1984) **8**:197–202.

28 SHUGAR MA, MAFEE MF, Diagnosis of carotid body tumors by dynamic computed tomography, *Head Neck Surg* (1982) **4**:518–21.

29 OLSON WL, BRANT-ZAWADZKI M, KELLY WM et al, MR imaging of paragangliomas, *AJNR* (1986) **7**:1039–42.

30 ENZINGER FM, WEISS SW, Soft tissue tumors (CV Mosby: St Louis 1983) 199–241.

31 SOM PM, SCHERL MP, RAO VM et al, Rare presentations of ordinary lipomas of the head and neck: a review, *AJNR* (1986) 7:657–64.

32 DOOMS CG, HRICAK H, SOLLITTO RA et al, Lipomatous tumors and tumors with fatty component: MR imaging potential and comparison of MR and CT results, *Radiology* (1985) 157:479–83.

33 LATACK JT, HUTCHINSON RJ, HYEN RM, Imaging of rhabdomyosarcomas of the head and neck, *AJNR* (1987) 8:353–9.

34 SOM PM, Lymph nodes of the neck, *Radiology* (1987) 165:593–600.

35 REEDE DL, BERGERON RT, WHELAN MA et al, Computed tomography of cervical lymph nodes, *RadioGraphics* (1983) 3:339–51.

36 REEDE DL, SOM P, Lymph nodes. In: Som P, Bergeron RT, eds, *Head and Neck Imaging*, 2nd edn (Mosby/Year Book: St Louis 1991) 558–77.

37 MANCUSO AA, HARNSBERGER HR, MURAKI AS et al, Computed tomography of cervical and retropharyngeal lymph nodes: normal anatomy, variants of normal, and applications in staging head and neck cancer. I. Normal anatomy, *Radiology* (1983) 148:709–14.

38 MANCUSO AA, HARNSBERGER HR, MURAKI AS et al, Computed tomography of cervical and retropharyngeal lymph nodes: normal anatomy, variants of normal and applications in staging head and neck cancer. II. Pathology, *Radiology* (1983) 148:715–23.

39 HARNSBERGER HR, The radiologic evaluation of squamous cell carcinoma nodal disease. In: *Handbooks in Radiology, Head and Neck Radiology* (Year Book Medical Publishers: Chicago in press).

40 RICE DH, SPIRO RH, *Current Concepts in Head and Neck Cancer* (American Cancer Society: USA 1989) 20.

41 LEE YY, VANTASSEL P, NAUERT C, Lymphomas of the head and neck: CT findings at initial presentation, *AJR* (1987) 149:575–81.

42 HARNSBERGER HR, BRAGG DG, OSBORN AG et al, Non-Hodgkin's lymphoma of the head and neck: CT evaluation of nodal and extranodal sites, *AJR* (1987) 149:785–91.

43 REEDE DL, BERGERON RT, Cervical tuberculous adenitis: CT manifestations, *Radiology* (1985) 154:701–4.

44 HOLLIDAY RA, COHEN WA, SCHINELLA RA et al, Benign lymphoepithelial parotid cysts and hyperplastic cervical adenopathy in AIDS risk patients: a new CT appearance, *Radiology* (1988) 168:439–41.

45 SWARTZ JD, YUSSEN PS, POPKY GL, Imaging of the neck: nodal disease, CRC *Crit Rev Diagn Imaging* (1991) 31:413–69.

46 CURTIN HD, Imaging of the larynx: current concepts, *Radiology* (1989) 173:1–11.

47 CURTIN H, The larynx. In: Som P, Bergeron RT, eds, *Head and Neck Imaging*, 2nd edn (CV Mosby-Year Book: St Louis 1991) 593–692.

48 MANCUSO A, HANAFEE WN, *Computed Tomography and Magnetic Resonance of the Head and Neck*, 2nd edn (Williams and Wilkins: Baltimore 1985) 241–357.

49 HANAFEE WN, Hypopharynx and larynx. In: Valvassori GE, Buckingham RA, Carter BL et al, *Head and Neck Imaging* (Thieme: New York 1988) 312–36.

50 LUFKIN RB, HANAFEE WN, Application of surface coils to MR anatomy of the larynx, *AJR* (1984) 146:483–9.

51 LUFKIN RB, HANAFEE WN, WORTHAM DG et al, Larynx and Hypopharynx: MR imaging with surface coils, *Radiology* (1986) 158:747–54.

52 STARK DD, MOSS AA, GAMSU G et al, MR imaging of the neck. I. Normal anatomy, *Radiology* (1984) 150:447–54.

53 CASTELIJNS JA, VAN HATTUM AH, SNOW GB, MR imaging of laryngeal cancer, *J Comput Assist Tomogr* (1987) 11:134–40.

54 CASTELIJNS JA, GERRITSEN GJ, KAISER MC et al, Invasion of laryngeal cartilage by cancer: comparison of CT and MR imaging, *Radiology* (1987) 166:199–206.

55 TERESI LM, LUFKIN RB, HANAFEE WN, Magnetic resonance imaging of the larynx, *Radiol Clin North Am* (1989) 27:393–406.

56 HARNSBERGER HR, ed, The larynx and hypopharynx. In: *Handbooks in Radiology, ENT Imaging* (Year Book Medical Publishers: Chicago in press).

57 SILVERMAN PM, BOSSEN EH, FISHER SR, Carcinoma of the larynx and hypopharynx: computed tomographic-histopathologic correlation, *Radiology* (1984) 151:697–702.

58 CASTELIJNS JA, GERRITSEN GJ, KAISER MC et al, MRI of normal and cancerous laryngeal cartilage: histiopathologic correlation, *Laryngoscope* (1987) **97**:1085–93.

59 LARSSON S, MANCUSO AA, HOOVER L et al, Differentiation of pyriform sinus cancer from supraglottic laryngeal cancer by computed tomography, *Radiology* (1981) **141**:427–32.

60 REID MH, Laryngeal carcinoma: high resolution computed tomography in thick anatomic sections, *Radiology* (1984) **151**:689–96.

61 LUFKIN RB, HANAFEE WN, WORTHAM D et al, Larynx and hypopharynx: MR imaging with surface coils, *Radiology* (1986) **158**:747–54.

62 NOMA S, NISHIMURA K, TOGASHI K et al, Thyroid gland: MR imaging, *Radiology* (1987) **164**:495–9.

63 NOMA S, KANAOKA M, MINAMI S et al, Thyroid masses: MR imaging and pathologic correlation, *Radiology* (1988) **168**:759–64.

64 GEFTER WB, SPRITZER CE, EISENBERG B et al, Thyroid imaging with high-field-strength surface-coil MR, *Radiology* (1987) **164**:483–90.

65 AUFFERMANN W, CLARK OH, THURNHER S et al, Recurrent thyroid carcinoma: characteristics on MR images, *Radiology* (1988) **168**:753–7.

66 TAKASHIMA S, MORIMOTO S, IKEZOE J et al, Primary thyroid lymphoma: comparison of CT and US assessment, *Radiology* (1989) **171**:439–43.

67 TAKASHIMA S, IKEZOE J, MORIMOTO S et al, Primary thyroid lymphoma: evaluation with CT, *Radiology* (1988) **168**:765–8.

68 CHARKES ND, MAURER AH, SIEGEL JA et al, MR imaging in thyroid disorders: correlation of signal intensity with Grave's Disease activity, *Radiology* (1987) **164**:491–4.

69 PECK WW, HIGGINS CB, FISHER MR et al, Hyperparathyroidism: comparison of MR imaging with radionuclide scanning, *Radiology* (1987) **163**:415–20.

70 STARK DD, GOODING GAW, MOSS AA et al, Parathyroid imaging: comparison of high-resolution CT and high-resolution sonography, *AJR* (1983) **141**:633–8.

71 SCHEIBLE W, DEUTSCH AL, LEOPOLD GR, Parathyroid adenoma: accuracy of preoperative localization by high-resolution real-time sonography, *JCU* (1981) **9**:325–30.

72 SIMEONE JF, MUELLER PR, FERRUCCI JT et al, High-resolution real-time sonography of the parathyroid, *Radiology* (1981) **141**:745–51.

73 DOPPMAN JL, KRUDY AG, BRENNAN MF et al. CT appearance of enlarged parathyroid glands in the posterior superior mediastinum, *J Comput Assist Tomogr* (1982) **6**:1099–102.

74 SOMMER B, WELTER HF, SPELSBERG WF et al, Computed tomography for localizing enlarged parathyroid glands in primary hyperparathyroidism, *J Comput Assist Tomogr* (1982) **6**:521–6.

75 OVENFORS CO, STARK D, MOSS A et al, Localization of parathyroid adenoma by computed tomography, *J Comput Assist Tomogr* (1982) **6**:1094–98.

76 OKERLUND MD, SHELDON K, CORPUZ S et al, A new method with high sensitivity and specificity for localization of abnormal parathyroid glands, *Ann Surg* (1984) **200**:381–7.

77 AUFFERMANN W, GOODING GAW, OKERLUND MD et al, Diagnosis of recurrent hyperparathyroidism: comparison of MR imaging and other imaging techniques, *AJR* (1988) **150**:1027–33.

78 KHAN A, RUMANCIK WM, ATTIE JN et al, Perladenomal vessel: an important MR imaging landmark for localization of parathyroid adenoma, *Radiology* (1990) **177**:157.

79 SPRITZER CE, GEFTER WB, HAMILTON R et al, Abnormal parathyroid glands: high-resolution MR imaging, *Radiology* (1987) **162**:487–91.

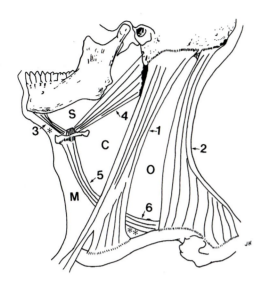

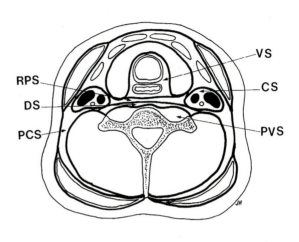

FIGURE 5.1

Lateral drawing of the neck depicting the cervical triangles. The sternocleidomastoid muscle demarcates the anterior triangle from the posterior triangle. The anterior triangle is subdivided into the submental (*) and submandibular triangles (S) in the suprahyoid region and into the carotid (C) and muscular (M) triangles in the infrahyoid regions. The posterior triangle is divided into the occipital (O) and subclavian (**) triangles. 1, Sternocleidomastoid muscle; 2, trapezius muscle; 3, anterior belly of digastric muscle; 4, posterior belly of digastric muscle; 5, superior belly of omohyoid muscle; 6, inferior belly of omohyoid muscle.

FIGURE 5.2

Transaxial drawing of the infrahyoid neck demonstrates the cervical spaces. VS, visceral space; CS, carotid space; PVS, pre-vertebral space; PCS, posterior cervical space; DS, danger space; RPS, retropharyngeal space.

A

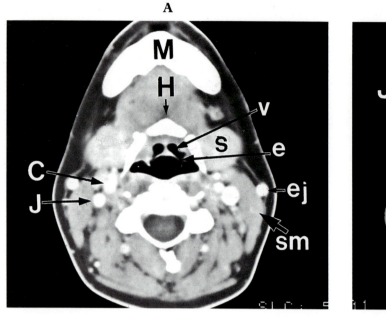

C

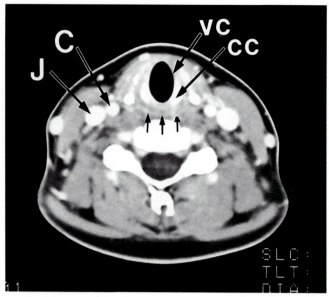

B

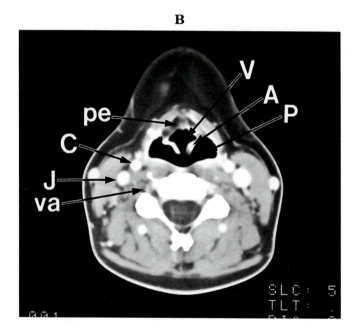

D

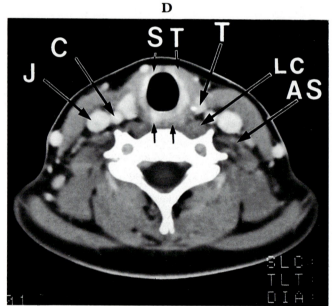

FIGURE 5.3

Normal CT anatomy. (**A**) Section at the level of the hyoid. H, hyoid; M, mandible; v, vallecula; S, submandibular gland; e, epiglottis; sm, sternocleidomastoid muscle; ej, external jugular vein; J, internal jugular vein; C, internal carotid artery. (**B**) Section at the supraglottic level. V, laryngeal vestibule; A, aryepiglottic fold; P, pyriform sinus; va, vertebral artery; J, internal jugular vein; C, common carotid artery; pe, pre-epiglottic space.

(**C**) Section at the level of the vocal cords. vc, vocal cords; cc, cricoid cartilage; J, internal jugular vein; C, common carotid artery; small arrows, hypopharynx. (**D**) Section at the cricoid ring. ST, strap muscles; T, thyroid gland; LC, longus colli muscles; AS, anterior scalene muscle; small arrows, post cricoid region; J, internal jugular vein; c, common carotid artery.

continued

E

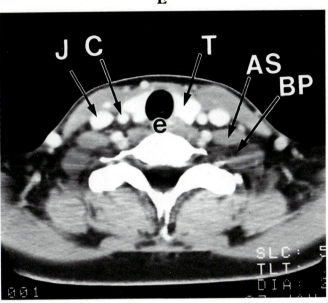

FIGURE 5.3 *(continued)*

(**E**) Section through the mid thyroid gland level. T,
thyroid gland; AS, anterior scalene muscle; BP,
brachial plexus; e, esophagus; t, trachea; C, common
carotid artery; J, internal jugular vein.

A

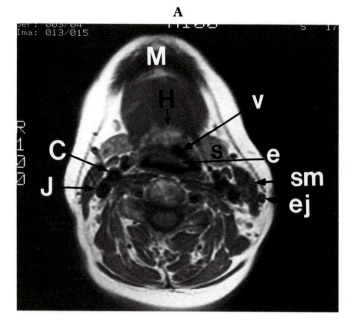

C

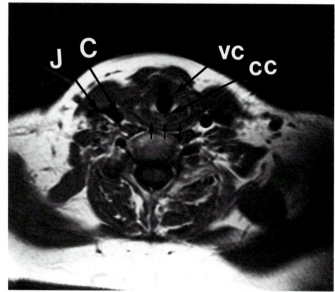

B

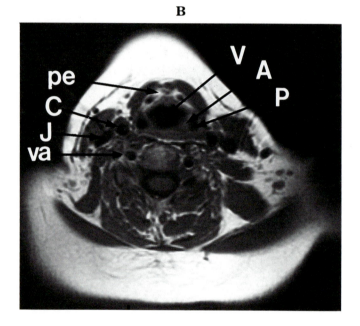

D

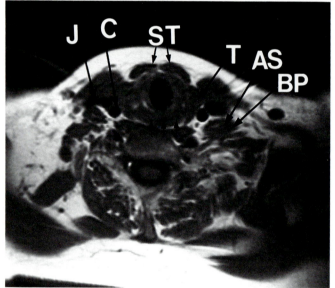

FIGURE 5.4

Normal axial MR anatomy of the neck on T1-weighted images (TR = 800 ms, TE = 12 ms). (**A**) Section at the level of the hyoid. H, hyoid; M, mandible; v, vallecula; S, submandibular gland; e, epiglottis; sm, sternocleidomastoid muscle; ej, external jugular vein; J, internal jugular vein; C, internal carotid artery. (**B**) Section at the supraglottic level. V, laryngeal vestibule: A, aryepiglottic fold; P, pyriform sinus; va, vertebral artery; J, internal jugular vein; C, common carotid artery; pe, pre-epiglottic space.

(**C**) Section at the level of the vocal cords. vc, vocal cords; cc, cricoid cartilage; J, internal jugular vein; C, common carotid artery; small arrows, hypopharynx. (**D**) Section at the cricoid ring level. ST, strap muscles; T, thyroid gland; AS, anterior scalene muscle; BP, brachial plexus; small arrows, postcricoid region; J, internal jugular vein; C, carotid artery.

continued

A

D

B

E

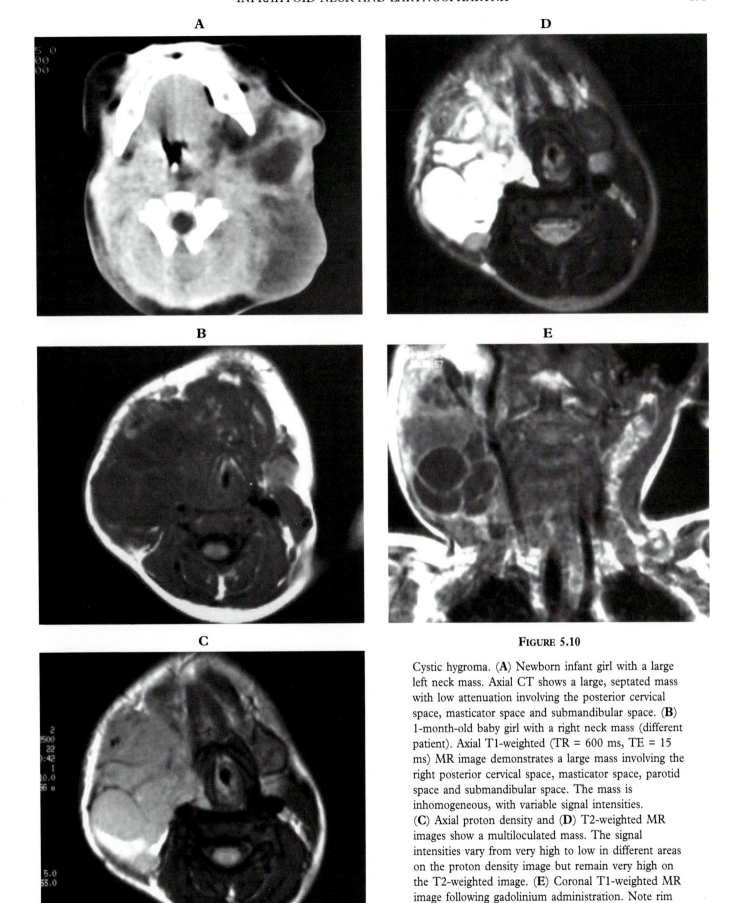

C

FIGURE 5.10

Cystic hygroma. (**A**) Newborn infant girl with a large left neck mass. Axial CT shows a large, septated mass with low attenuation involving the posterior cervical space, masticator space and submandibular space. (**B**) 1-month-old baby girl with a right neck mass (different patient). Axial T1-weighted (TR = 600 ms, TE = 15 ms) MR image demonstrates a large mass involving the right posterior cervical space, masticator space, parotid space and submandibular space. The mass is inhomogeneous, with variable signal intensities. (**C**) Axial proton density and (**D**) T2-weighted MR images show a multiloculated mass. The signal intensities vary from very high to low in different areas on the proton density image but remain very high on the T2-weighted image. (**E**) Coronal T1-weighted MR image following gadolinium administration. Note rim enhancement of the multiple loculations within the mass.

A

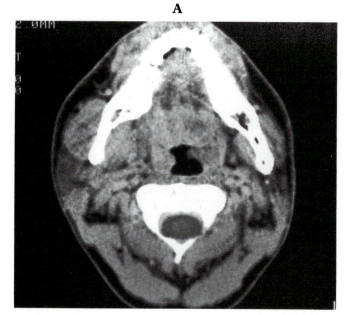

C

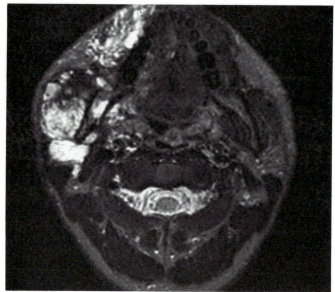

B

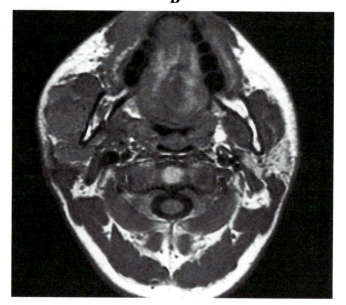

FIGURE 5.11

Hemangioma. 29-year-old man with right facial and neck prominence. (**A**) Axial CT scan shows enlargement of the right masseter muscle and medial pterygoid muscle. (**B**) Axial MR T1-weighted image (TR = 700 ms, TE = 20 ms) clearly demonstrates a mass infiltrating the right masticator and parotid space. The signal intensity of the mass is slightly higher than that of the muscle. (**C**) Axial T2-weighted (TR = 3000 ms, TE = 80 ms) image. The mass reveals high signal intensity. The mass infiltrates into the parapharyngeal space, soft tissues of the face and narrow space in the mandible.

A

C

B

D

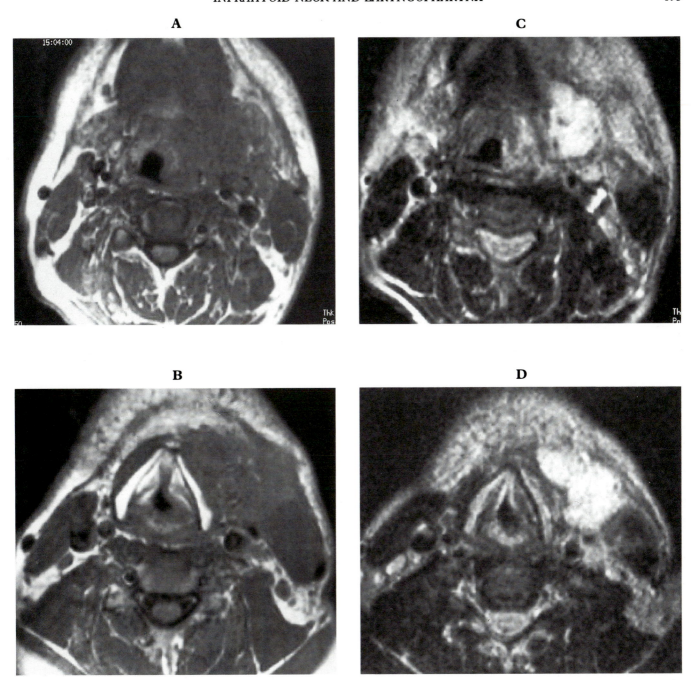

FIGURE 5.12

Abscess. 36-year-old man presented with swollen, painful neck mass following dental extraction. (**A,B**) T1-weighted (TR = 700 ms, TE = 15 ms) MR images show an ill-defined, intermediate signal mass in the submandibular space which extends into the infrahyoid neck. The left sternocleidomastoid muscle is enlarged. (**C,D**) T2-weighted axial (TR = 2400 ms, TE = 90 ms) MR images. The mass shows a high signal intensity.

A

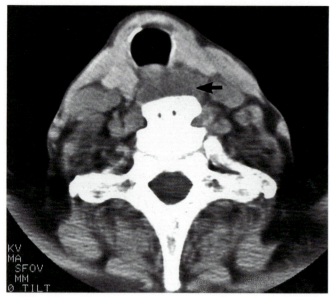

C

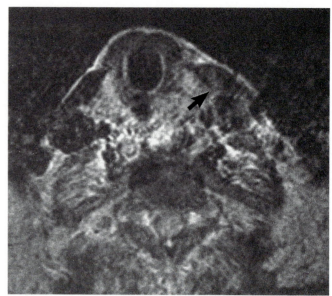

B

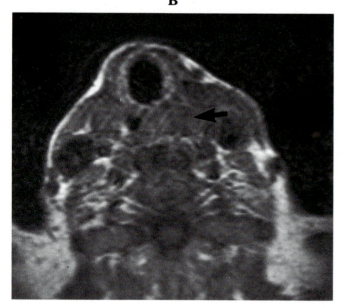

FIGURE 5.13

Pre-vertebral abscess. 77-year-old man with a low-grade fever, dysphagia and subacute bacterial endocarditis. (**A**) Axial unenhanced CT scan shows a low-density mass in the pre-vertebral space (arrow). The esophagus is displaced to the right. (**B**) Axial T1-weighted (TR = 700 ms, TE = 20 ms) MR image. The mass shows a low-intensity signal (arrow). (**C**) Axial T2-weighted (TR = 2000 ms, TE = 80 ms) MR image. The quality of the image is degraded by patient motion. The pre-vertebral mass (arrow) reveals a signal higher than that of muscles.

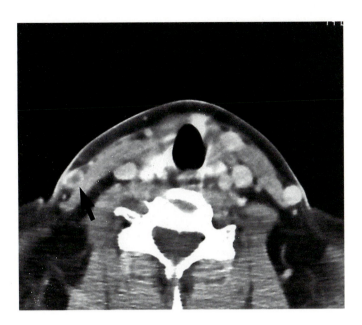

FIGURE 5.14

Venous thrombosis. Contrast-enhanced axial CT scan reveals a central lucency within the right external jugular vein (arrow). Swallowing artifact degrades the image.

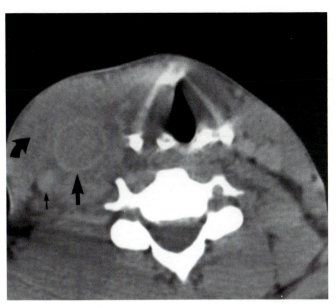

FIGURE 5.15

Venous thrombophlebitis. 26-year-old man with a history of drug abuse presented with a swollen right neck. Contrast-enhanced axial CT scan demonstrates rim enhancement of the right internal jugular vein with central lucency (arrow). The right sternocleidomastoid muscle (curved arrow) is enlarged. The fat planes in posterior cervical space are obscured. Also note reactive adenopathy (small arrow).

A

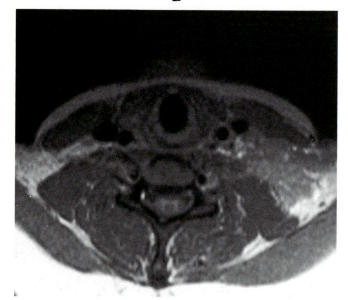

C

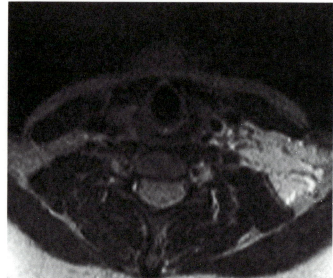

B

FIGURE 5.16

Plexiform neurofibroma. 20-year-old woman with a left neck mass. (**A**) Axial T1-weighted (TR = 600 ms, TE = 20 ms) MR image shows a lobulated mass in the left posterior cervical space, isointense with surrounding musculature. (**B**) Axial proton density (TR = 2000 ms, TE = 20 ms) and (**C**) T2-weighted MR images (TR = 2000 ms, TE = 80 ms). The mass is moderately hyperintense on T2-weighted image. The signal intensity is fairly characteristic of neural tumors.

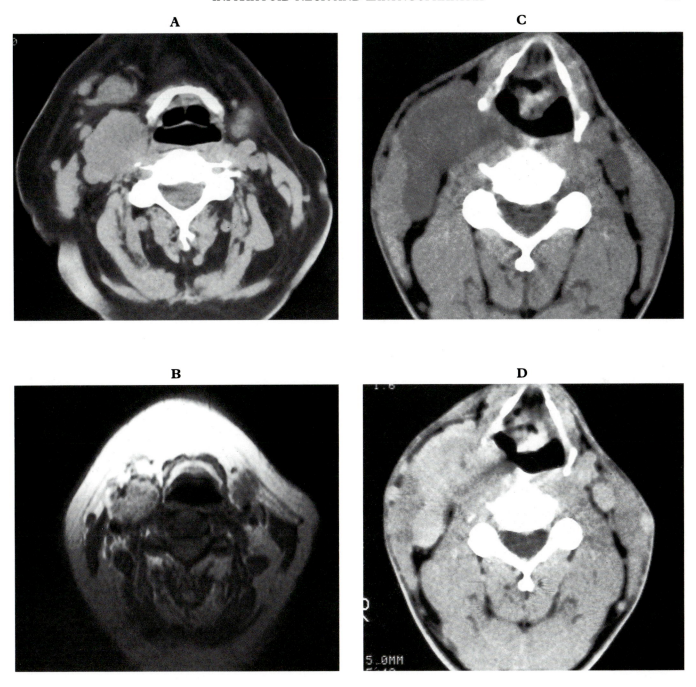

FIGURE 5.17

Carotid body tumor. 57-year-old man with a right neck mass. (**A**) CT scan shows a large soft tissue mass in the right neck at the level of the hyoid, which identifies the area of the carotid bifurcation. The mass displaces the internal jugular vein posteriorly and the submandibular gland anteriorly. (**B**) Proton density weighted MR image (TR = 2000 ms, TE = 30 ms). The mass reveals intermediate signal with multiple foci of signal void and splays the carotid bifurcation. The location and appearance is fairly characteristic of a carotid body tumor. (**C,D**) 32-year-old woman with a pulsatile right neck mass. Unenhanced axial CT scans (**C**) and contrast-enhanced CT scan (**D**) show an intense enhancement of the right neck mass, which is fairly typical of a carotid body tumor in this location.

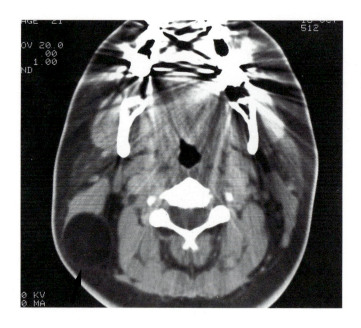

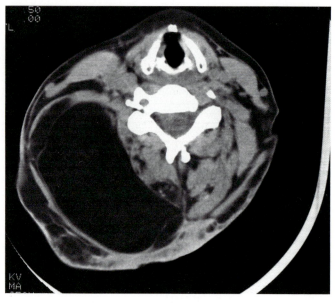

FIGURE 5.18

FIGURE 5.19

Lipoma. 35-year-old woman with a neck mass. Axial CT scan reveals a well-circumscribed, low-attenuation mass (arrow). The density of the mass is similar to that of subcutaneous fat.

Lipoma. 64-year-old woman with a right neck mass. Axial CT scan demonstrates a large, encapsulated, low-density right posterior neck mass. Note the fine septations within the mass and the medial displacement of the paraspinal muscles. The lipoma extends into the subcutaneous region.

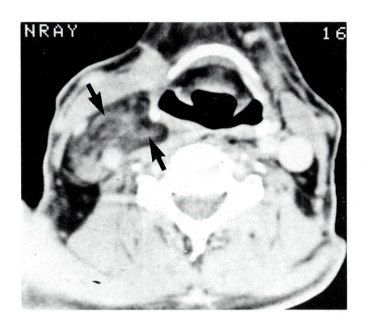

FIGURE 5.20

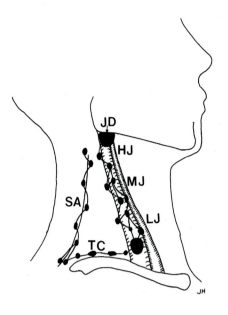

FIGURE 5.21

Liposarcoma. 67-year-old man with neck mass. Axial CT scan shows a right infiltrative neck mass with mixed attenuation (arrows). The neck vessels are displaced posteriorly and the sternocleidomastoid muscle is elevated.

Deep lateral cervical nodes. The deep lateral cervical chain is comprised of the internal jugular (JD, HJ, MJ, LJ), the spinal accessory chain (SA) and the transverse cervical chain (TC). The highest node in the internal jugular chain is called the jugulo-digastric node (JD). The internal jugular nodes are further divided into the high jugular (HJ), mid jugular (MJ) and low jugular (LJ). The HJ are above the hyoid level, MJ are between the hyoid and the cricoid level and LJ are below the cricoid cartilage. The superficial lateral cervical nodes course along the external jugular vein and are not depicted. Also not depicted are the anterior cervical nodes that course along the anterior jugular veins and include the juxta-visceral group of nodes.

A

D

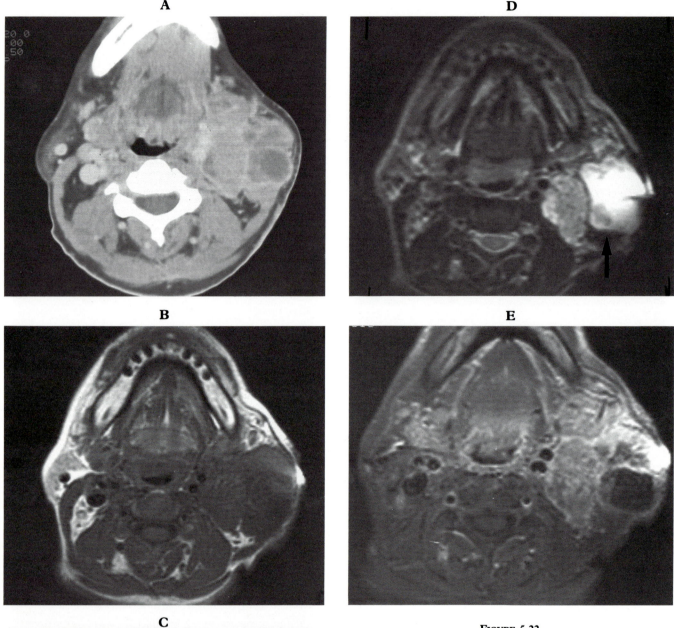

B

E

C

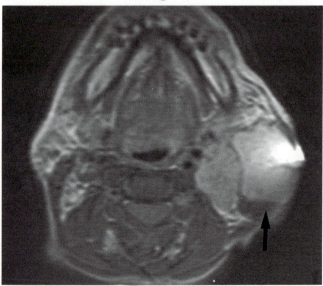

FIGURE 5.22

Metastatic adenopathy from posterior pharyngeal carcinoma. 65-year-old woman presented with a left neck mass. (**A**) Contrast-enhanced axial CT scan shows multiple masses with rim enhancement and varying regions of central necrosis. The masses are adherent to the left sternocleidomastoid muscles. The internal jugular vein and the internal carotid artery are displaced medially. (**B**) Axial T1 weighted MR image (TR = 450 ms, TE = 11 ms) demonstrates an inhomogeneous low signal intensity mass involving the left carotid space, parotid space, and the masticator space. (**C**) Axial proton density and (**D**) T2-weighted (TR = 2200 ms, TE = 30/80 ms) MR images reveal varying signal intensities with fluid-fluid level (arrow). The regions on CT yielding very low density correspond to the very high signal intensity on the T2-weighted image. (**E**) Axial T1-weighted MR image with fat suppression following gadolinium administration. A varying degree of enhancement is seen. The areas with very low signal correspond to the central necrotic debris.

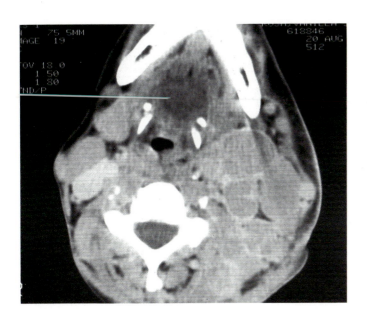

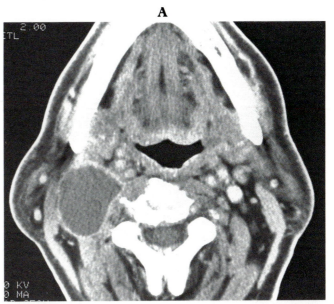

A

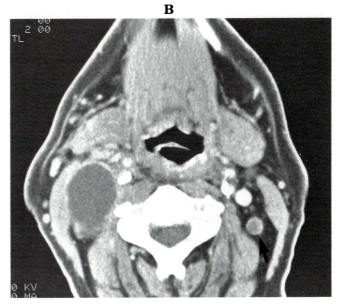

B

FIGURE 5.23

Metastatic squamous cell carcinoma. 37-year-old woman with tonsillar carcinoma. Contrast-enhanced axial CT scan shows multiple nodal masses with rim enhancement along the left jugular chain and spinal accessory chain.

FIGURE 5.24

Metastatic carcinoma from contralateral pyriform sinus squamous cell carcinoma. 50-year-old man presented with a neck mass and dysphagia. Axial CT scans (**A,B**) reveal a 4 cm low-density mass with thin rim enhancement. On (**B**) note another necrotic node in the left neck (arrow).

A   C

B   D

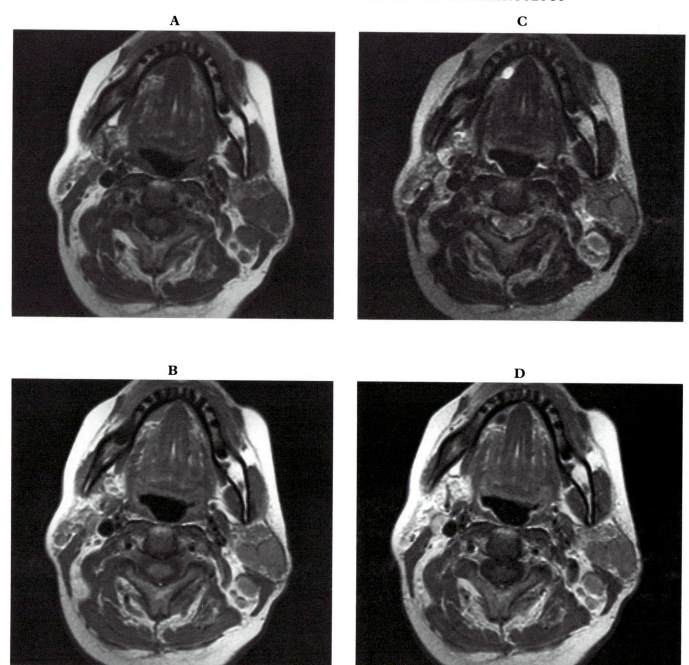

FIGURE 5.25

Lymphoma. 58-year-old woman with an enlarging left neck mass. (**A**) Axial T1-weighted MR image (TR = 600 ms, TE = 20 ms) reveals multiple low signal intensity masses in the left parotid gland and the posterior cervical space. (**B**) Axial proton density (TR = 2300 ms, TE = 20 ms) and (**C**) T2-weighted (TR = 2300 ms, TE = 80 ms) MR images. The masses are homogeneous in appearance and demonstrate intermediate signal intensity. (**D**) Axial T1-weighted image following gadolinium administration shows slight homogeneous enhancement.

A

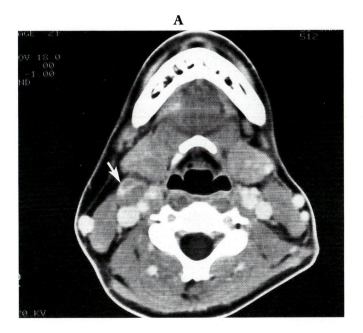

C

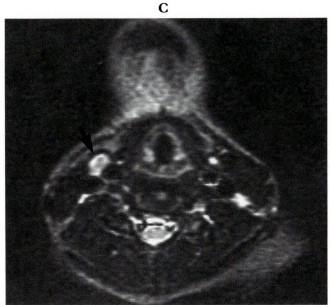

B

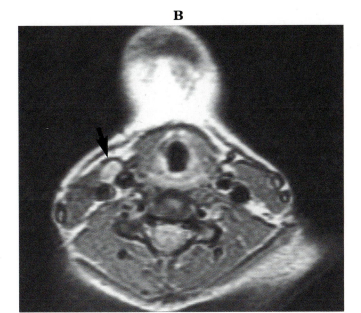

FIGURE 5.26

Hodgkin's disease. 20-year-old woman with a right neck mass. (**A**) Contrast-enhanced axial CT scan reveals a 1.5 cm mass, isodense with muscle, with peripheral enhancement (arrow). (**B**) Axial proton density (TR = 2000 ms, TE = 20 ms) and (**C**) T2-weighted (TR = 2000 ms, TE = 80 ms) MR images reveal high signal intensity within the mass (arrow).

A   A

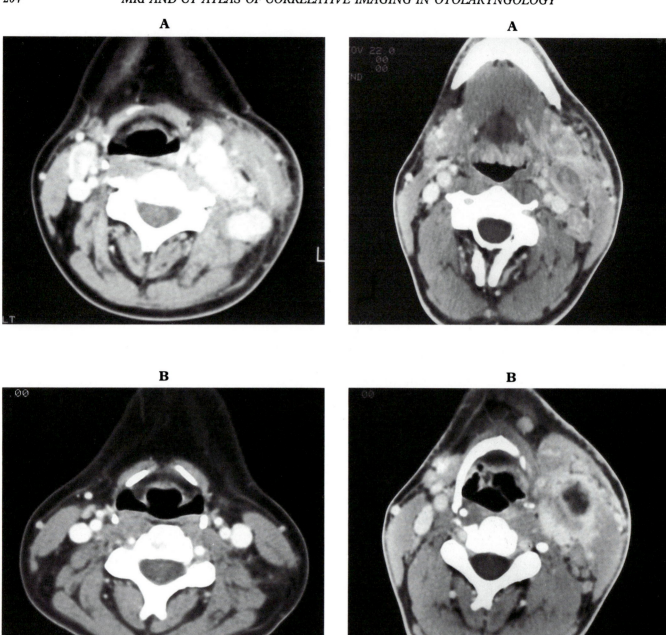

B   B

FIGURE 5.27

Hodgkin's disease. 33-year-old woman with neck
masses. (**A**) Contrast-enhanced axial CT scan reveal
multiple homogeneously enhancing nodal masses
bilaterally, more pronounced on the left.
(**B**) Contrast-enhanced axial CT scan 6 months post
chemotherapy shows almost total regression of
adenopathy.

FIGURE 5.28

Tuberculous adenitis. (**A,B**) Contrast-enhanced axial
CT scan shows multiple masses with central
necrosis. Note the thick, irregularly enhancing rim.
The platysma is thickened and the subcutaneous fat
is reticulated (courtesy of Peter Som, MD).

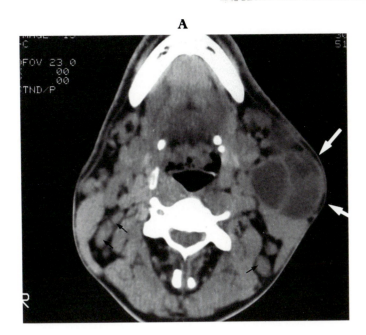

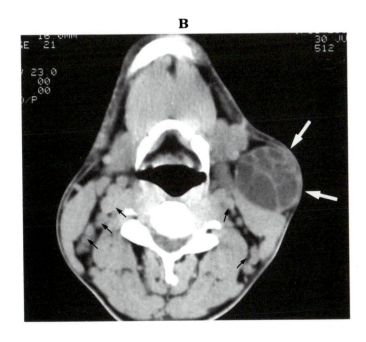

FIGURE 5.29

AIDS-acquired immune-related complex adenopathy. 24-year-old man with AIDS presented with an enlarging left neck mass. (**A,B**) Contrast-enhanced axial CT scans reveal diffuse bilateral cervical adenopathy (small arrows) in association with multiple parotid lymphoepithelial cysts (big arrows).

A

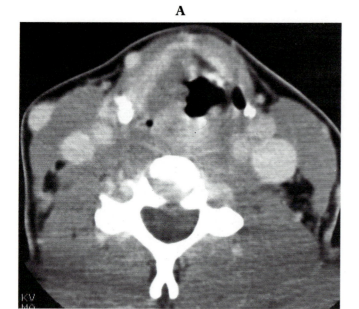

C

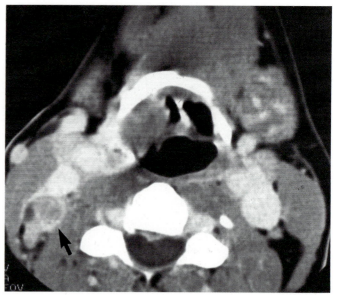

B

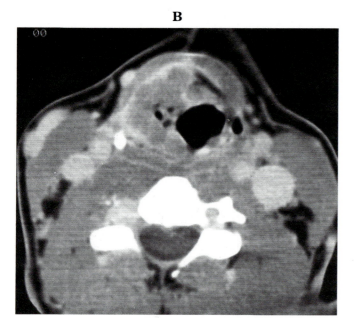

FIGURE 5.30

Supraglottic squamous cell carcinoma. (**A,B,C**) Contrast-enhanced axial CT scans show large, necrotic mass in the supraglottic region. The epiglottis is thickened. The tumor invades the pre-epiglottic space. The bulky tumor involves the right pharyngoepiglottic aryepiglottic folds and the paralaryngeal space. The tumor extends to the false cord on the right. Note necrotic nodes in the right neck (arrow).

A

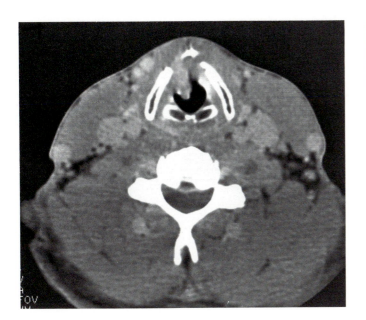

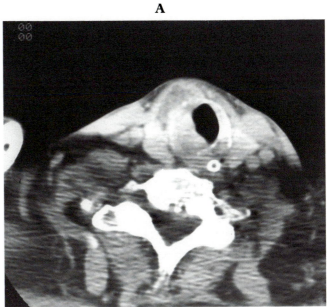

FIGURE 5.31

Glottic squamous cell carcinoma. Contrast-enhanced CT scan reveals a mass involving the right true vocal cord with extension to the anterior commissure and the left anterior true vocal cord.

B

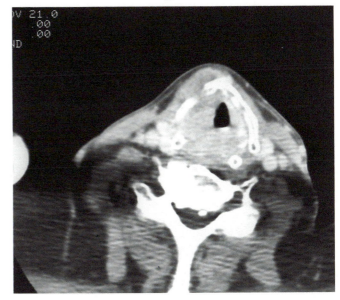

FIGURE 5.32

Subglottic squamous cell carcinoma. (**A**) Contrast-enhanced axial CT scans show subglottic extension of the right glottic carcinoma. (**B**) CT scan through the level of true cords demonstrates a large mass involving the right vocal cord with extension into the strap muscles and anterior neck. The thyroid lamina is eroded.

A

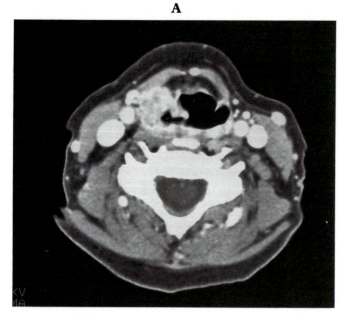

A

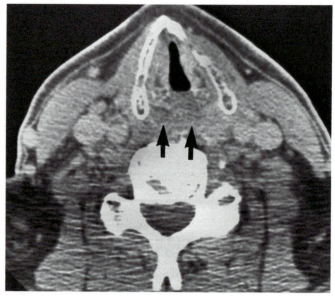

B

B

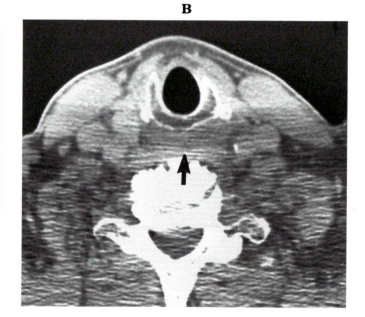

FIGURE 5.33

Pyriform sinus carcinoma. (**A**) Contrast enhanced axial CT scan shows large mass in the right pyriform sinus extending to the posterior pharyngeal margin. (**B**) Note intralaryngeal extension of tumor through the widened thyroarytenoid gap to involve the right true cord (arrow).

FIGURE 5.34

Hypopharyngeal squamous cell carcinoma. 51-year-old man presented with dysphagia. (**A,B**) Contrast-enhanced axial CT scan reveals a soft tissue mass along the posterior pharyngeal wall and postcricoid region (arrows), which was found by endoscopy to extend to the proximal esophagus.

A

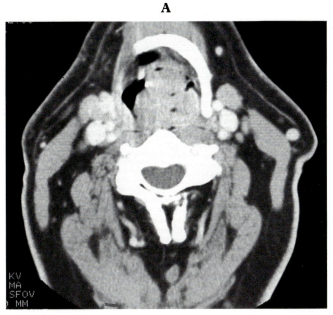

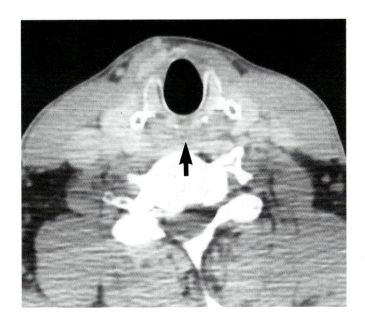

FIGURE 5.35

Postcricoid squamous cell carcinoma. 54-year-old man with a soft tissue mass in the postcricoid region (arrow). The esophagus was free of tumor.

B

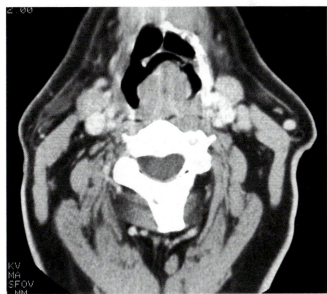

FIGURE 5.36

Malignant fibrous histiocytoma. 63-year-old man presented with a foreign body sensation. (**A,B**) Axial CT scans reveal a large, bulky mass with fairly homogeneous enhancement arising from the posterior pharyngeal margin.

A

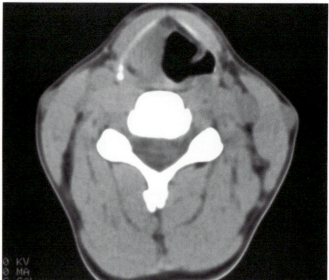

B

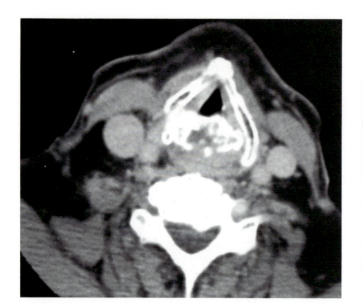

FIGURE 5.37

Cricoid chondrosarcoma. Axial CT scan
demonstrates a destructive soft tissue mass with the
epicenter at the cricoid cartilage.

FIGURE 5.38

Lymphoma. 27-year-old woman with hoarseness.
(**A,B**) Axial CT scans without contrast enhancement
show a soft tissue mass involving the right
supraglottic and glottic region. The pyriform sinus
was compressed, but free of tumor.

A

D

B

E

C

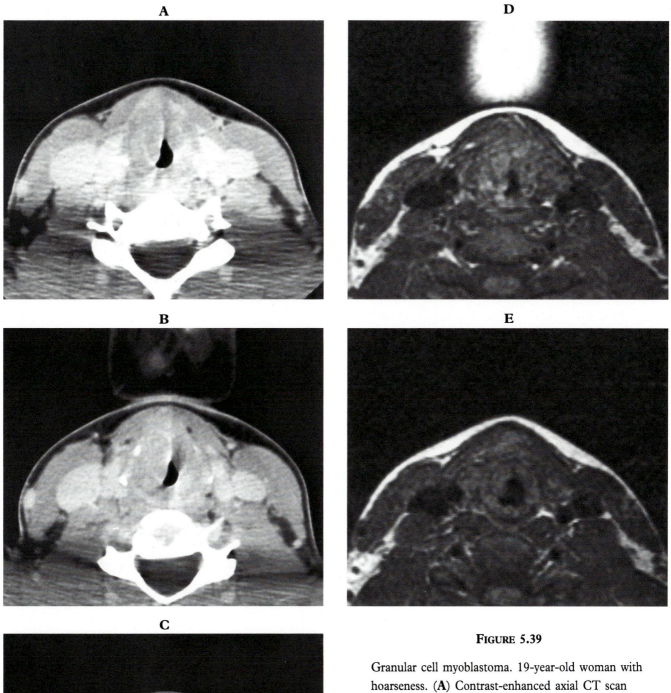

FIGURE 5.39

Granular cell myoblastoma. 19-year-old woman with hoarseness. (**A**) Contrast-enhanced axial CT scan reveals an extensive, circumferential glottic mass with extension anteriorly into the neck. Also note supraglottic extension (**B**) and subglottic extension (**C**) of the tumor. The tumor enhances homogeneously. No calcified thyroid cartilage is seen. (**D,E**) T1-weighted (TR = 500 ms, TE = 20 ms) axial MR images. The signal intensity of the transglottic mass is higher than that of muscle. Tumor extension into the strap muscles as well as into the subglottic region is well demonstrated (**E**).

continued

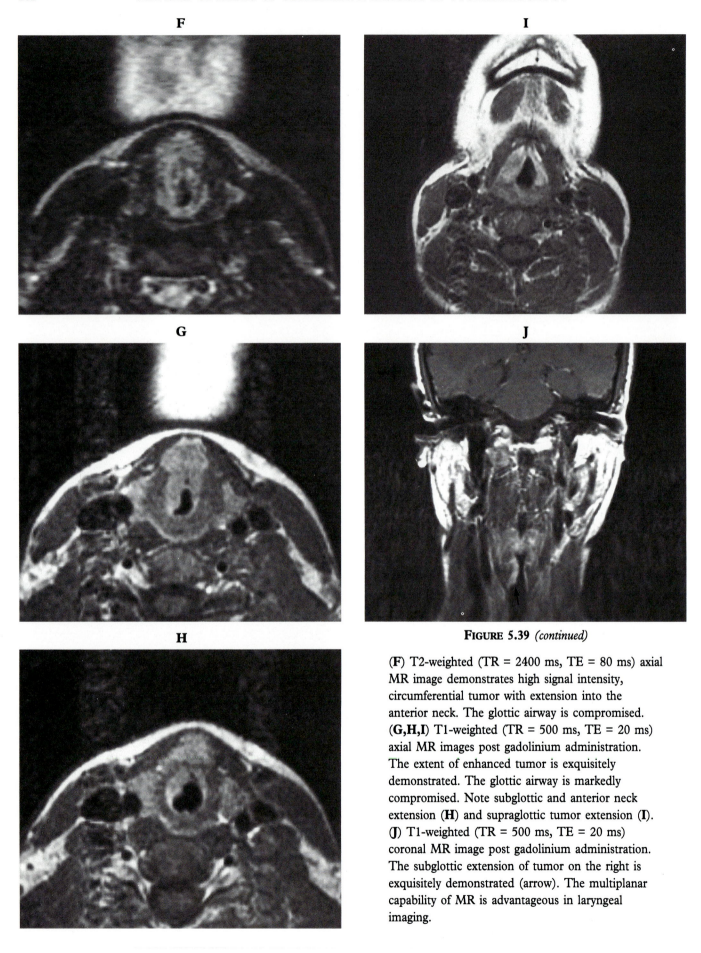

FIGURE 5.39 *(continued)*

(**F**) T2-weighted (TR = 2400 ms, TE = 80 ms) axial MR image demonstrates high signal intensity, circumferential tumor with extension into the anterior neck. The glottic airway is compromised. (**G,H,I**) T1-weighted (TR = 500 ms, TE = 20 ms) axial MR images post gadolinium administration. The extent of enhanced tumor is exquisitely demonstrated. The glottic airway is markedly compromised. Note subglottic and anterior neck extension (**H**) and supraglottic tumor extension (**I**). (**J**) T1-weighted (TR = 500 ms, TE = 20 ms) coronal MR image post gadolinium administration. The subglottic extension of tumor on the right is exquisitely demonstrated (arrow). The multiplanar capability of MR is advantageous in laryngeal imaging.

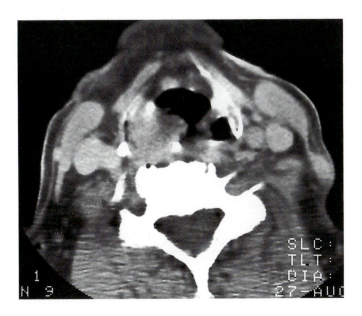

FIGURE 5.40

Supraglottic papilloma. Contrast-enhanced axial CT scan shows a large, lobulated, homogeneous mass involving the right ary-epiglottic fold. The appearance of this mass cannot be differentiated from that of carcinoma.

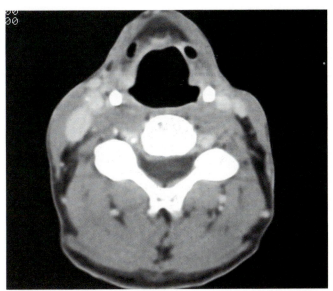

FIGURE 5.41

Laryngocele. Axial CT scan shows bilateral dilated laryngeal saccules consistent with small internal laryngoceles.

A

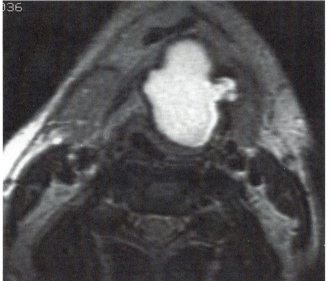

A

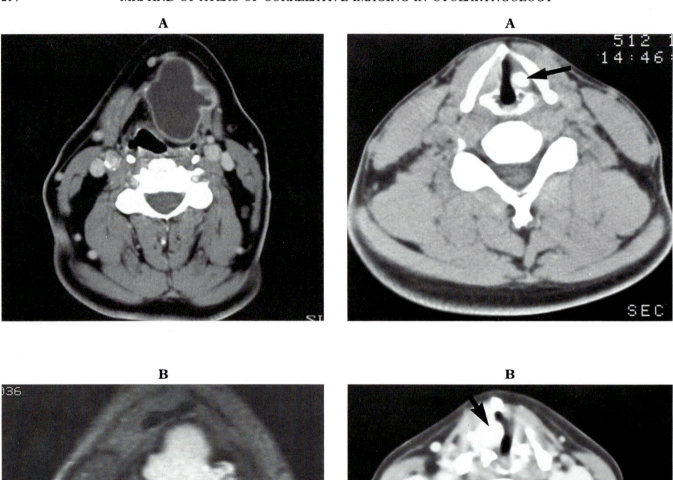

B

B

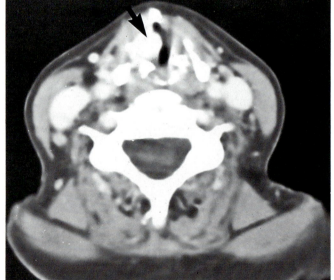

FIGURE 5.42

Laryngocele (saccular cyst). (**A**) Axial CT scan in a
56-year-old man reveals a large, low-density mass
with a thin rim, extending into the anterior neck
through the thyrohyoid membrane. The internal
component of the mass compresses the left pyriform
sinus and displaces the laryngeal vestibule. (**B**) T2-
weighted (TR = 2500 ms, TE = 80 ms) axial MR
image shows a high signal intensity mass consistent
with a fluid-filled laryngocele or a saccular cyst.

FIGURE 5.43

Vocal cord Teflon implant. (**A**) Axial CT scan in a
37-year-old man with paralyzed right vocal cord
shows dense radiopaque Teflon paste (arrow).
(**B**) 53-year-old woman with left vocal cord paralysis.
Axial CT scan demonstrates excessive amount of
Teflon paste in the left vocal cord (arrow) with slight
narrowing of the rima glottidis.

A

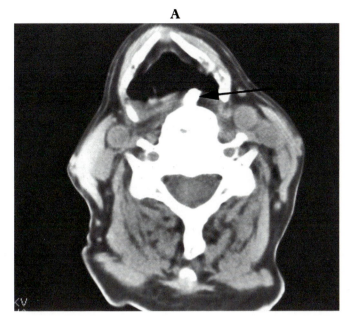

A

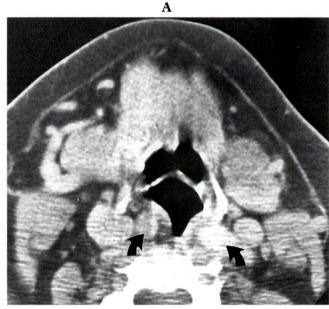

B

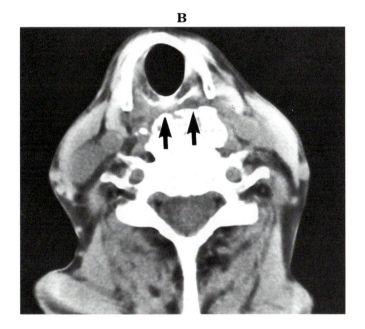

B

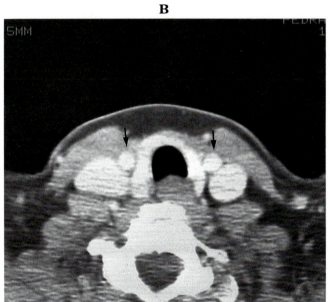

FIGURE 5.44

Cervical osteophytes. 75-year-old man with dysphagia. (**A,B**) Axial CT scan demonstrates large osteophytes (long arrow) impinging on the posterior pharyngeal margin. (**B**) Axial CT scan at the level of the cricoid cartilage shows extensive hypertrophic osteophytic changes compromising the post-cricoid region (arrows).

FIGURE 5.45

Aberrant carotid artery position. (**A**) Axial CT scan shows enhancing carotid artery in a medial position bilaterally, more prominent on the right and bulging into the posterior margin of the pharynx (curved arrows). (**B**) Axial CT scan at the level of the thyroid gland. The carotid arteries (small arrows) are located anterior to the jugular veins bilaterally. The normal location is medial to the jugular vein at this level.

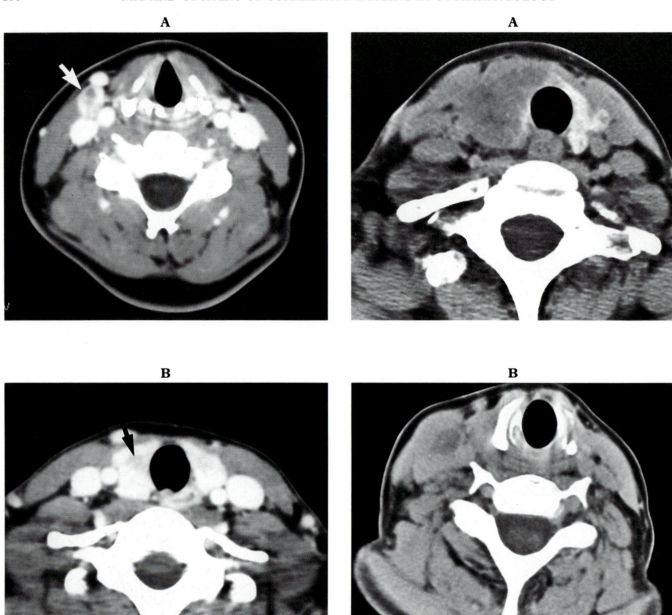

FIGURE 5.46

Papillary carcinoma of thyroid. 35-year-old woman presented with a neck mass. (**A**) Contrast-enhanced axial CT scan shows enhancing nodal metastases in the right neck (arrow). (**B**) Papillary carcinoma, the primary tumor, is seen as a small focus of low density in the right lobe of the thyroid gland (arrow).

FIGURE 5.47

Thyroid carcinoma. Contrast-enhanced axial CT scan. (**A**) The right lobe of the thyroid gland and isthmus are replaced by a low-density mass with ill-defined margins. (**B**) A low-density metastatic node is seen in the right midjugular region.

A

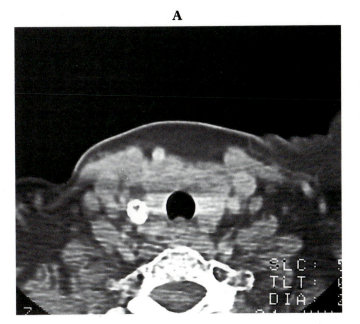

C

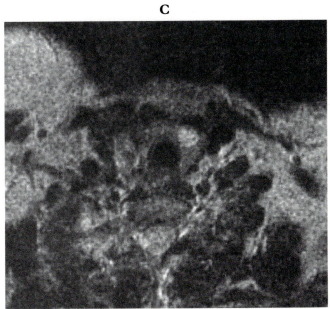

B

FIGURE 5.48

Adenomatous goiter with microscopic foci of papillary carcinoma in both lobes. (**A**) Contrast-enhanced CT scan shows a diffusely enlarged thyroid with a focus of ring-like calcification in the right lobe. (**B,C**) T1- and T2-weighted axial MR images (TR = 600 ms, TE = 20 ms and TR = 2000 ms, TE = 80 ms) reveal a diffusely enlarged, slightly inhomogeneous thyroid gland. T2-weighted image (**C**) shows several foci of high signal intensity. The lower signal focus in the right lobe represents calcification.

A

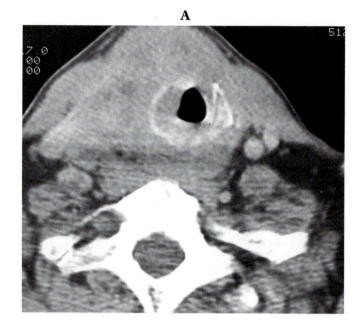

B

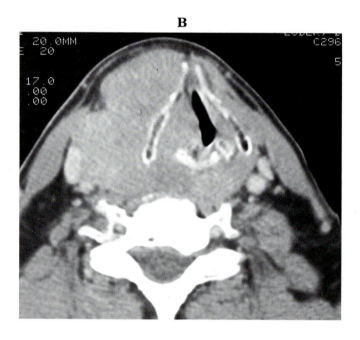

Thyroid lymphoma. (**A,B**) Contrast-enhanced axial CT scans show a large, circumferential homogeneous mass involving the thyroid gland with extension to the postcricoid region. Note intralaryngeal spread through the thyroarytenoid gap on the right (**B**).

A

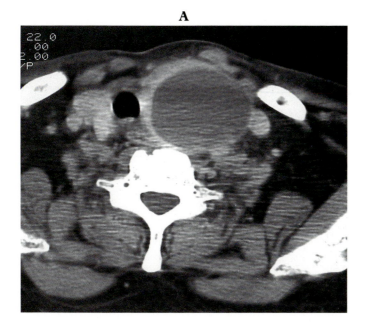

C

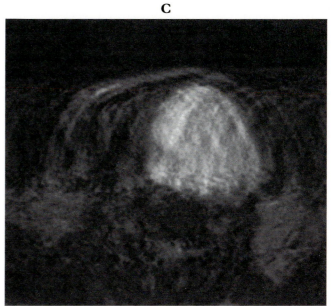

B

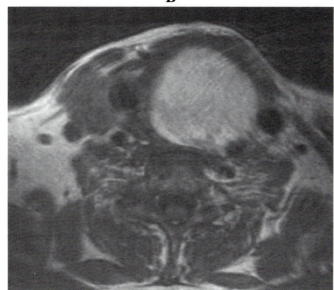

FIGURE 5.50

Thyroid cyst. (**A**) Contrast-enhanced axial CT scan demonstrates a large, well-circumscribed, low-density mass arising from the left thyroid lobe. The laryngeal skeleton is deviated to the right. The left jugular vein and carotid artery are displaced postero-laterally. (**B,C**) Axial T1-weighted (TR = 650 ms, TE = 15 ms) MR image reveals a large, cystic mass with high signal intensity. The T2-weighted image (**C**) (TR = 2100 ms, TE = 80 ms) was degraded by patient motion. The colloid cyst shows high signal intensity.

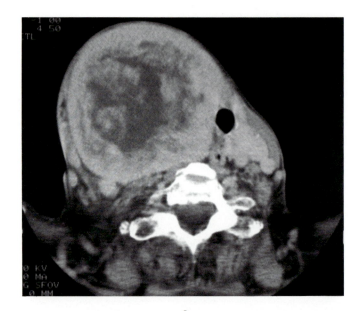

A

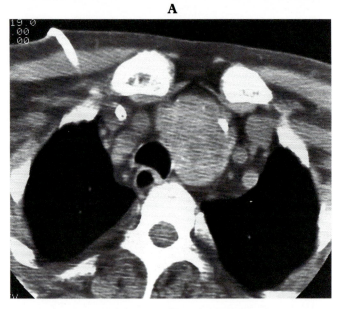

B

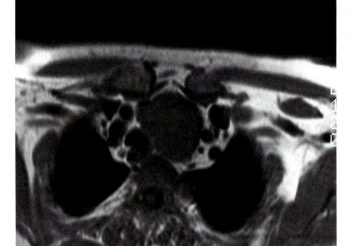

C

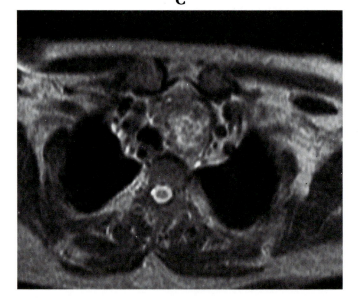

FIGURE 5.51

Multinodular goiter. Axial CT scan demonstrates a gigantic goiter involving predominantly the right thyroid lobe and the isthmus. Note inhomogeneity throughout the mass with central areas of low density. Cystic degeneration, hemorrhage and infarction were seen on histopathology. The trachea and esophagus are deviated to the left.

FIGURE 5.52

Substernal goiter. 65-year-old woman with tracheal deviation detected on a routine chest radiograph. (A) Axial CT scan shows a large inhomogeneous mass contiguous with the left lobe of the thyroid gland. Foci of high and low attenuation are noted. Speckled calcification is seen. The trachea and esophagus are deviated to the right. (B) Axial T1-weighted MR scan (TR = 700 ms, TE = 12 ms). The mediastinal mass is inhomogeneous and reveals low signal intensity with scattered foci of high signal. (C) Axial T2-weighted image (TR = 2000 ms, TE = 80 ms). The mass demonstrates a mixed signal pattern. The low-density areas on CT correspond to the high signal areas on this image.

A

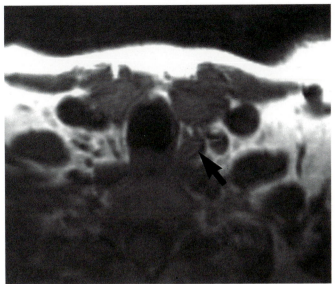

B

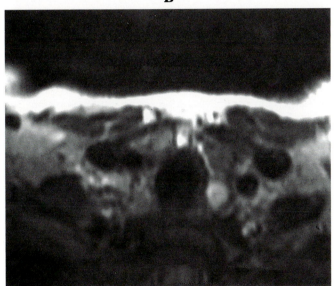

FIGURE 5.53

Parathyroid adenoma. (**A**) Axial T1-weighted (TR = 600 ms, TE = 25 ms) MR scan shows a well-circumscribed mass with low signal intensity in the left tracheo-esophageal groove (arrow). (**B**) Axial T2-weighted MR scan (TR = 2000 ms, TE = 70 ms). The mass shows high signal intensity.

A

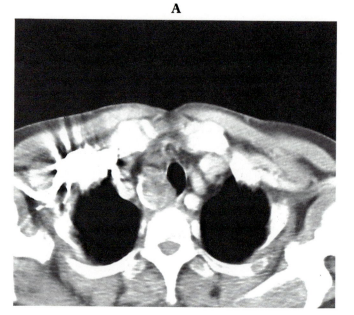

C

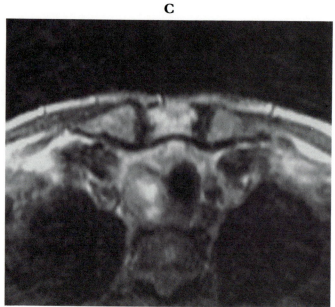

B

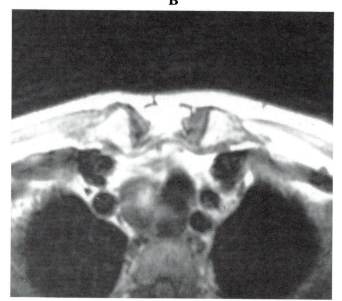

FIGURE 5.54

Parathyroid adenoma. (**A**) Axial CT scan shows a large right paratracheal mass in the substernal region with a peripheral calcific rim. (**B**) Axial T1-weighted MR scan (TR = 600 ms, TE = 20 ms) demonstrates a well-circumscribed mass of intermediate signal intensity with a few foci of high signal intensity. (**C**) Axial T2-weighted MR image (TR = 2000 ms, TE = 80 ms). Focal areas of hemorrhage show high signal intensity on both T1- and T2-weighted images.

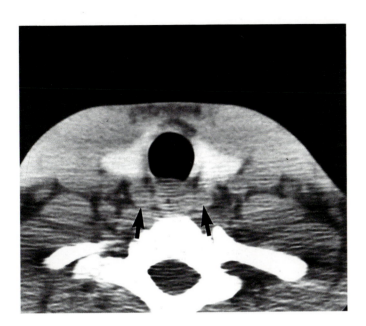

FIGURE 5.55

Parathyroid gland hyperplasia. 57-year-old woman with chronic renal failure and secondary hyperparathyroidism. Axial CT scan shows soft tissue masses measuring about 1 cm each in the tracheo-esophageal groove behind the thyroid gland bilaterally (arrows), representing hyperplastic parathyroid glands.

CHAPTER 6

TEMPOROMANDIBULAR JOINT

Introduction

Temporomandibular joint (TMJ) dysfunction, which is frequently accompanied by pain, is a common and significant clinical problem. Recent advances in imaging technology have greatly contributed to the understanding of diseases of the TMJ. Craniofacial pain related to the TMJ region affects approximately 28% of the population, with a striking predilection in women.[1] Common symptoms of TMJ dysfunction or internal derangement are headache, earache, joint clicking and periarticular pain. Clinical signs of TMJ dysfunction include audible clicking, decreased range of motion and pain to palpation.[2]

The TMJ is affected by a multitude of abnormalities with internal derangement the most common.[3–6] In most cases the exact cause of the internal derangement is, at best, obscure; however, a previous history of trauma is present in 25% of cases. Traumatically induced internal derangement is more common in men and children than in women. Iatrogenic cases are responsible for approximately 30% of trauma-induced internal derangement.[7] Procedures that necessitate jaw hyperextension, such as tonsillectomy, endoscopy and molar tooth extraction, are the most frequently implicated.

Imaging of the TMJ has been revolutionized with the advent of magnetic resonance (MR). The major advantage of MR is consistent visualization of internal joint architecture including the TMJ disk. Magnetic resonance also offers information on bony abnormalities of the articular eminence and mandibular condyle. Prior to the use of MR, plain films, plain film tomography, arthrography and arthro- tomography, and computed tomography (CT) were the modalities utilized in TMJ evaluation. In combination, these studies were capable of assessing the TMJ for pathology. Magnetic resonance imaging has now replaced these modalities as the imaging study of choice in the evaluation of TMJ-related symptoms.

Normal anatomy

The functional components of the TMJ include the TMJ disk and the articulating surfaces of the mandibular condyle and temporal bone (glenoid fossa and articular eminence). The TMJ is a synovial joint which is divided into superior and inferior joint compartments by the TMJ disk. The superior and inferior joint compartments do not communicate in the normal joint.

The TMJ disk is normally a biconcave fibrocartilaginous structure positioned between the articulating surfaces of the temporal bone superiorly and the mandibular condyle inferiorly. Dynamic stability is provided to the disk by several firm attachments. The posterior ligament (bilaminar zone) attaches the posterior band of the disk to the condyle and the temporal bone. These retrodiskal ligaments have a rich neurovascular supply and are the source of joint proprioception. The superior retrodiskal lamina is elastic and opposes the normal tension of the lateral pterygoid muscle. Fibers from the upper belly of the lateral pterygoid muscle attach to the anterior medial portion of the anterior band of the disk. Additional attachments to the joint capsule are present anteriorly, medially and laterally.[8] Normal disk morphology demonstrates three distinct segments. These include the anterior and posterior bands, which are thick, and a thin intermediate zone which joins the anterior and posterior segments. In the closed mouth position, the posterior band is normally situated at the 12 o'clock position relative to the mandibular condyle.

Normal TMJ function requires synchronized and coordinated motion of the disk, condyle, and the muscles of mastication. Temporomandibular joint motion is composed of two concurrent actions. With jaw opening, the disk rotates posteriorly on the condyle. Simultaneously, the condyle–disk complex translates anterior and inferior to a final position beneath the articular eminence of the temporal bone.[7] In the full open mouth position, the disk assumes a 'bow-tie' configuration, with the thin intermediate zone normally situated between the adjacent articulating surfaces of the mandibular condyle and the articular eminence (Fig. 6.1).

Imaging strategies

Radiologic imaging of the TMJ has greatly contributed to the development of the current concepts of normal and abnormal TMJ function. Magnetic resonance, which provides the most accurate assessment of the TMJ, has become the modality of choice in the initial evaluation of internal derangement.

There are five imaging modalities currently available for imaging of the TMJ. These are plain films, plain film tomography, arthrography, computed tomography and magnetic resonance imaging.

Plain radiography

Routine plain film examination of the TMJ consists of transcranial views of the TMJ in both the closed and open mouth positions. Plain films routinely demonstrate the glenoid fossa, the articular eminence, the mandibular condyle, and the relationship of these structures to each other. Positive plain film findings include decreased translation, spurring and eburnation (consistent with degenerative osteoarthritis) and less frequently, calcified loose bodies. The obvious disadvantage of plain film radiography is its inability to demonstrate internal joint architecture.

Arthrography

Prior to MR, arthrography was the standard in the evaluation of internal derangement. In the mid-1940s, Norgaard[9] pioneered the procedure which later became popular in the 1970s. Through the years, several TMJ arthrographic procedures have been developed and described.[10–17] In general, the procedure is performed under fluoroscopic guidance following local anesthesia. Using a pre-auricular approach, the posterior recess of the lower synovial compartment is punctured and opacified with approximately 0.5 ml of contrast media. Some radiologists advocate upper and lower compartment opacification. Static images, tomography, and video-fluoroscopy may be utilized to image the joint. Comparable and accurate information about disk position and shape is equally provided by arthrography as compared to MR. Arthrography is superior to MR in the detection of capsular adhesions and disk perforation. Disadvantages of arthrography include exposure to ionizing radiation, its invasive nature, indirect disk assessment and the expertise required to perform the study.[8,18–20]

Computed tomography

Prior to the advent of MR, the literature was replete with the use of CT in the evaluation of TMJ dysfunction. High resolution CT is preferable to plain film and pleuridirectional tomography as it allows better bone and soft tissue detail. The radiation dose to the skin with CT is comparable to that with plain film examination, and pleuridirectional tomography. Direct sagittal CT images of the TMJ are obtained by positioning the patient on a 45° lumbar sponge in the decubitus position. Disadvantages of CT include uncomfortable patient position, ionizing radiation and suboptimal resolution of the disk, particularly when compared to MR. Advantages, however, include its non-invasive nature and the ability to display bony detail. Magnetic resonance has replaced CT as the primary modality for imaging the TMJ.

Magnetic resonance imaging

Magnetic resonance offers direct visualization of the TMJ disk, is non-invasive, allows direct multiplanar imaging and does not utilize ionizing radiation.

Shortcomings which are inherent to MR include susceptibility to motion and other artifacts and the lack of bony detail. Magnetic resonance routinely demonstrates the TMJ disk and condylar translation. Modern MR imaging of the TMJ requires the use of surface coils. Small diameter coils are preferable as the signal-to-noise ratio (SNR) varies inversely with coil diameter. Dual surface coils allow simultaneous bilateral imaging which significantly decreases examination time.

Routine examination of the TMJ consists of T1-weighted spin-echo coronal or axial localizer and T1-weighted spin-echo sagittal images in closed and open mouth positions. Short TR/TE (T1-weighted) spin-echo pulse sequences allow maximum utilization of inherent soft tissue contrast by enhancing differences in T1 relaxation times present in the TMJ region. The TMJ disk reveals low signal intensity in contrast to the high signal from the fibrofatty tissue in the bilaminar zone (Fig. 6.2).

When the TMJ is affected by inflammation, infection or tumor, additional information can be obtained utilizing long repetition time (TR)/echo delay time (TE) spin-echo and gradient-echo pulse sequences. The long TR/TE pulse sequence will increase signal intensity from abnormal tissues with high water content. Joint effusions, pannus and edema become quite apparent.

Gradient-echo techniques utilize small flip angles and allow 'rapid' or 'fast' scanning. Although this technique is highly sensitive to intra-articular fluid, magnetic susceptibility, chemical shift and blood flow artifacts are prominent, leading to reduced diagnostic quality of the image.[21] The conventional long TR/TE spin-echo technique remains the most sensitive in the detection of joint fluid. Recent investigators recommend long TR with both short and long TE spin-echo closed mouth sagittal images combined with gradient-echo closed and open mouth views whenever inflammatory disease of the TMJ is suspected.[22]

The gradient-echo technique can offer information on the dynamic nature of common abnormalities such as meniscal recapture. In this technique, static images are obtained at progressive increments of mouth opening. These images are sequentially placed in video memory and then displayed in a back-and-forth closed cine-loop. The information gained from the cine-loop is often complementary to the conventional spin-echo study.[21]

Three-dimensional volume acquisition gradient-echo imaging can produce ultrathin contiguous slices with a high SNR which can potentially enhance resolution but suffers from magnetic susceptibility artifact. Rao et al utilized a short TE of 5–7 ms, using nearly symmetrical data acquisition to minimize the susceptibility artifact, and compared the images obtained with conventional spin-echo images. It was concluded that spin-echo images were superior.[23] In a later study, high-resolution T1-weighted thin slice (1.8 mm slice thickness) spin-echo images were shown to be preferable to conventional T1-weighted 3 mm thick SE sections.[24] The TMJ disk was better visualized and on a greater number of sections without penalty in additional imaging time with the high resolution technique.[24]

Currently MR of the TMJ is recommended as the initial imaging study for the evaluation of internal derangement. However, multimodality imaging is often helpful in the evaluation of TMJ-related symptoms. Plain films can provide additional information in the detection of inflammatory arthritis, tumors, post-traumatic deformity, and congenital malformations. Disk perforations and disk dynamics are best demonstrated with arthrography, although there is a 20% false positive rate for disk perforation.[25] Finally, CT may add exquisite bony detail in those cases where plain films are inadequate or inconclusive.

Pathology

Internal derangement

Internal derangement is defined as an abnormal relationship of the TMJ disk to the mandibular condyle, articular eminence and glenoid fossa. This disorder is three to five times more common in women with symptoms typically appearing in the fourth decade of life.[25] The exact etiology of internal derangement is unclear, although a recent trauma history can sometimes be elicited.

Internal derangement has been classically categorized progressing from least to most severe.[3,4,26] The categories are: (A) anterior or anteromedial disk displacement with recapture on mouth opening (Fig. 6.3); (B) anterior or anteromedial displacement without recapture on mouth opening (Fig. 6.4); and (C) chronic anterior or anteromedial disk displacement with perforation at the posterior attachment of the disk to the bilaminar zone or in the bilaminar zone itself. The disk may occasionally be displaced medially. Clinically, patients also manifest a typical history of sequential progression from one category to the next. The 'popping' or 'clicking' is a manifestation of disk recapture and is typical of category A, internal derangement. Although this clicking is reciprocal (present on both opening and closing), it is most pronounced on mouth opening. Translation is typically normal.

As the elastic fibers in the bilaminar zone become stretched and lose elasticity, the disk no longer recaptures with jaw opening and it remains anteriorly displaced (category B). These patients will have some degree of diminished translation or no translation (closed lock). Usually, there is no complaint of clicking at this stage. Chronic disk displacement may lead to perforation, usually at the posterior attachment or in the bilaminar zone (category C). The disk remains far forward displaced and no longer causes mechanical interference with the condylar translation. Thus, there may not be decreased range of motion. Direct friction between the condyle and articular eminence predisposes these patients to degenerative changes of the temporomandibular joint.

Arthropathies

Temporomandibular joint arthritis is a relatively common clinical problem. Many patients with TMJ arthritis have osteoarthritis, usually as the result of internal derangement. Other causes of TMJ arthritis include the rheumatoid arthropathies, gout,[27] calcium pyrophosphate dihydrate crystal deposition disease[28] and infection.[29]

Osteoarthritis

Osteoarthritis of the TMJ may result in narrowing, erosion, eburnation, osteophytosis and remodeling. Osteophytes typically develop at the margins of the articular surfaces of the mandibular condyle and the glenoid fossa.

Osteoarthritis of the TMJ is not necessarily a disease of the aging process. It is well recognized that many cases of TMJ osteoarthritis are the result of internal derangement.[30–33] As many as 20% of patients with internal derangement have osteoarthritis at the time of initial presentation.[33] Osteoarthritis becomes more common with increasing duration of internal derangement and is closely associated with disk dislocation, locking and perforation (Fig. 6.5). An association between the hypoplastic, pointed or regressively remodeled condyle and internal derangement is reported.[34]

Rheumatoid arthritis

Rheumatoid arthritis involving the TMJ is not uncommon and sometimes patients with rheumatoid arthritis initially seek dental help due to the TMJ-related symptoms. Radiographic changes of rheumatoid arthritis include erosions, osteoporosis, narrowing, decreased range of motion and flattening of the glenoid fossa and condylar head. These radiographic changes are more apparent on CT than on routine radiographs. Magnetic resonance imaging is helpful in demonstrating joint effusions, pannus formation, position and morphology of the disk (Fig. 6.6).

Rheumatoid arthritis, psoriatic arthritis, ankylosing spondylitis and systemic lupus erythematosis may all affect the TMJ and they may be clinically and radiographically indistinguishable.[3]

Infectious arthritis

Infections of the TMJ may be pyogenic or granulomatous. These disorders are rare.[29] Most commonly, infection of the TMJ is the result of direct extension of oral infection, or following surgery of the TMJ. Although the radiographic appearance of TMJ infection closely resembles that of rheumatoid arthritis, the rapid clinical course and physical examination should suggest the diagnosis.

Avascular necrosis and osteochondritis dissecans

Avascular necrosis (AVN) and osteochondritis dissecans (OCD) of the mandibular condyle are not uncommon, although they frequently go unrecognized.[18,35–39] These two entities share several features. Both involve the articular surfaces of joints and they both may represent a spectrum of the same patho-physiology.[39] Avascular necrosis describes large areas of cortical and medullary infarction with subsequent structural weakening. Osteochondritis dissecans is often the result of a transchondrial fracture with failure of the depressed cortical fragment to heal or reunite. Avascular necrosis and OCD may be clinically indistinguishable and both may be associated with underlying hematologic disorders, skeletal dysplasias, exogenous steroids, chemotherapy, trauma and familial predisposition.[40–43] In many cases of AVN and OCD, a prior history of trauma, surgery or inflammatory arthropathy is present.[22,39,44]

Magnetic resonance imaging has been established as a highly sensitive and accurate procedure for the diagnosis of early AVN and OCD.[39] The typical MR appearance of acute AVN is due to the vascular congestion with resultant fluid transudation into the medullary space. This increase in medullary fluid causes prolongation of T1 and T2 relaxation times, producing decreased T1-weighted signal intensity and increased T2-weighted signal intensity. Magnetic resonance is more accurate than nuclear scintigraphy in detecting these early changes of AVN.[42,45,46] With chronic AVN, the normal fat-containing marrow is replaced by hypointense fibrous tissue and sclerotic bone. This change results in the loss of the normal marrow signal. Computed tomography in AVN is characterized by irregularity and flattening of the mandibular condyle. Increased sclerosis and subchondral cyst formation may be apparent (Figs 6.7 and 6.8).

Acute OCD on MR imaging typically exhibits a hypointense central fragment surrounded by a zone of increased signal on both T1- and T2-weighted images. Variable marrow signal can be seen with longstanding OCD.

Tumors

Tumors of the TMJ are rare[47,48] and malignant tumors are particularly rare.[49,50] Most malignant tumors of the temporomandibular joint are secondary extensions of a mandibular tumor, such as an osteosarcoma or metastasis (Figs 6.9–6.11). Osteochondromas of the TMJ regions are the most common benign tumors (Fig. 6.12). Other benign tumors include osteomas, giant cell tumors, fibrous cortical defects and nonossifying fibromas (Figs 6.13 and 6.14).

Miscellaneous

Non-neoplastic synovial processes may affect the temporomandibular joint. Disease entities such as synovial osteochondromatosis,[51] pigmented villonodular synovitis and ganglion cysts[52] have been described involving the TMJ. These entities are similar in clinical presentation and radiographic appearance when compared with other more commonly involved joints in the body. Ganglion cysts of the TMJ may clinically mimic internal derangement. This is a rare entity with only 10 reported prior cases. The MR appearance of ganglion cysts of the TMJ has been described (Fig. 6.15).[52]

Congenital malformations of the TMJ are uncommon and often associated with anomalies of the external auditory canal and middle ear structures. Malformations of the mandibular condyle may be confused with some of the benign bone tumors. Figure 6.16 is an example of a congenital bifid condyle which mimics an osteochondroma (see Fig. 6.12).

Diffuse bony processes such as fibrous dysplasia, Paget's disease and osteogenesis imperfecta may affect the skull base and often involve the TMJ. Figure 6.17 demonstrates fibrous dysplasia of the temporal bone involving the articular eminence.

Postoperative TMJ

Commonly performed procedures in the management of internal derangement include diskal plication with repositioning of the disk substance to its normal position, and simple diskectomy with or without the placement of a diskal implant. In most cases, diskectomy is followed by the placement of a diskal implant in order to reduce the probability of osteoarthritis, adhesions, and recurrent pain and dysfunction. Various alloplastic and autogenous implants can be utilized. Alloplastic materials include non-porous teflon, silicone and silastic. Autogenous implants include fascial, dermal and rib grafts (Fig. 6.18). The synthetic implants are diamagnetic substances and therefore demonstrate absent signal on all MR pulse sequences.[2] In more advanced cases of internal derangement, condylectomy and reduction osteotomy of the articular eminence (eminectomy) may be necessary.

Magnetic resonance imaging provides direct and noninvasive evaluation of the postoperative TMJ. Magnetic resonance is able to clearly demonstrate postoperative granulation tissue, joint fluid, adhesions and meniscal implants.[37] Magnetic resonance also demonstrates failed TMJ implants which may be the result of foreign body reactions.[38] These destructive reactions have been described with a variety of implant materials and are characterized by erosions which are similar in appearance to those seen in infectious and rheumatoid arthropathies. Plain films are helpful as an adjunctive study in distinguishing joint calcification from hypointense scar tissue and in distinguishing postoperative bony remodeling from ordinary osteoarthritis.

There is a poor correlation between the postoperative clinical symptoms and the appearance of the postoperative TMJ. Although the postoperative MRI demonstrates little if any change when compared with the preoperative MRI, patients often report remarkable improvement in their symptoms.[53]

References

1   Harms SE, Wilk RM, Magnetic resonance imaging of the temporomandibular joint, *Radiographics* (1987) **7**:521.

2   Hasso AN, Christiansen EL, Alder ME, The temporomandibular joint, *Radiol Clin North Am* (1989) **27**:301–14.

3   Murphy WA, The temporomandibular joint. In: Resnick D, Niwayama G, eds., *Diagnosis of bone and joint disorders*, 2nd edn (WB Saunders: Philadelphia 1988) 1816–63.

4   Manzione JV, Katzberg RW, Manzione TF, Internal derangement of the temporomandibular joint. 1. Normal anatomy, physiology, and pathophysiology, *Int J Periodontol Rest Dent* (1984) **4**:9–27.

5   Solberg WK, Woo MW, Houston JB, Prevalence of mandibular dysfunction in young adults, *J Am Dent Assoc* (1979) **98**:25–34.

6   Morgan DH, The great imposter: disease of the temporomandibular joint, *J Am Med Assoc* (1976) **235**:2395 (comment).

7   Sherry CS, Harms SE, The temporomandibular joint. In: Bassett LW, Gold RH, Seeger LL, eds, *MR atlas of the musculoskeletal system* (M. Dunitz: London 1989) 59–94.

8   Katzberg RW, Temporomandibular joint imaging, *Radiology* (1989) **170**:297–307.

9   Norgaard F, Arthrography of the temporomandibular joint, *Acta Radiol (Diagn) (Stockh)* (1987) **25**:679–85.

10   Lynch TP, Chase DC, Arthrography in the evaluation of the temporomandibular joint, *Radiology* (1987) **126**:667–72.

11   Katzberg RW, Dolwick MF, Bales DJ et al, Arthrotomography of the TMJ: new technique and preliminary observations, *AJR* (1979) **132**:949–55.

12   Murphy WA, Arthrography of the temporomandibular joint, *Radiol Clin North Am* (1981) **19**:365–78.

13   Dolwick MF, Katzberg RW, Bales DJ et al, Arthrotomographic evaluation of the temporomandibular joint, *J Oral Maxillofac Surg* (1979) **37**:793–800.

14   Westesson PL, Rohlin M, Diagnostic accuracy of double-contrast arthrotomography of the temporomandibular joint: correlation with post-mortem morphology, *AJNR* (1984) **5**:463–8.

15   Campbell RL, Alexander JM, Temporomandibular joint arthrography: negative pressure, non-tomographic techniques, *Oral Surg Oral Med Oral Pathol* (1983) **55**:121–6.

16   Bell KA, Walters PJ, Video fluoroscopy during arthroscopy of the temporomandibular joint, *Radiology* (1983) **147**:879.

17   Jacobs JM, Manaster BJ, Digital subtraction arthrography of the temporomandibular joint, *AJR* (1987) **148**:344–6.

18   Schellhas KP, Wilkes CH, Omile MR, Diagnosis of temporomandibular joint disease: two compartment arthrography and MR, *AJNR* (1988) **151**:341–50.

19   Kaplan PA, Helms CA, Current status of temporomandibular joint imaging for the diagnosis of internal derangement, *AJR* (1989) **152**:697–705.

20   Rao VM, Farole A, Karasick D, Temporomandibular joint dysfunction: correlation of MR imaging, arthrography and arthroscopy, *Radiology* (1990) **174**:663–7.

21 BURNETT KR, DAVIS CL, READ J, Dynamic display of the temporomandibular joint meniscus by using 'fast-scan' MR imaging, *AJR* (1987) **149**:959–62.

22 SCHELLHAS KP, WILKES CH, Temporomandibular joint inflammation: comparison of MR fast scanning with T1- and T2-weighted imaging techniques, *AJR* (1989) **153**:93–8.

23 RAO VM, VINITSKI S, BABARIA A, Comparison of SE and short TE three dimensional gradient echo imaging of the temporomandibular region, *Radiology* (1989) **173(P)**:99 (abst).

24 RAO VM, VINITSKI S, TOM BM, High resolution spin echo imaging of TMJ, *Radiology* (1990) **177(P)**:126 (abst).

25 HELMS CA, KAPLAN PA, Diagnostic imaging of the various techniques, *AJR* (1990) **154**:319–22.

26 PALACIOS E, VALVASSORI GE, SHANNON M, Internal derangement and other pathology. In: Palacios E, Valvassori GE, Shannon M, Reed CF, eds, *Magnetic Resonance of the Temporomandibular Joint* (Thieme Medical Publishers: New York 1990) 75–121.

27 CHUN HH, Temporomandibular joint gout, *J Am Med Assoc* (1973) **226**:253 (letter to ed).

28 GOOD AE, UPTON LG, Acute temporomandibular arthritis in a patient with bruxism and calcium pyrophosphate deposition disease, *Arthritis Rheum* (1982) **25**:353–5.

29 CHUE PWY, Gonococcal arthritis of the temporomandibular joint, *Oral Surg* (1975) **39**:572–7.

30 TOLLER PA, Osteoarthrosis of the mandibular condyle, *Br Dent J* (1973) **134**:223.

31 WEINBERG LA, Practical evaluation of the lateral temporomandibular joint radiograph, *J Prosthet Dent* (1984) **51**:676–85.

32 ANDERSON QN, KATZBERG RW, Pathologic evaluation of disk dysfunction and osseous abnormalities of the temporomandibular joint, *Maxillofac Surg* (1985) **43**:947.

33 KATZBERG RW, KEITH DA, GURALNICK WC, Internal derangements and arthritis of the temporomandibular joint, *Radiology* (1983) **146**:107–12.

34 RAO VM, BABARIA A, MANDHARAN A ET AL, Altered condylar morphology associated with disk displacement in TMJ dysfunction: observations by MRI, *Magn Reson Imaging* (1990) **8**:231–5.

35 REISKIN AB, Aseptic necrosis of the mandibular condyle: a common problem? *Quintessence Int* (1979) **2**:85–9.

36 BEHRMAN SJ, Complications of saggital osteotomy of the mandibular ramus, *J Oral Surg* (1972) **30**:554–61.

37 SCHELLHAS KP, WILKES CH, DEEB M, Temporomandibular joint: MR imaging of internal derangements and post-operative changes, *AJNR* (1987) **8**:1093–101; *AJR* (1988) **150**:381–9.

38 SCHELLHAS KP, WILKES CH, DEEB M, Permanent proplast temporomandibular joint implants: MR imaging of destructive complications, *AJR* (1988) **151**:731–5.

39 SCHELLHAS KP, WILKES CH, FRITTS HM, MR of osteochondritis dissecans and avascular necrosis of the mandibular condyle, *AJNR* (1989) **152**:551–60.

40 TOTTY WG, MURPHY WA, GANZ WI, Magnetic resonance imaging of the normal and ischemic femoral head, *AJR* (1984) **143**:1273–80.

41 GILLESPY T III, GENANT HK, HELMS CA, Magnetic resonance imaging of osteonecrosis, *Radiol Clin North Am* (1986) **24**:193–208.

42 MITCHELL DG, RAO VM, DALINKA MK, Femoral head avascular necrosis, correlation of MR imaging, radiographic staging, radionuclide imaging, and clinical findings, *Radiology* (1987) **162**:709–15.

43 SWEET DE, MADEWELL JE, Pathogenesis of osteonecrosis. In: Resnick DK, Niwayama G, eds, *Diagnosis of bone and joint disorders* (WB Saunders: Philadelphia 1988) 3188–237.

44 SCHELLHAS KP, Temporomandibular joint injuries, *Radiology* (1989) **173**:211–16.

45 MITCHELL MD, KUNDEL HL, STEINBERG ME, Avascular necrosis of the hip: comparison of MR, CT, and scintigraphy, *AJR* (1986) **147**:67–71.

46 BELTRAN J, HERMAN LJ, BURK JM, Femoral head avascular necrosis: MR imaging with clinical-pathologic and radionuclide correlation, *Radiology* (1988) **166**:215–20.

47 NWOKU ALN, KOCH H, Temporomandibular joint: a rare localization for bone tumors, *J Maxillofac Surg* (1974) **2**:113.

48 THOMAS KH, Tumors of the condyle and temporomandibular joint, *Oral Surg* (1954) **7**:1091.

49 HARTMAN GL, ROBERTSON GR, SUGG JR, WE, Metastatic carcinoma of the mandibular condyle: report of case, *J Oral Surg* (1973) **31**:716–19.

50   RICHTER KJ, FREEMAN NS, QUICK CA, Chondrosarcoma of the temporomandibular joint: report of case, *J Oral Surg* (1974) **32**:777–81.

51   BLANKESTIJN J, PANDERS AK, VERNEY A, Synovial chondromatosis of the temporomandibular joint. Report of three cases and review of the literature, *Cancer* (1985) **55**:479.

52   TOM BM, RAO VM, FAROLE A, Bilateral temporomandibular ganglion cysts: CT and MR characteristics, *AJNR* (1990) **11**:746–9.

53   RAO VM, FAROLE A, TOM BM, Comparison of pre- and postoperative MR imaging of internal derangement of the temporomandibular joint: correlation with clinical symptoms, *Radiology* (1990) **177(P)**:127.

A

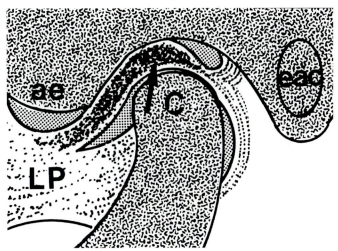

B

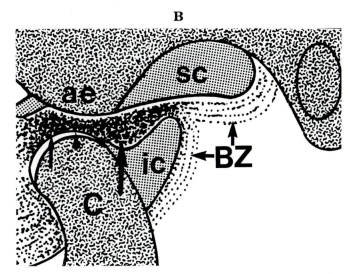

FIGURE 6.1

Normal anatomy of the TMJ. (**A**) In the closed mouth position, the mandibular condyle (C) is situated within the glenoid fossa. The posterior band of the temporomandibular joint disk (large arrow) is normally situated at the 12 o'clock position relative to the condyle. (**B**) With jaw opening, the mandibular condyle (C) translates anteriorly and is located beneath the articular eminence (ae) of the temporal bone. The TMJ disk assumes a 'bow-tie' configuration, with the thin intermediate zone (arrowhead) interposed between the articulating surfaces of the condyle and the articular eminence. Also note the graphic illustration of the bilaminar zone (BZ) which attaches the posterior band of the disk to the condyle and the posterior glenoid fossa. The lateral pterygoid muscle (LP) is depicted with fibers inserting on the anterior band of the disk (small arrow). The superior and inferior synovial joint compartments (sc) and (ic) are also illustrated. eac, external auditory canal.

A

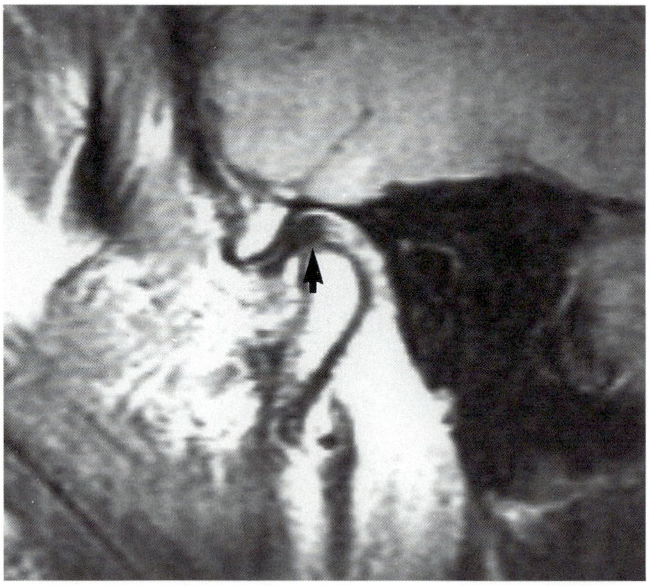

B

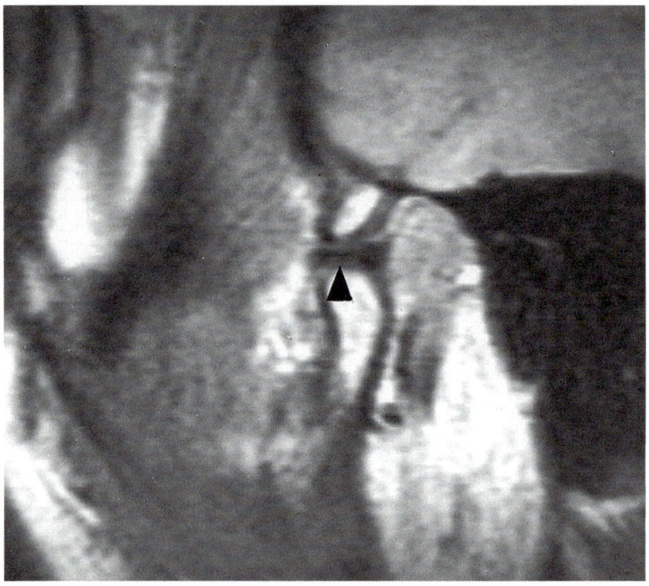

A

B

FIGURE 6.2

Magnetic resonance of the normal TMJ. (**A,B**) Sagittal MR images (TR = 1000 ms, TE = 25 ms) of the right TMJ in the closed and open mouth positions. In the closed mouth orientation, the posterior band of the TMJ disk is normally situated at the 12 o'clock position relative to the mandibular condyle (arrow). With jaw opening, the TMJ disk assumes a 'bow-tie' configuration, with the thin intermediate zone (arrowhead) normally interposed between the mandibular condyle and the articular eminence.

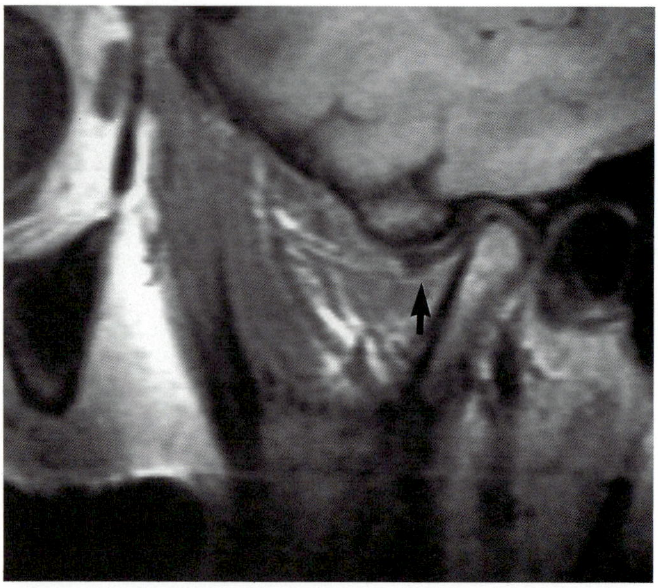

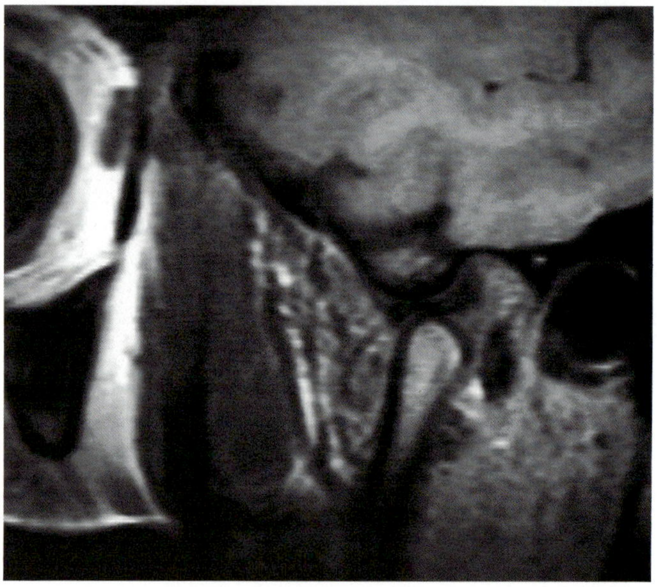

FIGURE 6.3

Internal derangement: anterior displacement with recapture. (**A,B**) Sagittal MR images (TR = 400 ms, TE = 20 ms) of the right TMJ in the closed and open mouth positions. In the closed mouth orientation the TMJ disk (arrow) is anteriorly displaced. With jaw opening, the TMJ disk assumes its normal position.

A

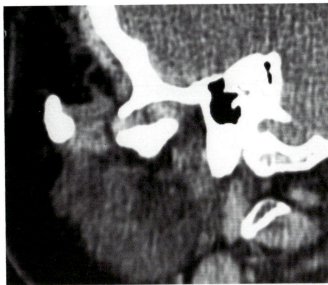

B

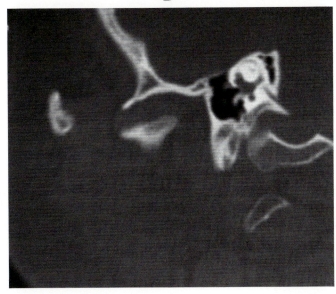

C

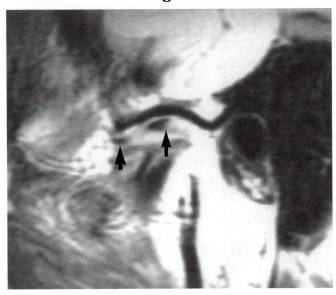

D

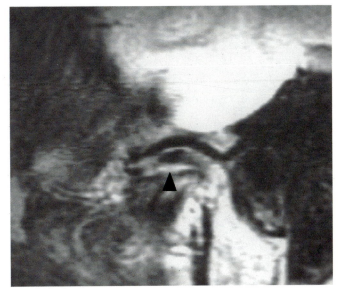

FIGURE 6.6

Computed tomography and MR in rheumatoid arthritis. (**A,B**) Soft tissue and bone window direct sagittal CT of the TMJ. These images demonstrate erosion and flattening of the mandibular condyle. Also note the shallow glenoid fossa. The TMJ disk is not readily apparent on these images. (**C,D**) Sagittal, double-echo T2-weighted images (TR = 2000 ms, TE = 20/80 ms) of the TMJ. The TMJ meniscus is well visualized (arrows), is normally situated, and morphologically intact. The MR again demonstrates the condylar erosion and shallow glenoid fossa. (**D**) Note the pannus (arrowhead) on the long TR/TE sequence.

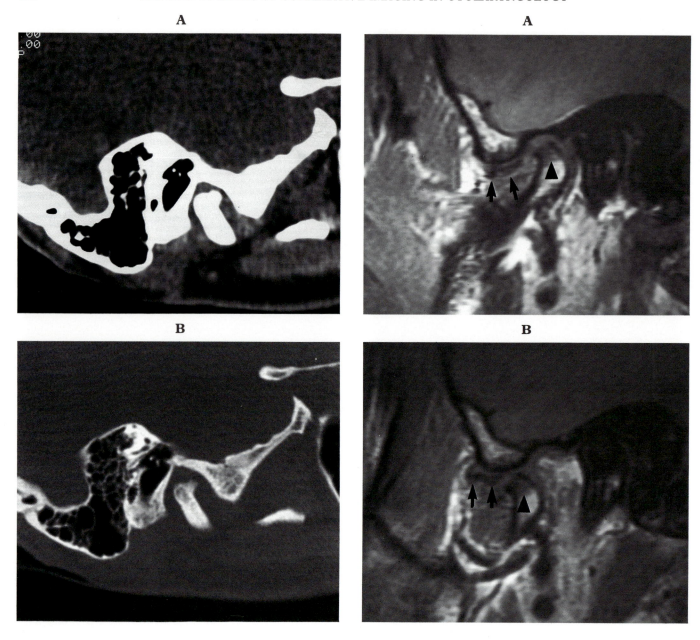

FIGURE 6.7

Avascular necrosis of the left mandibular condyle. (A,B) Soft tissue and bone window settings of the left TMJ demonstrate cortical irregularity and flattening of the mandibular condyle suggesting possible AVN. The exact position and morphology of the TMJ disk is difficult to ascertain.

FIGURE 6.8

Avascular necrosis associated with internal derangement. Sagittal MR images (TR = 700 ms, TE = 25 ms) of the left TMJ. (A) In the closed mouth position, the TMJ disk is anteriorly displaced (arrows). Note the decreased marrow signal in the subchondral bone of the mandibular condyle (arrowhead). (B) With jaw opening, the disk remains anterior (arrows). Again note the decreased marrow signal in the mandibular condyle (arrowhead).

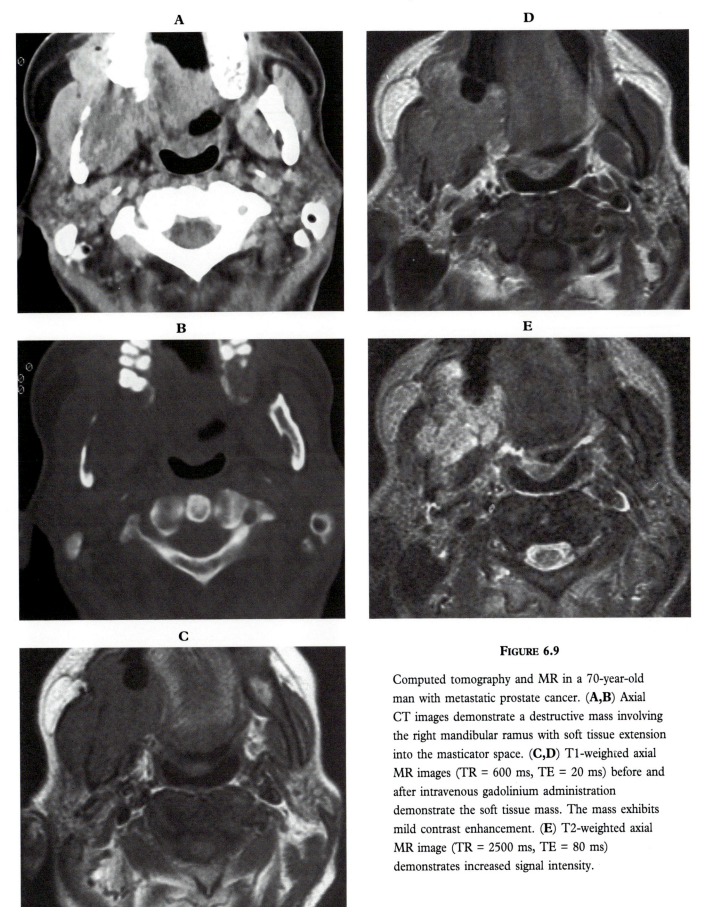

A

B

C

D

E

FIGURE 6.9

Computed tomography and MR in a 70-year-old
man with metastatic prostate cancer. (**A,B**) Axial
CT images demonstrate a destructive mass involving
the right mandibular ramus with soft tissue extension
into the masticator space. (**C,D**) T1-weighted axial
MR images (TR = 600 ms, TE = 20 ms) before and
after intravenous gadolinium administration
demonstrate the soft tissue mass. The mass exhibits
mild contrast enhancement. (**E**) T2-weighted axial
MR image (TR = 2500 ms, TE = 80 ms)
demonstrates increased signal intensity.

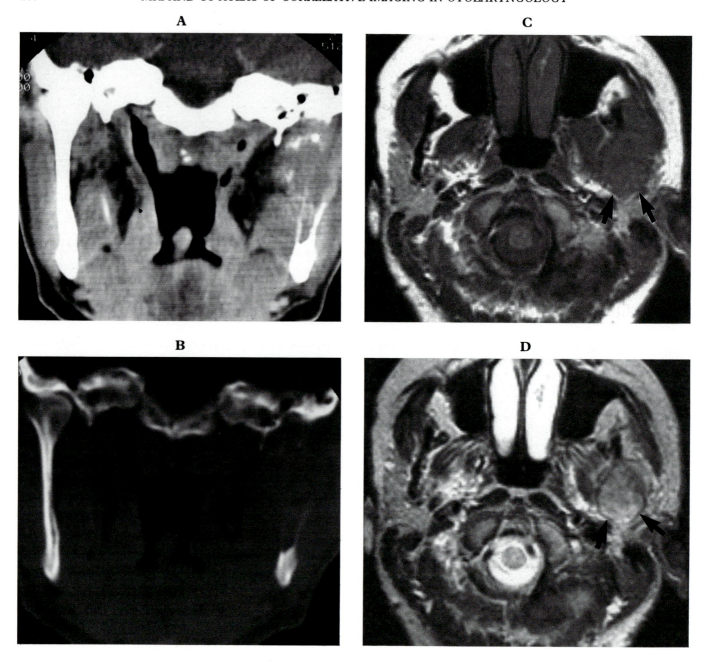

FIGURE 6.10

Leiomyosarcoma of the mandible in a 53-year-old woman. (**A,B**) Coronal CT images demonstrate an expansile lytic mass involving the left mandibular ramus and condyle. (**C,D**) Axial T1-weighted (TR = 500 ms, TE = 30 ms) and T2-weighted (TR = 2000 ms, TE = 80 ms) images reveal an expansile mass (arrows) which is isointense with muscle on the T1-weighted image and slightly hyperintense on the T2-weighted image. The left mandibular ramus and condyle demonstrate cortical destruction as well as marrow replacement by tumor.

A

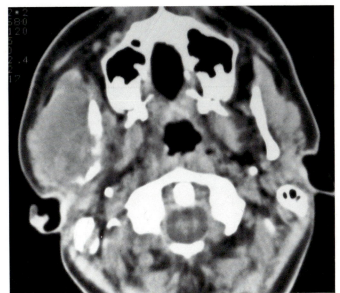

B

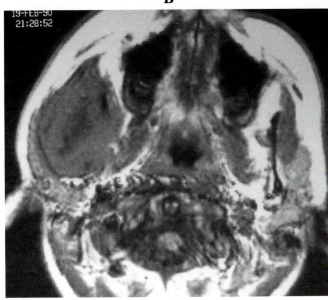

FIGURE 6.11

Undifferentiated sarcoma in a 14-year-old adolescent. (**A**) Axial CT demonstrates a large destructive mass involving the left mandibular ramus and condyle. The soft tissue planes within the masticator space are obliterated. (**B**) Axial T1-weighted image (TR = 600 ms, TE = 15 ms) demonstrates a large intermediate signal mass with regions of lower signal intensity, possibly the result of necrosis. (Courtesy of Dr Robert Zimmerman, Children's Hospital of Philadelphia.)

A

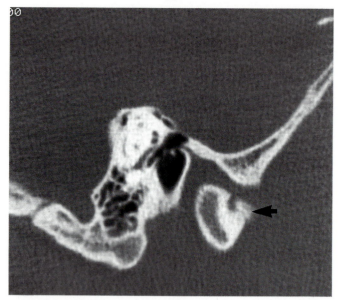

C

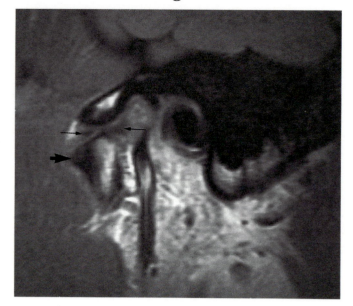

B

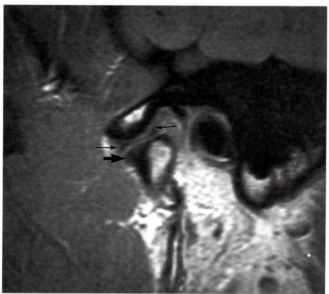

FIGURE 6.12

Osteochondroma in a 32-year-old man. (**A**) Direct sagittal CT image of the left TMJ demonstrates an anterior bony exostosis emanating from the condylar neck (arrow). (**B,C**) Sagittal T1-weighted images (TR = 1000 ms, TE = 25 ms) in the closed and open mouth positions demonstrate no evidence of internal derangement (smaller arrows). There is, however, a focal area of low signal intensity emanating from the condylar neck (large arrow), which corresponds to the bony exostosis appreciated on the CT image.

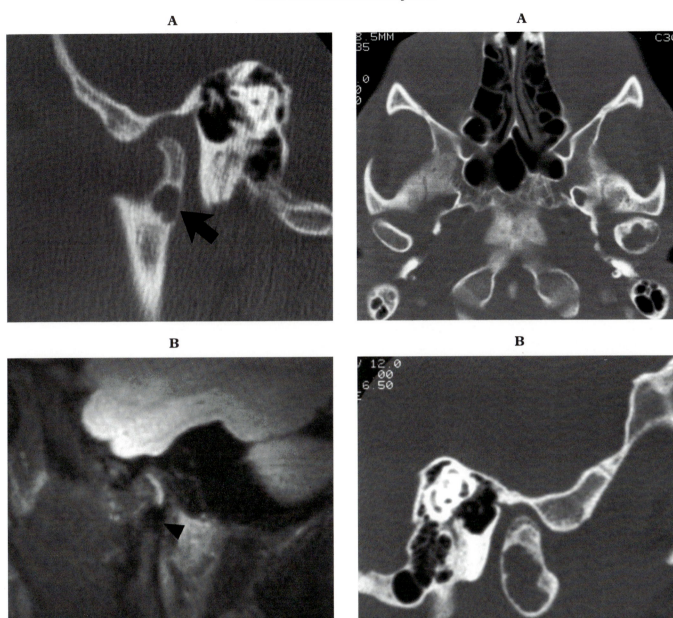

A

A

B

B

FIGURE 6.13

Fibrous cortical defect. (**A**) Sagittal CT of the right TMJ reveals a lytic, slightly expansile lesion of the condylar neck (arrow). (**B**) Sagittal T2-weighted image (TR = 2000 ms, TE = 70 ms) in the closed mouth position demonstrates a 1 cm circular focus of low signal intensity in the condylar neck (arrowhead). The TMJ meniscus is normally positioned with no evidence of internal derangement.

FIGURE 6.14

Nonossifying fibroma. (**A,B**) Direct sagittal and axial images. There is an expansile and lytic lesion in the mandibular condyle which extends into the subcortical region of the condyle. The articular surface is intact.

A

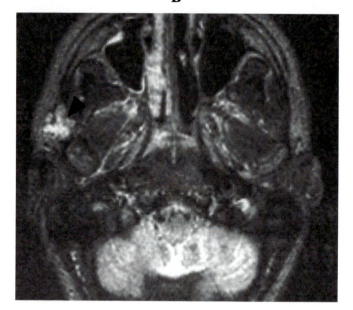

C

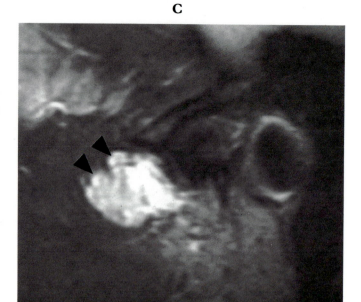

B

FIGURE 6.15

Right TMJ ganglion cyst. (**A**) Postarthrogram CT of the right TMJ demonstrates an opacified cystic structure (arrow) slightly anterior and medial to the mandibular condyle. (**B,C**) Axial and sagittal T2-weighted MR images (TR = 2000 ms, TE = 80 ms) demonstrate a high signal intensity cystic structure (arrowheads) in close proximity to the right TMJ.

A

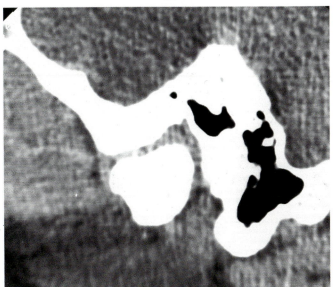

B

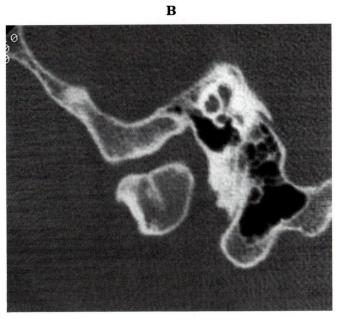

FIGURE 6.16

Congenital bifid condyle. (**A,B**) The mandibular condyle is flattened and takes a bifid configuration. Congenital bifid condyle may mimic benign bone lesions such as an osteochondroma.

A

C

B

D

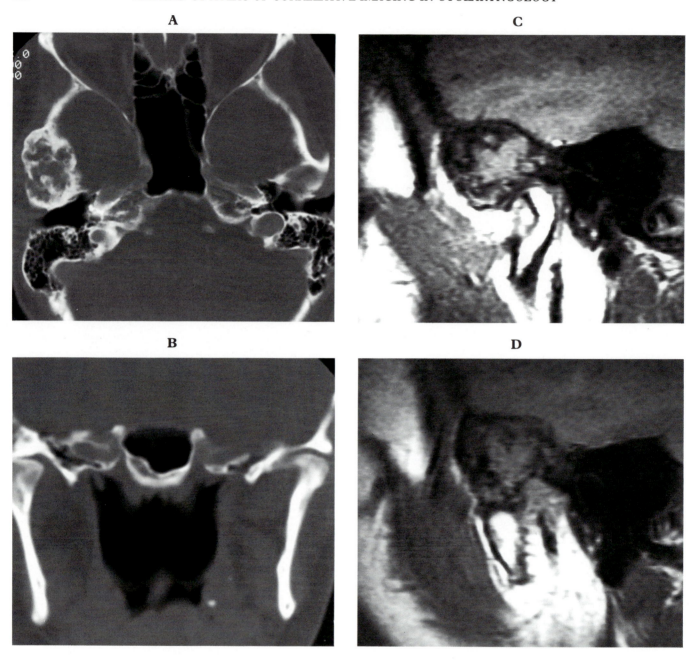

FIGURE 6.17

Fibrous dysplasia right articular eminence. (**A,B**) Axial and coronal CT images demonstrate a bubbly expansile lesion of the right temporal bone. The lesion involves the right TMJ.

(**C,D**) T1-weighted MR images (TR = 600 ms, TE = 23 ms) of the right TMJ in the closed and open mouth positions demonstrate no evidence of internal derangement. The articular eminence is

continued

E

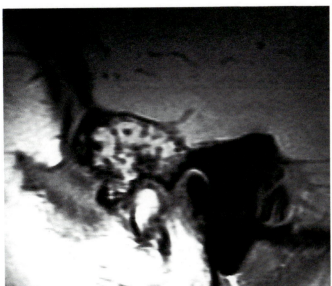

A

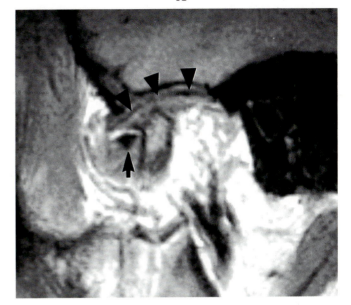

FIGURE 6.18

Postoperative TMJ (postdiskectomy and eminectomy) with Silastic prosthesis in place. Sagittal T1-weighted MR image (TR = 750 ms, TE = 25 ms) of the right TMJ. There is a Silastic TMJ implant (arrowheads) in place. The prosthesis typically appears as a thin band of low signal intensity. The low signal focus (arrow) represents fibrosis in the pterygoid fascia. Note also the degenerative remodeling of the mandibular condyle.

F

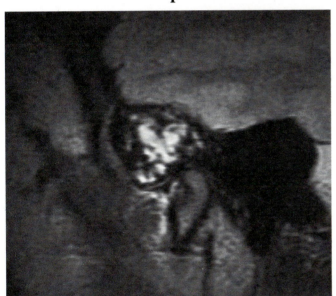

FIGURE 6.17 *(continued)*

expanded and demonstrates an inhomogenous appearance predominantly consisting of intermediate signal intensity interspersed with foci of low signal intensity. (**E,F**) T2-weighted MR images (TR = 2000 ms, TE = 20/80 ms) demonstrate increased signal intensity within the articular eminence.

CHAPTER 7

TEMPORAL BONE

Introduction

The advent of computed tomography (CT) and magnetic resonance imaging (MRI) within the past two decades has completely revolutionized imaging of the temporal bone. With such rapid and dynamic changes in the imaging field, the radiologist needs to work together with the otolaryngologist to ensure the most efficient, noninvasive and cost-containing imaging protocol individualized for each patient depending upon the clinical presentation. In general, however, CT provides high-resolution images of the temporal bone with emphasis on bone detail and is the mainstay of diagnosis in detecting congenital anomalies and middle ear diseases. Magnetic resonance imaging is superior to CT in the evaluation of central lesions, internal auditory canal and cerebellopontine angle (CPA) masses. The choice of imaging modality thus depends on the clinical presentation of the patient and the suspected location of the pathology.

In patients with asymmetric sensorineural hearing loss who are suspected of having an acoustic neuroma, contrast-enhanced MRI is the modality of choice. Magnetic resonance imaging has also made great advances in vascular imaging and is showing promise in the detection of vascular loops, which may compress the 7th and 8th nerve complex at the porus acusticus. For patients with conductive hearing loss, CT is the appropriate initial imaging modality. When intracranial complications arising from middle ear disease are suspected, MRI serves as a complementary study to CT.

Evaluation of fractures, ossicular injury and facial nerve injury in patients with a history of trauma is primarily done by CT. However, MRI is complementary to CT in the evaluation of intracranial complications.

If a vascular mass is suspected, the imaging should begin with high-resolution CT to detect any vascular anomalies, variants or masses. With glomus tumor, MRI can aid in confirming the diagnosis. In patients with pulsatile tinnitus without a mass on otoscopic examination, a similar protocol should be used. However, if CT and MRI fail to demonstrate a lesion, angiography should be done to detect lesions such as dural arteriovenous malformation or vascular anomalies.

To adequately evaluate CT or MR images of the temporal bone, one should be familiar with the anatomy of this compact but seemingly complex region.

Normal anatomy

Each temporal bone comprises five parts: (1) squamous portion; (2) petrous portion; (3) tympanic portion; (4) mastoid portion; and (5) styloid process. The squamous portion forms the lateral wall of the middle cranial fossa and gives origin to the temporalis muscle. The zygomatic process of the squamous portion fuses with the temporal process of the zygoma to complete the zygomatic arch. The zygomatic muscle arises from the medial aspect of the zygomatic process. At the posterior end of the zygomatic process, a tuberosity projects anteriorly which forms the articular eminence of the glenoid fossa.

The petrous portion is pyramidal in shape and forms an angle of 45° with the sagittal plane at the skull base. It houses the inner ear structures. The middle cranial fossa lies in front of the petrous pyramid, while the posterior fossa is behind it. The opening of the internal auditory canal along the posterior surface is called the porus acusticus. The concavity along the anterior surface of the petrous pyramid is called Meckel's cave in which lies the gasserian ganglion. The superior margin of the petrous pyramid shows a slight bulge called the arcuate eminence which serves as a landmark for localizing the superior semicircular canal. The entrance to the carotid canal and jugular fossa lies along the inferior surface. The petrous apex is separated from the clivus by the petro-occipital fissure.

The tympanic portion (tympanic ring) is small, crescent-shaped and forms most of the inferior and posterior portion of the bony external auditory canal. Anteriorly, the petrotympanic fissure (glaserian fissure) forms the passage for the tympanic branch of the internal maxillary artery and the chorda tympani, a branch of the 7th cranial nerve. Posteriorly, the tympanic bone merges with the squamous and mastoid portions at the tympanomastoid fissure. The lower border of the tympanic bone encompasses the root of the styloid process.

The mastoid portion contains a large network of air cells which interconnect. The largest air cell is the mastoid antrum, which connects with the epitympanum (attic) via the aditus ad antrum. Koerner's septum, a remnant of the petrosquamous suture, projects into the superior portion of the mastoid antrum and forms a surgical landmark.

The styloid bone is an elongated narrow process that projects inferiorly just anterior to the stylomastoid foramen. The styloid process gives origin to several muscles and ligaments extending to the pharynx, the larynx and the tongue.

Imaging strategies

High-resolution CT is the modality of choice for imaging the osseous component of the temporal bone.[1-6] Magnetic resonance is superior in demonstrating the soft tissues and is the preferred modality for evaluation of the cerebello-pontine angle lesions and the 7th and 8th nerve complex.

Computed tomography technique consists of obtaining 1–1.5 mm thick, contiguous or overlapping sections in the axial and coronal planes. Direct sagittal sections can also be obtained if needed. The raw data are saved and images are reconstructed and geometrically enlarged under bone algorithms for maximum detail.

Computed tomography anatomy

Figures 7.1 and 7.2 depict the normal anatomy in the axial and coronal planes.

External ear

The auricle and the external auditory canal constitute the external ear. The lateral one-third portion of the external auditory canal is fibrocartilaginous and the medial two-thirds is osseous. The tympanic membrane marks the medial boundary of the external auditory canal.

Middle ear

The middle ear cavity (tympanic cavity) is divided into three parts: epitympanum or attic, mesotympanum or tympanic cavity proper and hypotympanum. The lateral margin of the middle ear is defined by the tympanic membrane. The tympanic membrane attaches to the scutum superiorly and the tympanic annulus inferiorly. The medial margin of the middle ear is marked by the bony labyrinth consisting of the cochlea, vestibule, and the semicircular canals. The round window and oval window are situated along this surface. Superiorly, the middle ear is separated from the middle cranial fossa by a bony plate called the tegmen tympani. The inferior boundary of the middle ear is formed by the jugular bulb in the jugular fossa and the carotid artery as it enters the carotid canal.

The epitympanum lies above a line extending from the scutum to the geniculate ganglion. It is shaped like an inverted triangle. The head of the malleus and the body of the incus with the short process are located in this space. Posteriorly it connects to the mastoid antrum through an opening called the aditus ad antrum. The roof of the epitympanum, the tegmen tympani, separates the middle ear from the middle cranial fossa. Prussak's space is limited laterally by the lateral attic wall and the scutum, medially by the incus and malleus, superiorly by the lateral mallear ligament and inferiorly by the pars flaccida.

The mesotympanum lies below the epitympanum. The inferior extent is defined by a line extending from the inferior aspect of the external auditory canal to the bottom of the cochlear promontory. The ossicles extend from the epitympanum into the mesotympanum. The long process of the malleus, incus and the stapes are located in this space. The foot plate of stapes attaches to the oval window along the medial boundary of the middle ear. Along the posterior wall of the mesotympanum lies the bony surgical landmark, the pyramidal eminence which contains the belly of the stapedius muscle. The tendon of the muscle attaches to the stapes. Lateral to the pyramidal eminence is the facial recess. The sinus tympani lies medial to the pyramidal eminence. The stapedius muscle is innervated by the facial nerve. Two important structures lie along the anterior aspect of the mesotympanum. The eustachian tube connects from the mesotympanum to the nasopharynx. Slightly above and parallel to the eustachian tube lies the semicanal containing the tensor tympani muscle. The tensor tympani muscle hooks around the cochleariform process to insert on the head of the malleus and is innervated by the 5th cranial nerve.

The ossicular chain consists of the malleus, the incus and the stapes and lies in the epitympanum and mesotympanum. The head of the malleus and the body and short process of the incus lie in the epitympanum. The malleus is the most anterior ossicle with the incus behind it. Several suspensory ligaments provide stability to the ossicular chain. The malleus articulates with the incus, which in turn articulates with the stapes. The malleus is also attached to the tympanic membrane. The manubrium of the malleus and the long process of the incus are parallel in location. The head of the malleus articulates with the body of the incus at the incudomallear joint. These ossicles form an 'ice-cream cone' appearance in the epitympanum on axial CT scans. The lenticular process of the incus forms a right angle turn at the tip of the long process and forms the incudostapedial joint. This lenticular process is better seen on coronal CT sections while the stapes is visualized better on axial CT scans.

The hypotympanum lies below the mesotympanum.

The inferior wall of the hypotympanum is formed by the carotid canal anteriorly and the jugular fossa posteriorly. The bony wall of the carotid canal or the jugular fossa can be dehiscent congenitally and may be the cause of pulsatile tinnitus.

Inner ear
The inner ear lies medial to the middle ear and comprises the otic capsule and the internal auditory canal in the petrous pyramid. The otic capsule contains the cochlea (the organ of hearing) and the vestibular system (the organ of balance). The membranous labyrinth containing endolymph is enclosed within the osseous labyrinth which contains the perilymph.

The normal cochlea is spiral-shaped, consisting of two and a half to two and three-quarter turns. The first turn, also called the basal turn, opens into the vestibule. It begins at the round window through which a potential communication with the tympanic cavity exists. The round window is, however, covered by a membrane. The bony protuberance formed by the basal turn in the tympanic cavity is referred to as the promontory. The tympanic nerve plexus formed by the Jacobson's nerve (branch of the glossopharyngeal nerve) and the Arnold's nerve (branch of the vagus nerve) lies on the surface of the promontory. The cochlear aqueduct connects the cochlear perilymph to the subarachnoid cerebrospinal fluid (CSF) space in the posterior fossa. The cochlear aqueduct is a bony canal that lies parallel and inferior to the internal auditory canal (IAC). It is lined by connective tissue and forms a semipermeable barrier for exchange of perilymph and CSF. It also forms a potential route for meningeal spread of middle ear infections.

The vestibular system consists of the three semicircular canals and the vestibule. The membranous components of the vestibule (saccule and utricle) consist of endolymph and are not visualized by CT separately. The endolymphatic duct arises from the utricle and saccule and lies within a bony duct called the vestibular aqueduct. The vestibular aqueduct is visualized in axial and sagittal CT sections and opens in the posterior fossa. There is no exchange of the endolymph and the CSF. All three semicircular canals (lateral, superior and posterior) arise and terminate in the utricle. The posterior and superior semicircular canals join to form the common crus which is in close proximity to the endolymphatic duct. The superior semicircular canal forms a little bulge along the superior aspect of petrous pyramid called the arcuate eminence.

The internal auditory canal provides passage to both the 7th and 8th cranial nerves. In the lateral portion of the IAC, there is a ridge along the anterior surface known as the crista falciformis. In the same region, a thin bony plate called Bill's bar is present in a vertical plane and separates the facial nerve from the exit point of the superior vestibular nerve. The 7th nerve lies in the anterior and superior portion of the internal auditory canal. The cochlear nerve courses through the anterior and inferior aspect of the canal. The superior and inferior divisions of the vestibular nerve pass through the superior and inferior posterior portions of the IAC, respectively. The facial nerve takes a complicated course through the temporal bone. Computed tomography and MR are extremely useful in outlining the course of the 7th nerve.[7,8] The 7th cranial nerve should be carefully inspected along the entire course and divided into the following segments: (1) intracranial extending from the brainstem to the IAC, (2) intracanalicular, (3) labyrinthine, (4) intratympanic (horizontal), (5) mastoid, and (6) parotid. The 7th nerve enters the IAC through the porus acusticus. At the fundus of the IAC, it courses between the cochlea and vestibule as the labyrinthine portion into the region of the geniculate ganglion. At the ganglion it forms a hairpin bend and the horizontal portion goes through the tympanic cavity below the lateral semicircular canal in its own bony canal. The bony canal, however, is often dehiscent. At the geniculate ganglion, the greater superficial petrosal nerve courses forward and joins the deep petrosal nerves to form the vidian nerve. The tympanic portion of the facial nerve makes a second bend down at the posterior wall and becomes the vertical or the descending or the mastoid portion. This nerve finally exits the mastoid through the stylomastoid foramen at the skull base. The chorda tympani nerve branches from the vertical portion and courses through the middle ear between the long process of the incus and the manubrium of the malleus to exit

anteriorly through the glaserian fissure. It then joins the lingual nerve to provide taste sensation to the anterior two-thirds of the tongue. Another small branch of the vertical portion of the 7th nerve innervates the stapedius muscle.

Jugular fossa

The jugular fossa, which is located at the base of the skull is divided by a fibrous or bony septum into two compartments: (1) a smaller anteromedial portion, the pars nervosa, and (2) a larger posterolateral portion, the pars vascularis. The pars nervosa contains the 9th cranial nerve, and the pars vascularis contains the jugular bulb, and the 10th and the 11th cranial nerves.[7] The right jugular foramen is usually larger than the left in size.[8] The cortical margins are smooth and intact. The roof of the jugular bulb abuts the floor of the hypotympanum, although separated by a bony plate. When the bulb extends above the level of the inferior tympanic ring, it is referred to as a high riding jugular bulb.[9] Complete or partial absence of the jugular roof indicates a dehiscent jugular bulb.

Magnetic resonance imaging anatomy

Magnetic resonance imaging has established its superiority over CT in the evaluation of cerebellopontine angle masses and intracanalicular anatomy and pathology due to superb soft tissue resolution. The middle ear anatomy cannot be adequately evaluated by MRI because of the lack of signal from air and the cortical bone.

The standard MR technique utilizes spin-echo imaging in the axial and coronal planes with T1- and T2-weighted pulse sequences (Figs 7.3 and 7.4). Other pulse sequences such as 3DFT MR imaging using thin slices and short echo delay time (TE) better demonstrate soft tissues of the otic capsule and the endolymphatic duct.[10] Gadolinium is now routinely utilized in the evaluation of cerebellopontine angle tumors, dizziness, vertigo, facial nerve palsy and other cranial neuropathies. The MR examination can be tailored to look for vascular flow and vascular lesions.

Magnetic resonance angiography (MRA) has become a clinically useful technique in the evaluation of the carotid arteries, intracranial vessels, arteriovenous malformations and venous pathology such as sagittal sinus thrombosis.

Pathology

Congenital malformations

The incidence of congenital malformation of the ear is approximately 1 in 3800 live births.[11] The malformations are unilateral in over 90% of the cases and bilateral in less than 10%. Malformations of the external and middle ear are more common than those of the inner ear.

The external and middle ear malformations often coexist because of the common embryologic development from the first and second branchial arches, the first branchial cleft and the first pharyngeal pouch. The clinical manifestations include cosmetic deformity and conductive hearing loss.

Atresia or hypoplasia of the external auditory canal is common. The atretic plate may be bony or membranous and is easily assessed with high-resolution computed tomography. Severe degrees of external auditory canal agenesis are often associated with auricular anomalies such as extreme microtia, a tissue tag or a pit. The tympanic cavity often reveals varying degrees of hypoplasia. The ossicles are typically deformed, either fused or rudimentary but rarely absent. There may be a bony strut between the ossicles and the tegmen tympani. The facial nerve canal is usually placed in a more anterior position than normal. Hypoplasia of the mandibular condyle in the glenoid fossa often coexists. The mastoid pneumatization is also easily assessed with computed tomography. Computed tomography is essential prior to corrective surgery to assess: (1) the atretic plate; (2) the ossicular status; (3) the size of the middle ear cavity; (4) the course of the facial nerve canal; and (5) the inner ear (Fig. 7.5).[11]

Inner ear anomalies include malformations of the cochlea, vestibule, semicircular canals and the cochlear or the vestibular aqueducts. The inner auditory canal develops separately from the labyrinth but it may also be abnormal.

The cochlea may reveal aplasia or varying degrees of hypoplasia. The classic Mondini defect described in 1791 implies partial cochlear aplasia with an intact basal turn and a common cavity between the middle and apical turns. The semicircular canals may also demonstrate varying degrees of anomalies. The lateral semicircular canal is frequently affected and shows dilatation. It is often discovered as an incidental finding in combination with a dilated vestibule (Fig. 7.6). Vestibular aqueduct dilatation is described in association with 'vestibular aqueduct syndrome' in which the major clinical manifestation is sensorineural hearing loss.[12,13] Dilated cochlear aqueduct is reported to be often associated with stapes foot plate gusher.[5,13] Marked narrowing of the internal auditory canal may occur in association with sensorineural hearing loss.[14] Dilatation of the internal auditory canal is described in association with neurofibromatosis due to dural ectasia.[15] Duplication anomaly of the IAC is rare.[16,17]

The facial nerve bears a complex relationship to both the middle and inner ear structures. The facial nerve canal may be anomalous in course either in conjunction with the other parts of the temporal bone or as an isolated anomaly. Careful evaluation of the facial nerve canal by CT is essential prior to any surgical intervention in the temporal bone.

Vascular anomalies

Congenital vascular anomalies in the temporal bone may present as pulsatile tinnitus. An aberrant internal carotid artery (ICA) is the most common anomaly. Computed tomography reveals a soft tissue mass in the middle ear cavity anterior to the cochlear promontory which is contiguous with the horizontal portion of the carotid canal. A defect in the posterolateral margin of the vertical carotid canal is clearly visualized by CT and confirms the diagnosis.[18] A dehiscent jugular bulb, a high riding jugular vein or jugular diverticulum are also easily evaluated by high resolution CT (Fig. 7.7).

Inflammatory

Malignant external otitis

Malignant external otitis (MEO) is classically secondary to *Pseudomonas* infection and occurs predominantly in older patients with uncontrolled diabetes or in patients who are immunocompromised. The external otitis usually begins at the junction of the cartilaginous and bony portions of the external auditory canal and is referred to as 'malignant' because of its aggressive nature. Uncontrolled infection may lead to mastoiditis with involvement of the facial nerve, osteomyelitis of the base of the skull, sigmoid sinus thrombosis and meningitis. The infection may also spread inferiorly into the nasopharynx, masticator and parotid spaces. Involvement of the 9th, 10th, 11th and 12th cranial nerves may occur in the advanced stages of this disease.[19] Direct extension of the inflammatory process into the middle ear cleft is rare. Computed tomography is the modality of choice for evaluation of the extent of MEO. Contrast-enhanced CT shows a soft tissue mass with enhancement and bone erosion (Figs 7.8 and 7.9). The radiographic findings, however, cannot be distinguished from that of aggressive carcinoma. The clinical setup of the patient and culture of the appropriate pathogens provide the diagnosis. Gallium scans have been utilized in following the progress of disease during patient management.[20]

Keratosis obturans

Keratosis obturans is a relatively rare condition and is also referred to as invasive keratosis or canal cholesteatoma. It is characterized by accumulation of plugs of exfoliated keratin in the bony portion of the external canal. The margins of the bony canal are often remodeled. It is usually seen in patients under 40 years of age. The etiology is not known but it is often associated with a history of bronchiectasis or sinusitis. It is often bilateral. Patients may present with acute pain and hearing loss. Computed tomography shows soft tissue mass with bone resorption and widening of the external auditory canal.[21]

Acute otomastoiditis

Acute otitis media and mastoiditis is a bacterial infection that is clinically evident and does not routinely require imaging. However, if complications are suspected, imaging can be very useful.

Coalescent mastoiditis shows erosion of the mastoid air cell septae and formation of empyema cavity (Fig. 7.10). Other complications include subperiosteal or neck abscess secondary to the perforation of the external mastoid cortex. Intracranial complications such as dural sinus thrombosis, lepto-meningitis, epidural or subdural abscess may occur in the presence of perforation of the internal mastoid cortex.[22]

In the early stage, coalescent mastoiditis is best imaged by CT; however, the intracranial complications are better studied by MRI.

Gradenigo's syndrome may result if the infection progresses towards the petrous apex. The syndrome refers to apical petrositis with 6th nerve palsy, deep facial pain along the 5th nerve distribution and otitis media (Fig. 7.11).

Chronic otomastoiditis

Chronic otitis media and mastoiditis are secondary to eustachian tube dysfunction. This entity incorporates a broad spectrum of manifestations which include cholesteatoma, granulation tissue, fibrous tissue, and fluid.[23,24] Computed tomography is the primary imaging modality for middle ear diseases to define the extent of the disease and assess bone or ossicular erosions. Nondependent soft tissue masses such as cholesteatoma, granulation tissue or fibrous tissue cannot be distinguished from each other by their density on CT (Fig. 7.12). Enhanced MRI may play a role in characterizing the nondependent soft tissue masses based on signal intensities and enhancement pattern.[25] Unlike cholesteatoma, granulation tissue enhances following gadolinium.[25] Magnetic resonance imaging is also useful in evaluation of intracranial complications. Magnetic resonance imaging is particularly helpful in postmastoidectomy cases where recurrent disease and fibrosis have to be differentiated from meningoencephalocele.

Fibrous tissue formation in the middle ear secondary to chronic otomastoiditis may lead to ossicular fixation resulting in conductive hearing loss. Punctate calcifications in soft tissue debris and the tympanic membrane, referred to as tympanosclerosis, are also easily identified by CT.[26]

Focal erosion of the ossicular chain may occur in noncholesteatomatous otitis media. The tympanic cavity may be normally pneumatized but reveal minor ossicular erosion, particularly involving the long process of the incus and region of the incudostapedial articulation. Such erosions are best visualized on axial CT scans.[27]

Cholesteatoma

Cholesteatoma is a mass composed of stratified squamous epithelium and exfoliated keratin. Two types of cholesteatomas are described: congenital and acquired. The majority of middle ear cholesteatomas are of the acquired type.[28-30] The acquired cholesteatoma is associated with a history of previous middle ear infections and may arise from the pars flaccida or from the pars tensa. The pars flaccida cholesteatomas usually begin in Prussak's space. There are several different theories that attempt to explain the etiology of acquired cholesteatomas. The three popular ones are: (1) proliferation of the squamous epithelium that migrates into the middle ear through a perforated tympanic membrane; (2) encystment of retraction pockets of the tympanic membrane; and (3) squamous metaplasia of middle ear mucosa following chronic inflammation. Congenital cholesteatoma in the middle ear is rare and is not associated with a history of previous ear infections. Cholesteatomas are diagnosed at CT by the presence of a nondependent soft tissue mass in a location appropriate for the origin of the cholesteatoma (Fig. 7.13). These findings are not by any means pathognomonic, however, and a consideration of clinical findings and radiographic findings is often diagnostic. Complete radiographic evaluation includes analysis of the bony structures, scutum, ossicles, integrity of the tympanic cavity as well as any anatomic variants. Almost all of the complications of cholesteatoma are secondary to bony erosion. Local complications include labyrinthine fistula, erosion of the facial nerve canal and ossicular destruction (Figs 7.14–7.16). Intracranial complications include epidural or brain abscess, sigmoid sinus thrombosis, meningitis, and all are usually secondary to infected cholesteatomas.[31] The first imaging study should be high-resolution CT. If intracranial complications are suspected, the workup should include MRI.

Cholesterol granuloma

Cholesterol granuloma is an entity totally distinct from cholesteatoma. Cholesterol granuloma refers to a subtype of granulation tissue in the middle ear resulting as a foreign body response to cholesterol crystals. While cholesteatoma is lined by keratinized squamous epithelium, cholesterol granuloma has a fibrous connective tissue lining and no epithelial or neoplastic cells. The cholesterol granuloma may present as a bluish-red mass behind the tympanic membrane due to the hemorrhagic nature of this mass. The hemorrhagic products lend the characteristic MR appearance—bright signal intensity on both T1- and T2-weighted sequences.[32,33] Cholesteatoma reveals low to intermediate signal intensity on T1- and variable signal intensity on T2-weighted images.

Giant cholesterol cyst

Giant cholesterol cyst, often referred to as cholesterol granuloma, presents as an expansile mass in the petrous apex, usually in the presence of a normally pneumatized mastoid and middle ear. A giant cholesterol cyst is lined by fibrous connective tissue and contains brownish liquid and cholesterol crystals. Magnetic resonance imaging reveals hyperintense signal on both T1- and T2-weighted images (Fig. 7.17). This entity should not be confused with congenital cholesteatoma (also known as epidermoid) (Fig. 7.18).[34]

Labyrinthitis

The etiology of labyrinthitis may be a viral infection, suppurative (bacterial), toxic (ototoxic drug) or serous (reactive following chronic otitis or surgery). Magnetic resonance imaging may reveal enhancement of the vestibular system following gadolinium administration (Fig. 7.19).[35] Longstanding suppurative labyrinthitis may lead to ossification of the membranous labyrinth and is referred to as labyrinthitis ossificans.

Facial palsy

The facial nerve is subject to disease at any point from its origin in the cerebral cortex to the motor endplate in the face. The term peripheral facial nerve paralysis implies injury to the facial nerve from the level of the brain stem nucleus to the motor endplates, resulting in paralysis of the ipsilateral muscles of facial expression. On the other hand, central facial paralysis indicates a supranuclear injury which results in paralysis of the contralateral muscles of facial expression with sparing of the muscles of the forehead. The cause of facial nerve paralysis includes trauma (temporal bone fracture or surgical injury to the nerve), neoplasms (CPA tumors or facial nerve schwannoma), infection (otitis media, herpes zoster oticus) or idiopathic (Bell's palsy). Bell's palsy is probably the most common cause of peripheral, unilateral paralysis of the facial nerve. In patients suspected of Bell's palsy, imaging is not routinely performed in the initial phase. However, if surgical decompression of the nerve is warranted, MR imaging with gadolinium can be helpful in identifying the enhancing segment of the facial nerve (Fig. 7.20). Enhancement of the facial nerve may be seen along the entire intratemporal course in Bell's palsy.[36]

Neoplasms

Paraganglioma

In the temporal bone, paragangliomas arise from nonchromaffin tissue. The glomus tympanicum tumors are located adjacent to the cochlear promontory in the middle ear while the glomus jugulare tumors arise from the adventitial tissues of the jugular bulb. In addition, glomus tumors may arise along the inferior tympanic canaliculus (nerve of Jacobson) and mastoid canaliculus (nerve of Arnold). All of the above may be grouped together as the jugulo-tympanic paragangliomas.[37] In the middle ear, the most common neoplasm is glomus tympanicum. The jugulo-tympanic paragangliomas are benign tumors and are more common in women over the age of 30 years. Presenting symptoms include pulsatile tinnitus because of tumor vascularity, conductive hearing loss due to the tumor mass and vertigo if the inner ear is involved.[37] Patients with glomus jugulare may present with jugular fossa syndrome (involvement of 9th, 10th and 11th cranial nerves) or hypoglossal nerve involvement. Cavernous sinus and middle cranial fossa invasion may lead to symptoms related to 3rd through 6th cranial neuropathy. These tumors are usually locally invasive and distant metastases are rare.

Contrast-enhanced high-resolution CT is desirable as the first imaging study. An enhancing soft tissue mass in the middle ear cavity adjacent to the cochlear promontory is consistent with glomus tympanicum (Fig. 7.21). The glomus jugulare tumors are located in the jugular fossa and may reveal extensive bone erosion. Extension into the middle ear cavity is common. Computed tomography demonstrates the extent of local invasion by the tumor. Magnetic resonance imaging appearance on T1-weighted image is that of an intermediate signal intensity mass with areas of signal void due to the vascularity of the tumor.[38] The tumors reveal slightly high signal on T2-weighted image and the signal void areas persist. These tumors show moderately intense enhancement following gadolinium administration (Figs 7.22 and 7.23). Angiography provides a road map for the surgeon, determines the collateral arterial and venous circulation of the brain, and helps in preoperative embolization of the tumor.

Acoustic neurinoma (vestibular schwannoma)

Acoustic schwannoma arises from the vestibulocochlear nerve (8th cranial nerve) and is the most common neoplasm of the cerebellopontine angle. Since the majority of the so-called 'acoustic neuromas' arise from the schwann cells of the superior vestibular nerve, they are more accurately known as vestibular schwannomas. They usually occur in patients over the age of 50 years. Clinical symptoms are due to compression of cochlear nerve resulting in sensorineural hearing loss. Vertigo and dizziness are relatively infrequent. About 15% of patients present with a history of sudden onset of hearing loss, probably secondary to hemorrhage within the tumor. Bilateral acoustic neuromas are associated with neurofibromatosis type II.

Small acoustic neuromas can be surgically removed with preservation of hearing.[39] If, however, the tumor extends to the fundus of the internal auditory canal, microscopic extension into the cochlea and vestibule becomes more likely. Acoustic neuromas are seen as homogeneously enhancing masses in the internal auditory canal or CPA, depending on the size.

Approximately 5% of the acoustic neuromas are accompanied by an arachnoid cyst in the CPA. Large tumors may show cystic areas secondary to necrosis. On MRI, these tumors are isointense with the brain and are of higher signal intensity compared to the CSF in the CPA on T1-weighted images. T2-weighted MR images are less sensitive since acoustic neuromas are bright on T2-weighted images and may blend with the signal intensity of surrounding CSF.[40,41] Acoustic neuromas show intense enhancement with gadolinium. Magnetic resonance imaging with contrast is the most sensitive noninvasive imaging modality for the detection of intracanalicular acoustic neuromas (Figs 7.24–7.26).[42] However, all enhancing lesions within the IAC are not tumors. Enhancement can be seen with non-neoplastic diseases such as viral neuritis, Bell's palsy or Ramsay Hunt syndrome.[43]

Meningioma

Meningioma is the second most common tumor in the CPA. Meningiomas are well-encapsulated, benign tumors that occur along the dural surfaces. These tumors are more common in women and manifest in the 40–70 year age group. Meningiomas arising from the posterior surface of the petrous bone may present with 5th, 7th or 8th cranial nerve deficits. Meningiomas appear as broad-based masses that may show increased density on unenhanced CT scans. Intense enhancement with contrast is typically seen. Hyperostosis of adjacent bone may occur. Calcification in the tumor aids in the diagnosis of meningioma. By MRI, meningiomas may appear isointense with the brain on both T1- and T2-weighted images.[44] Another appearance of meningiomas is described with intermediate signal intensity on T1-weighted images but high signal intensity on T2-weighted images.[45] Intense enhancement occurs following gadolinium administration. Although the mass is dural based and outside the IAC, linear enhancement extending into the canal may be noted and has been described as 'the tail sign' (Figs 7.27 and 7.28).

Epidermoid (congenital cholesteatoma)

Epidermoid is a congenital lesion resulting from intracranial or intraosseous inclusion of ectoderm during early development. The epidermoid is a sac lined by squamous epithelial cells and contains exfoliated keratin debris and solid cholesterol crystals. Epidermoid is the third most common tumor in the CPA and usually manifests between 20 and 50 years of age. There is a slight male predilection. The clinical symptoms relate to compression of the adjacent structures.

Computed tomography demonstrates a low density mass that is pliable and does not enhance with contrast.[46] There is expansion of bone at the petrous apex. Epidermoids reveal variable signal but usually are of low signal intensity on T1-weighted images and of high signal intensity on T2-weighted images (Fig. 7.29).

Metastases

Metastases may involve the temporal bone or clivus and present as an erosive mass. Frequent primary sites are breast and lung carcinomas (Figs 7.30 and 7.31).

Facial nerve neurinoma

Facial nerve schwannomas may occur anywhere along the course of the facial nerve from its origin in the pons until it exits at the stylomastoid foramen.[47]

There is a predilection for the occurrence of the facial schwannomas in the region of geniculate ganglion. These tumors usually cause facial palsy by compression of the nerve rather than by invasion. The facial nerve schwannomas that arise along the proximal portion may cause sensorineural hearing loss and mimic acoustic neuromas.

Tumors arising from the tympanic portion of the facial nerve may cause conductive hearing loss due to compression of the ossicular chain. In less than 5% of the patients with facial palsy, a facial schwannoma is found to be the cause.[47]

The segment of the facial nerve involved by schwannoma is easily detected by CT and MRI. Computed tomography demonstrates a moderately enhancing homogeneous mass. Facial neuromas are usually isointense with the brain on T1-weighted images and hyperintense on T2-weighted images. These tumors reveal intense enhancement following administration of gadolinium.

Facial neuromas arising from the cisternal or intracanalicular segment may mimic an acoustic neuroma. Facial neuromas originating at the geniculate ganglion demonstrate enlargement and erosion in the region of the geniculate ganglion (Fig. 7.32). Facial neuromas that occur along the tympanic segment demonstrate soft tissue mass in the middle ear, medial to the ossicles and enlargement or erosion of the facial canal. Neuromas that arise from the descending portion of the facial nerve usually demonstrate expansion of the facial canal, erosion of the mastoid air cells and scalloping of the mastoid bone (Fig. 7.33).

Jugular fossa neurinoma

Schwannomas arising from the nerve sheaths of the 9th, 10th or the 11th cranial nerves can present as masses in the jugular fossa. Smooth enlargement of the jugular fossa with or without scalloping accompanied by an enhancing mass is suggestive of a neurogenic tumor. The MRI signal intensity of neurinomas is quite variable, but is typically intermediate on T1-weighted images and high on T2-weighted images. Enhancement with gadolinium is usually intense. Small tumors tend to be homogeneous in appearance but large tumors may reveal inhomogeneity due to areas of necrosis.

Hypoglossal neurinoma

Although hypoglossal neurinoma does not occur in the temporal bone, it is in close proximity and is therefore included in this chapter. Hypoglossal schwannoma may arise anywhere along the course of the 12th cranial nerve. If the proximal portion of the nerve is abnormal, enlargement of the hypoglossal canal may be seen. Clinically, patients may show tongue atrophy or deviation towards the involved side. The CT and MRI characteristics are similar to the acoustic or jugular fossa schwannomas (Fig. 7.34).

Trigeminal neurinoma

Schwannomas of the trigeminal nerve can occur anywhere along the course of the 5th nerve. These neurinomas can get very large and present as large dumbbell-shaped masses that extend into the cavernous sinus and also extend posteriorly into the CPA. As the 5th nerve is compressed, the tumor may cause progressive facial numbness, pain or paraesthesias (Fig. 7.35).

Chordoma

Chordomas arise from notochordal cell rests and occur in the clivus. These tumors are characteristically midline with erosion of the clivus. Computed tomography reveals a slightly dense mass, often with calcifications, that enhances moderately. The MRI signal intensity is usually intermediate on T1-weighted images and bright on T2-weighted images. Magnetic resonance imaging is the preferred imaging modality because it demonstrates the full extent of the tumor at the skull base.

Bone neoplasms

Cartilaginous tumors (chondromas and chondrosar-comas) usually arise near the spheno-occipital and basi-sphenoid synchondrosis at the skull base. Chondrosarcomas can cause extensive bone erosion and present with adjacent cranial neuropathies. Computed tomography demonstrates a soft tissue mass with aggressive bone erosion at the skull base. In the jugular fossa region, these masses may mimic glomus jugulare tumors (Fig. 7.36). Magnetic resonance imaging may show intermediate signal on T1-weighted images and variable signal on T2-weighted images. Osteosarcomas similarly show aggressive bone erosion at the skull base. The differential diagnostic considerations include chondrosarcoma, paraganglioma and metastatic disease (Fig. 7.37).

The chondromas and osteochondromas are benign masses that may show a chondroid matrix on CT. Exostosis or osteomas may occur along the petrous apex and may cause stenosis of the porus acusticus.

External auditory canal neoplasms

The most common neoplasms arising in or near the external auditory canal include squamous cell carcinoma, basal cell carcinoma and adenoid cystic carcinoma (Fig. 7.38).[48] Malignant melanomas and metastases may also be encountered. Squamous cell carcinoma usually arises from the skin of the external canal or rarely may arise in the middle ear or mastoid complex (Fig. 7.39). The basal cell carcinoma commonly begins on the pinna or in the retroauricular sulcus and then infiltrates into the external canal. Tumors of salivary gland origin may begin in the canal or extend from the parotid gland (Fig. 7.40). These tumors usually occur in older age groups. Computed tomography and MRI are complimentary in defining the extent of the tumors.

Osteodysplasias

Fibrous dysplasia

Fibrous dysplasia is an inherited disorder of unknown etiology, in which the involved bones show progressive enlargement. Fibrous dysplasia is classified into sclerotic, cystic and pagetoid types. The sclerotic type is the most common. The temporal bone is enlarged and shows variable encroachment upon the external auditory canal. The otic capsule and the internal auditory canal are generally spared. Computed tomography appearance is usually diagnostic in sclerotic and cystic types. Magnetic resonance appearance is more variable. The sclerotic type tends to show low signal intensity on both T1- and T2-weighted images. However, the other two types (cystic and pagetoid) are inhomogeneous in appearance and may show variable signal intensities ranging from low to high with different pulse sequences (Fig. 7.41).

Paget's disease

Paget's disease is an inherited disease that primarily affects the axial skeleton. It is characterized by an imbalance between the formation and resorption of bone, usually with excessive bone formation. The otic capsule may reveal diffuse demineralization and result in sensorineural or mixed hearing loss. The temporal bone involvement is usually accompanied by changes in the skull (Fig. 7.42).

Otosclerosis

Otosclerosis is characterized by replacement of enchondral bone in the otic capsule by foci of spongy bone in the early stages and dense ossific plaques in the later stages when the decalcified foci recalcify. Two types of otosclerosis are described: fenestral and cochlear.[49,50] Fenestral otosclerosis is the most common type (80–90%). Cochlear otosclerosis, when present, is almost always associated with fenestral disease. Otosclerosis is usually bilateral and more common in women. The conductive hearing loss in fenestral disease is purely mechanical. The sensorineural hearing loss in cochlear otosclerosis is believed to be secondary to diffusion of cytotoxic enzymes into the fluid of the membranous labyrinth. The most common CT finding in fenestral disease is new bone plaque formation along the anterior margin of the oval window, and subsequently plaques along the posterior margin and the round window. In the early lytic phase, the oval window may appear to be enlarged because of bone resorption along its margins. In the sclerotic phase, there may be obliteration of the oval and round windows by proliferative bone. The CT findings in the early phase of cochlear otosclerosis include foci of demineralization in the otic capsule surrounding the cochlear turns. In the latter phase of cochlear otosclerosis, the diagnosis is less obvious because the density of these plaques may approach that of the normal otic capsule. Imaging is not routinely performed in patients with otosclerosis.

Osteogenesis imperfecta

Osteogenesis imperfecta (OI) describes a classic triad of fragile bones, blue sclera and hearing loss. Two types of OI are described; congenita and tarda. Death usually occurs in infants with osteogenesis imperfecta congenita, in utero or shortly after birth. Patients with the tarda variety of OI have a normal life expectancy. Computed tomography reveals proliferation of undermineralized bone involving all or part of the otic capsule; the round and oval windows may be obliterated. The facial nerve canal may be encroached upon by the dysplastic process. The CT appearance is similar to that of otosclerosis in the temporal bone (Fig. 7.43), but is usually more severe.

Trauma

Temporal bone fractures are seen in 6–8% of patients with severe head trauma. Up to 30% of temporal bone fractures can be bilateral. These fractures are typically described as longitudinal, transverse, and mixed. The longitudinal fractures run along the long axis of the petrous bone and account for about 80% of all temporal bone fractures (Figs 7.44 and 7.45). The transverse fractures run at right angles to the longitudinal axis and account for about 20% of all temporal bone fractures (Fig. 7.46). Fractures with both components are described as complex or mixed (Fig. 7.47). Imaging of temporal bone trauma remains in the domain of CT. For complete evaluation, in addition to the fracture lines, special note should be made of the following: (1) ossicular injury, (2) facial nerve injury, (3) integrity of tegmen tympani, (4) bony labyrinth, (5) mastoid air cells, and (6) carotid canal.

Clinically, patients may present with a 'battle sign' (hemorrhage and ecchymosis overlying the mastoid process), particularly with longitudinal fractures. Other manifestations include hearing loss, CSF otorrhea or otorhinorrhea, tympanic membrane disruption, facial nerve palsy and vestibular dysfunction.

Longitudinal fractures are the most common type of temporal bone fractures and usually result from a lateral blow to the temporo-mastoid region. The longitudinal fractures are subdivided into an anterior and a posterior type. The anterior type course along the anterior aspect of the squamous temporal bone and extend along the roof of the external canal, tegmen tympani and end in the region of geniculate ganglion. The posterior type course along the posterior aspect of the squamous temporal bone and extend through the mastoid air cells, posterior wall of the external canal, through the tympanic cavity and terminate in the region of the geniculate ganglion.

Conductive hearing loss commonly accompanies the longitudinal fracture which may be transient due to hemotympanum or ruptured tympanic membrane. However, ossicular injury may occur in about 50% of patients and result in persistent conductive hearing loss. The most easily dislocated ossicle is the incus resulting from disruption of the incudo-stapedial joint. The incudomallear dislocation is less common. Facial nerve injury occurs in only 10–20% of patients with longitudinal fractures.[51,52]

Transverse fractures are subdivided into a lateral and a medial type. The lateral type extends across the vestibule, basal turn and promontory of the cochlea, posterior and lateral semicircular canals. The medial type extends across the fundus of the IAC.

Transverse fractures are almost always accompanied with sensorineural hearing loss, either due to transection of the cochlear nerve or cochlear injury. Vertigo, dizziness and tinnitus may result from injury to vestibular nerves, the vestibule, the semicircular canals and the vestibular aqueduct with transverse fractures. Facial nerve injury may occur in 30–50% of patients with transverse fractures.[51,52] Immediate facial nerve paralysis is usually indicative of nerve transection or severe compression by fracture fragments. Delayed onset of facial nerve paralysis may be secondary to facial canal fracture, with contusion, edema or intraneural hematoma.

Other complications of trauma include CSF otorhinorrhea, perilymph fistula, post-traumatic meningocele, and meningo-encephalocele. Cerebrospinal fluid otorrhinorrhea is usually due to dural tear from fractures of the tegmen, the mastoid, the IAC and the petrous air cells. High resolution CT cisternography is the most useful study for the localization of the site of CSF leak.

References

1 BROGAN M, CHAKERES DW, Computed tomography and magnetic resonance imaging of the normal anatomy of the temporal bone, *Semin Ultrasound CT MR* (1989) **10**:178–94.

2 SWARTZ JD, *Imaging of Temporal Bone, A Text/Atlas* (Thieme Medical Publishers, Inc: New York 1986).

3 SWARTZ JD, High resolution CT of the middle ear and mastoid. Parts I, II, III, *Radiology* (1983) **148**:449–64.

4 BERGERON RT, In: Bergeron RT, Osborn AG, Som PM, eds *The Temporal Bone* (Mosby-Year Book: St Louis 1984) 728–846.

5 HARNSBERGER H, Temporal bone. In: *Head and Neck Imaging* (Year Book Medical Publishers: Chicago 1990) 290–328.

6 MAY M, Anatomy of the facial nerve for the clinician. In: May M, ed., *The Facial Nerve* (Thieme Medical Publishers: New York 1986) 21–2.

7 DANIELS DL, WILLIAMS AL, HAUGHTON VM, Jugular foramen: Anatomic and computed tomography, *AJR* (1984) **142**:153–8.

8 LO WWM, SOLTI-BOHMAN LG, High resolution CT of the jugular foramen: anatomy and vascular variants and anomalies, *Radiology* (1984) **150**:743–7.

9 REMLEY KB, HARNSBERGER HR, JACOBS JM et al, The radiologic evaluation of pulsatile tinnitus and the vascular tympanic membrane, *Semin Ultrasound CT MR* (1989) **10**(3):236–50.

10 BROGAN M, CHAKERES DW, SCHMALBROCK P, High-resolution 3DFT MR imaging of the endolymphatic duct and soft tissues of the otic capsule, *AJNR* (1991) **12**:1–11.

11 SWARTZ J, FAERBER EN, Congenital malformations of the external and middle ear. High resolution CT findings of surgical import, *AJR* (1985) **144**:501–6.

12 VALVASSORI GE, CLEMIS JD, The large vestibular aqueduct syndrome, *Laryngoscope* (1978) **5**:723–8.

13 SWARTZ J, The inner ear. In: Swartz J, ed., *Imaging of the Temporal Bone: A Text/Atlas* (Thieme Medical Publishers: New York 1986) 117–60.

14 EELKEMA EA, CURTIN HD, Congenital anomalies of the temporal bone, *Semin Ultrasound CT MR* (1989) 10(3):195–212.

15 EGELHOFF JC, BALL WS, TOWBIN RB, Dural ectasia as a cause of widening of the internal auditory canals in neurofibromatosis, *Pediatr Radiol* (1987) 17:7–9.

16 CURTIN HD, MAY M, Double internal auditory canal associated with progressive facial weakness, *Am J Otol* (1986) 7:275–81.

17 WEISSMAN JL, ARRIAGE M, CURTIN HD et al, Duplication anomaly of the internal auditory canal, *AJNR* (1991) 12(5):867–9.

18 LO WMM, SOLTI-BOHMAN LG, MCELVEEN JT, Aberrant carotid artery: radiologic diagnosis with emphasis on high resolution computed tomography, *Radiographics* (1985) 5:985–93.

19 CURTIN HD, WOLFE P, MAY M, Malignant external ottitis: CT evaluation, *Radiology* (1982) 145:383–8.

20 MENDELSON DS, SOM PM, MENDELSON MH et al, Malignant external otitis: the role of computed tomography and radionuclides in evaluation, *Radiology* (1983) 149:745–9.

21 PIEPERGERDES JC, KRAMER BM, BEHNKE EE, Keratosis obturans and external canal cholesteatoma, *Laryngoscope* (1980) 88: 420–34.

22 MAFEE MF, SINGLETON EL, VALVASSORI GE et al, Acute otomastoiditis and its complications: role of CT, *Radiology* (1985) 155:391–7.

23 MAFEE MF, AIMI K, KAHEN HL et al, Chronic otomastoiditis. A conceptual understanding of CT findings, *Radiology* (1986) 160:193–200.

24 SWARTZ JD, GOODMAN RS, RUSSELL KB et al, High resolution computed tomography of the middle ear and mastoid. Part II: Tubotympanic disease, *Radiology* (1983) 148:455–9.

25 MARTIN N, STERKERS O, NAHUM H, Chronic inflammatory disease of the middle ear cavities: Gd DTPA-enhanced MR imaging, *Radiology* (1990) 176:399–405.

26 SWARTZ JD, WOLFSON RJ, MARLOWE FI et al, Post-inflammatory ossicular fixation: CT analysis with surgical correlation, *Radiology* (1985) 154:697–700.

27 SWARTZ JD, BERGER AS, ZWILLENBERG S et al, Ossicular erosions in the dry ear: CT diagnosis, *Radiology* (1987) 163:763–5.

28 MAFEE MF, LEVIN BC, APPLEBAUM EL et al, Cholesteatoma of the middle ear and mastoid: a comparison of CT scan and operative findings, *Otolaryngol Clin North Am* (1988) 21:265–93.

29 JOHNSON DW, VOORHEES RL, LUFKIN RB et al, Cholesteatomas of the temporal bone: role of computed tomography, *Radiology* (1983) 143:733–7.

30 KOLTAI PJ, EAMES FA, PARNES SM et al, Comparison of computed tomography and magnetic resonance imaging in chronic otitis media with cholesteatoma, *Arch Otolaryngol Head Neck Surg* (1989) 115:1231–3.

31 SILVER AJ, JANECKA I, WAZEN J et al, Complicated cholesteatomas: CT findings in inner ear complications of middle ear cholesteatomas, *Radiology* (1987) 164:47–51.

32 GREENBERG JJ, OOT RF, WISMER GL et al, Cholesterol granuloma of the petrous apex: MR and CT evaluation, *AJNR* (1988) 9:1205–14.

33 MARTIN N, STERKERS O, MOMPOINT D et al, Cholesterol granulomas of the middle ear cavities: MR imaging, *Radiology* (1989) 172:521–5.

34 SATALOFF RT, MYERS DL, ROBERTS BR et al, Giant cholesterol cysts of the petrous apex, *Arch Otolaryngol Head Neck Surg* (1988) 114:451–3.

35 SELTZER S, MARK AS, Contrast enhancement of the labyrinth on MR scans in patients with sudden hearing loss and vertigo: Evidence of labrynthine disease, *AJNR* (1991) 12:13–16.

36 DANIELS DL, CZERVIONKE LF, MILLEN SJ, MR imaging of facial nerve enhancement in Bell palsy or after temporal bone surgery, *Radiology* (1989) 171:807–9.

37 LO WMM, SOLTI-BOHMAN LG, LAMBERT PR, High resolution CT in the evaluation of glomus tumors of the temporal bone, *Radiology* (1984) 150:737–42.

38 HASSO AN, LEDINGTON JA, Imaging modalities for the study of the temporal bone, *Otolaryngol Clin North Am* (1988) 21:219–44.

39 HASSO AN, SMITH DS, The cerebellopontine angle, *Semin Ultrasound CT MR* (1989) 10(3):280–301.

40   DANIELS DL, MILLEN SJ, MEYER GA et al, MR detection of tumor in the internal auditory canal, *AJR* (1987) **148**:1219–22.

41   VALVASSORI GE, MARATES FG, PALACIOS E et al, MR of the normal and abnormal internal auditory canal, *AJNR* (1988) **9**:115–19.

42   HAUGHTON VM, RIMM AA, CZERVIONKE LF et al, Sensitivity of Gd-DTPA-enhanced MR imaging of benign extraaxial tumors, *Radiology* (1988) **166**:829–33.

43   HAN MH, JABOUR BA, ANDREWS JC et al, Nonneoplastic enhancing lesions mimicking intracanalicular acoustic neuroma on gadolinium-enhanced MR images, *Radiology* (1991) **179**:795–6.

44   SPAGNOLI MV, GOLDBERG HI, GROSSMAN RI et al, Intracranial meningiomas: high field MR imaging, *Radiology* (1986) **161**:369–75.

45   ZIMMERMAN RD, FLEMING CA, SAINT-LOUIS LA et al, Magnetic resonance imaging of meningiomas, *AJNR* (1985) **6**:149–57.

46   LATACK JT, KARTUSH JM, KEMINK JL et al, Epidermoidomas of the cerebellopontine angle and temporal bone: CT and MR aspects, *Radiology* (1985) **157**:361–6.

47   LATACK JT, GABRIELSEN TO, KNAKE JE et al, Facial neuromas: radiologic evaluation, *Radiology* (1983) **149**:731–9.

48   HEADINGTON JT, Epidermal carcinomas of the integument of the nose and ear. In: Batsakis JG, ed., *Tumors of the Head and Neck* (Williams and Wilkins: Baltimore 1979) 420–30.

49   SWARTZ JD, The otodystrophies, In: Swartz JD, ed., *Imaging of the Temporal Bone, A Text/Atlas* (Thieme Medical Publishers, Inc: New York 1986) 161–78.

50   TABOR EK, CURTIN HD, HIRSCH, BE et al, Osteogenesis imperfecta tarda: appearance of the temporal bones at CT, *Radiology* (1990) **175**:181–3.

51   JOHNSON DW, HASSO AN, STEWART III CE et al, Temporal bone trauma: high-resolution computed tomographic evaluation, *Radiology* (1984) **151**:411–15.

52   HASSO AN, LEDINGTON JA, Traumatic injuries of the temporal bone, *Otolaryngol Clin North Am* (1988) **21**:295–316.

A

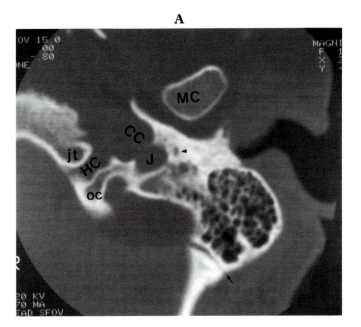

C

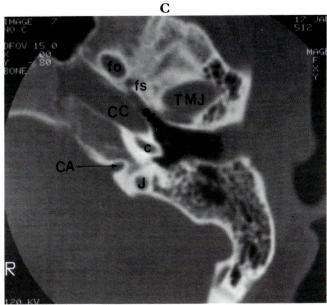

B

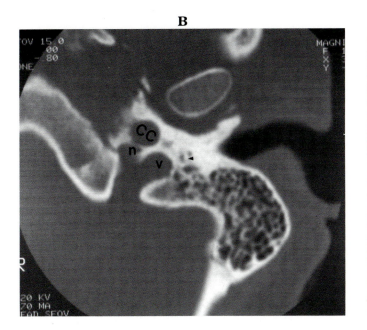

D

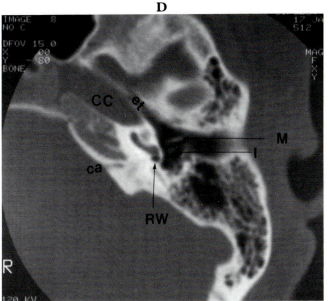

FIGURE 7.1

Axial CT scans of a temporal bone extending from skull base to the top of the petrous bone demonstrating normal anatomy. (**A**) Section through the hypoglossal canal. jt, jugular tubercle; HC, hypoglossal canal; oc, occipital condyle; CC, carotid canal; J, jugular fossa; MC, mandibular condyle; arrowhead, facial canal; arrow, occipito-mastoid suture. (**B**) Section through the jugular fossa. CC, carotid canal; n, pars nervosa; v, pars vascularis (two components of the jugular fossa); arrowhead, facial canal. (**C**) Section through basal turn of cochlea. fo, foramen ovale; fs, foramen spinosum; TMJ, temporomandibular joint; et, eustachian tube; CC, carotid canal; J, jugular fossa; c, cochlea (basal turn); CA, cochlear aqueduct; eac, external auditory canal; M, malleus. (**D**) Section through the round window. CC, carotid canal; et, eustachian tube; ca, cochlear aqueduct; M, malleus (long process); I, incus (long process); RW, round window.

continued

E

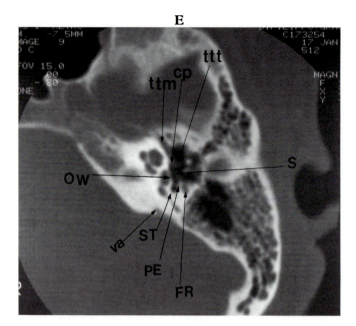

G

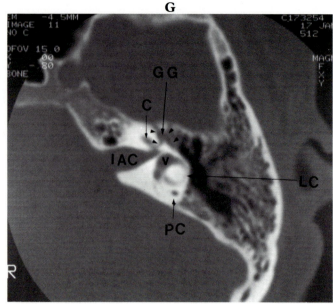

F

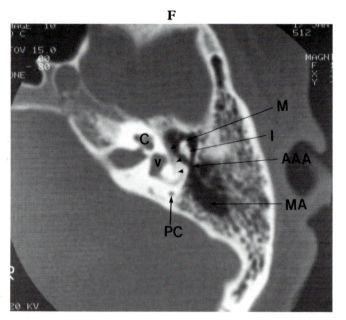

H

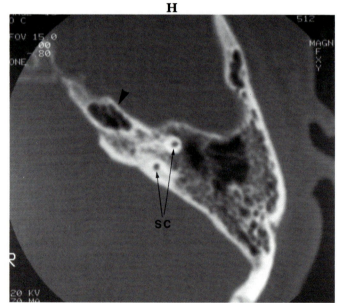

FIGURE 7.1 *(continued)*

(**E**) Section through oval window. ttm, tensor tympani muscle in the semicanal; cp, cochleariform process; ttt, tendon of tensor tympani muscle; S, stapes; OW, oval window; ST, sinus tympani; PE, pyramidalis eminence; FR, facial recess; Va, vestibular aqueduct. (**F**) Section through the internal auditory canal. C, cochlea; v, vestibule; arrowheads, tympanic portions of facial nerve canal; M, malleus head; I, incus body; AAA, aditus ad antrum; MA,

mastoid antrum; PC, posterior semicircular canal. (**G**) Section through the genu of facial nerve canal. C, cochlea; IAC, internal auditory canal; GG, geniculate ganglion; arrowheads, labyrinthine and tympanic portion of facial nerve canal; LC, lateral semicircular canal; PC, posterior semicircular canal; v, vestibule. (**H**) Section through the superior semicircular canal. SC, superior semicircular canal; large arrowhead, air cells in petrous apex.

A

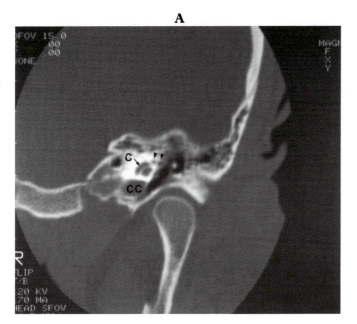

C

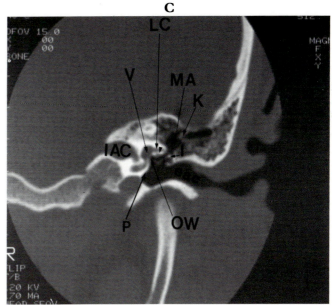

B

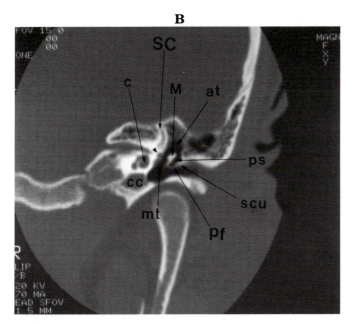

D

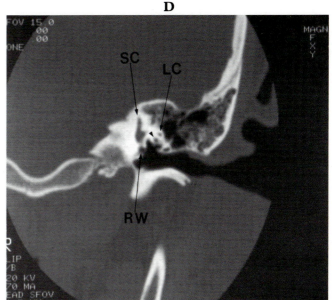

FIGURE 7.2

Coronal CT scans of temporal bone extending from an anterior to posterior direction depicting normal anatomy. (**A**) Section through cochlea. C, cochlea; CC, carotid canal; arrowheads, labyrinthine and tympanic portions of facial nerve canal. (**B**) Section partially through IAC. C, cochlea; CC, carotid canal; SC, superior semicircular canal; M, malleus; at, attic (epitympanum); ps, Prussak's space; scu, scutum; pf, pars flaccida; mt, mesotympanum; arrowhead, tympanic portion of facial nerve canal. (**C**) Section through the oval window. IAC, internal auditory canal; v, vestibule; LC, lateral semicircular canal; MA, mastoid antrum; K, Koerner's septum; I, incus; OW, oval window; P, promontory; eac, external auditory canal; arrowhead, labyrinthine and tympanic portion of facial nerve canal. (**D**) Section through the round window. SC, superior semicircular canal; LC, lateral semicircular canal; RW, round window; arrowhead, tympanic portion of facial nerve canal.

continued

E

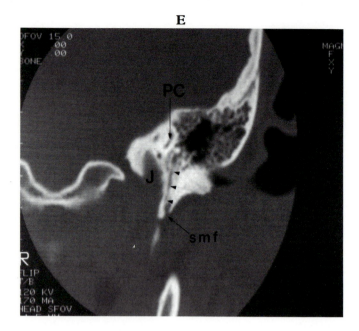

FIGURE 7.2 *(continued)*

(**E**) Section through the vertical facial canal. PC, posterior semicircular canal; J, jugular fossa; arrowheads, vertical portion of facial nerve canal; smf, stylomastoid foramen. (**F**) Section through the hypoglossal canal. J, jugular fossa; jt, jugular tubercle; hc, hypoglossal canal; oc, occipital condyle.

F

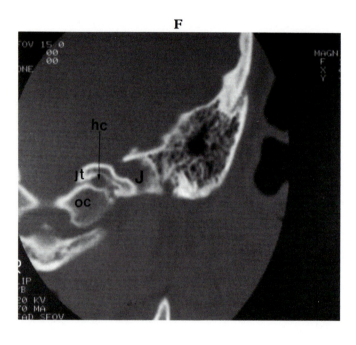

A

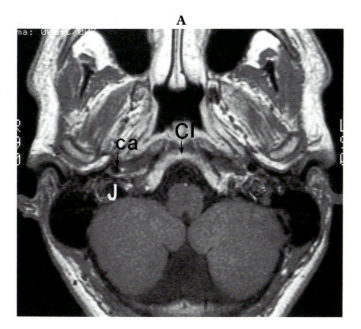

C

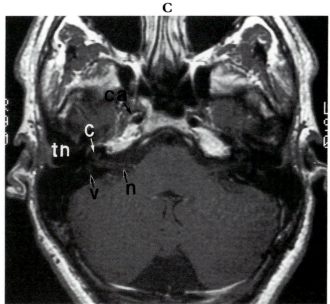

B

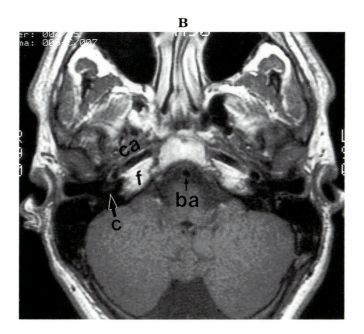

D

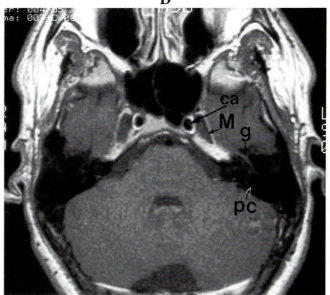

FIGURE 7.3

Normal MRI anatomy in axial plane. T1-weighted MR image (repetition time TR=500 ms, echo delay time TE=20 ms). (**A**) Section through the jugular fossa. J, jugular vein; Ca, carotid artery; Cl, clivus with high signal marrow. (**B**) Section through the basal turn of cochlea. Ca, carotid artery; c, cochlea (basal turn); ba, basilar artery; f, petrous apex fatty marrow. (**C**) Section through the internal auditory canal. Ca, carotid artery; c, cochlea; v, vestibule; tn, tympanic portion of facial nerve; n, 7th–8th nerve complex in the internal auditory canal. (**D**) Section at the genu of the facial nerve. Ca, carotid artery; M, Meckel's cave; G, geniculate ganglion; pc, posterior semicircular canal.

A

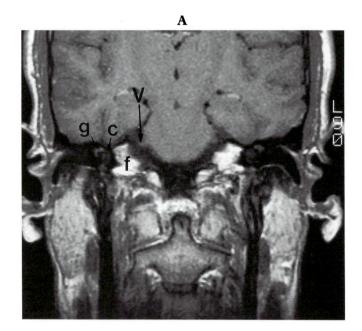

C

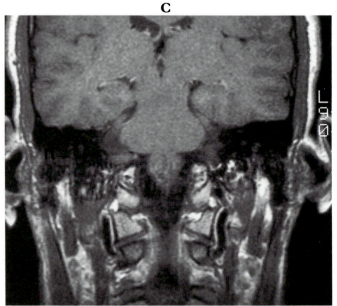

B

FIGURE 7.4

Normal MRI anatomy in the coronal plane from anterior to posterior direction. (**A**) Section through the cochlea. c, cochlea; g, genu of the facial nerve; V, 5th nerve (preganglionic segment); f, fatty marrow in the petrous apex. (**B**) Section through the IAC. n, 7th and 8th nerve complex in the internal auditory canal; cpa, cerebellopontine angle cistern; J, jugular vein; hc, hypoglossal canal. (**C**) Section through the vertical (mastoid) facial canal. n, vertical portion of the facial nerve canal. Note the lack of signal from the bony septae and air in the mastoid cells.

A

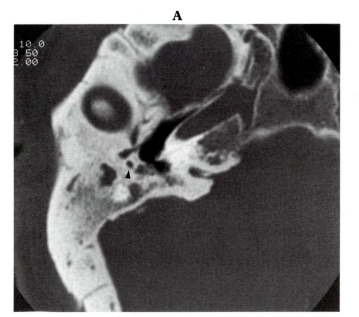

C

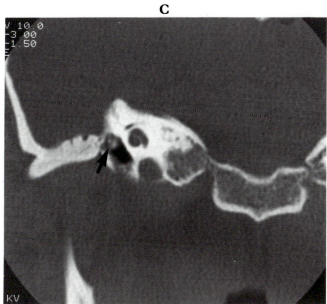

B

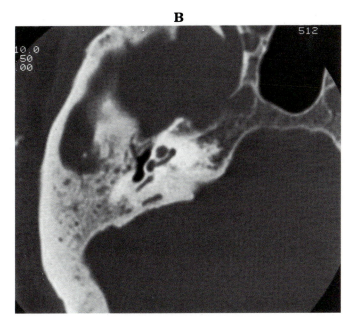

D

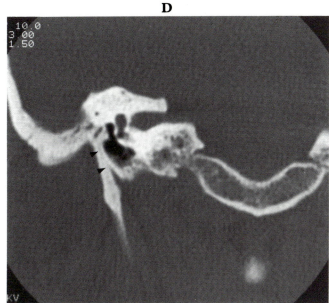

FIGURE 7.5

Atresia of external auditory canal. (**A, B**) Axial CT scans demonstrate complete atresia of the external auditory canal. The facial nerve canal is located anteriorly (arrowhead). The middle ear cavity is hypoplastic. (**C, D**) Coronal CT scans confirm the atretic external canal and hypoplastic tympanic cavity. The ossicles are malformed (arrow). The facial nerve canal is placed anterior and medial (arrowheads). The inner ear structures are unremarkable.

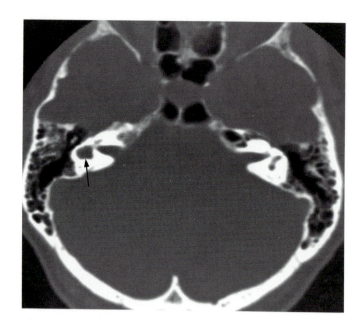

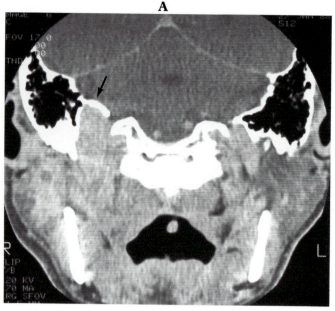

A

FIGURE 7.6

Inner ear malformation. Axial CT scan demonstrates dilatation of the right lateral semicircular canal that forms a single cavity with the vestibule (long arrow).

B

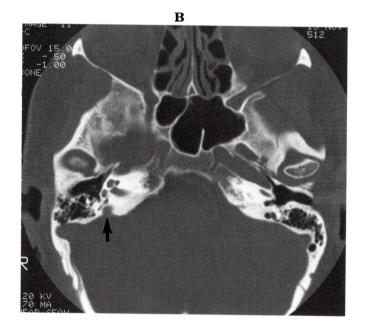

FIGURE 7.7

Normal variants. (**A**) Coronal CT scan shows a high riding right jugular vein (arrow). The right parotid gland shows increased density due to inflammatory disease. (**B**) Axial CT scan (different patient) demonstrates a small jugular diverticulum on the right (arrow).

A

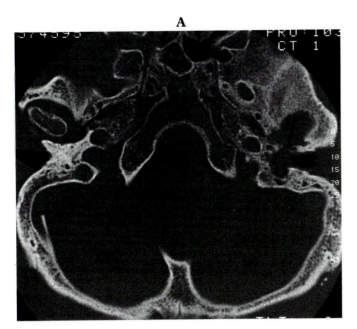

C

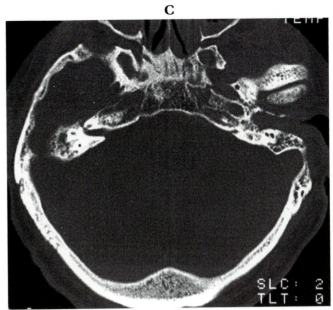

B

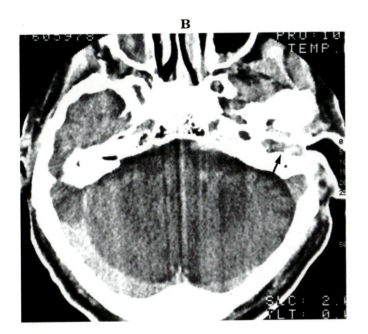

FIGURE 7.8

Malignant external otitis. (**A**) Axial CT scan reveals opacification of the left external canal and middle ear cavity. The anterior wall of the external canal and TMJ fossa are eroded (arrow). The CT appearance is indistinguishable from that of squamous cell carcinoma. (**B, C**) Axial CT scans (different patient) demonstrate an enhancing soft tissue mass (arrow) in the external auditory canal and bony erosion.

A

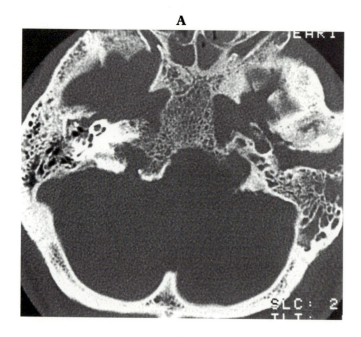

A

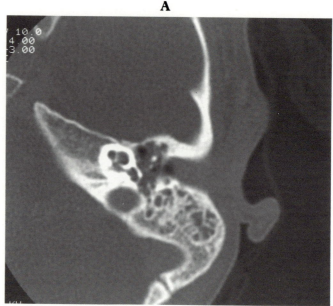

B

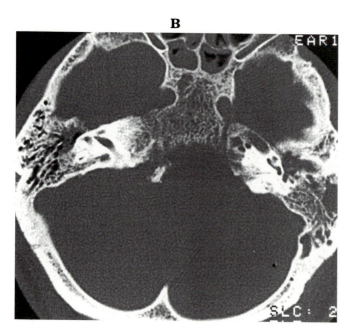

B

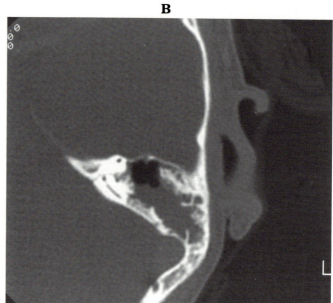

FIGURE 7.9

Osteomyelitis. (**A, B**) Axial CT scans demonstrate extensive osteomyelitis involving the skull base. The clivus is eroded, as are the petrous bones bilaterally. Note opacification of the middle ears bilaterally and left external canal. There is erosion of the external mastoid cortex and opacification of mastoid air cells.

FIGURE 7.10

Acute otomastoiditis. 11-year-old with persistent otorrhea. (**A**) Axial CT scan at the level of the tympanic cavity demonstrates almost complete opacification of the middle ear cavity and mastoid air cells. The ossicles are intact. (**B**) Axial CT scan shows erosion of the septae of the mastoid air cells and an empyema cavity with an air fluid level.

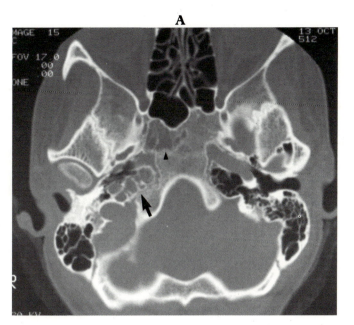

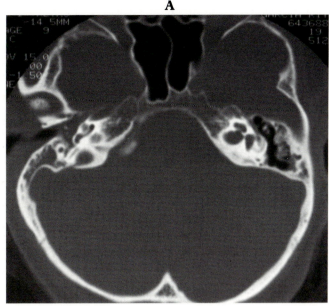

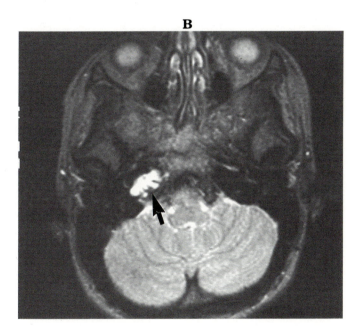

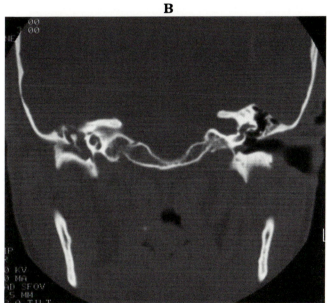

FIGURE 7.11

Apical petrositis. 28-year-old woman with resolving otitis media. (**A**) Axial CT scan reveals soft tissue opacification of the petrous air cells on the right (arrow). Incidentally noted is fibrous dysplasia at the skull base (arrowhead). (**B**) Axial T2-weighted MR image (TR=2000 ms, TE=80 ms). Note the very high signal intensity compatible with inflammatory disease in the petrous apex (arrow).

FIGURE 7.12

Granulomatous otomastoiditis. (**A, B**) Axial and coronal CT scans demonstrate complete opacification of the right middle ear cavity and mastoid air cells. The tympanic membrane is bulging laterally. The scutum and ossicles are intact. Differential diagnosis includes granulation tissue, polyp or cholesteatoma. Pathology revealed tuberculous granulomas in the middle ear.

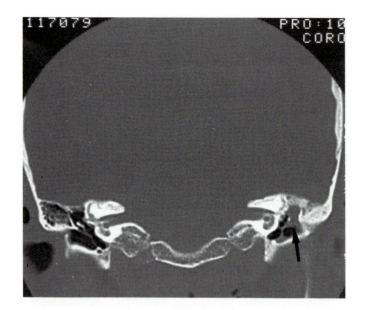

A

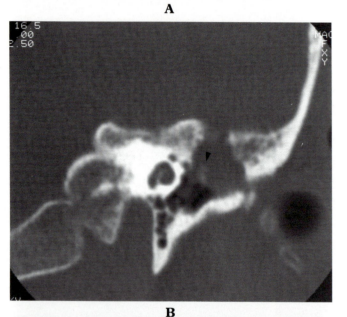

B

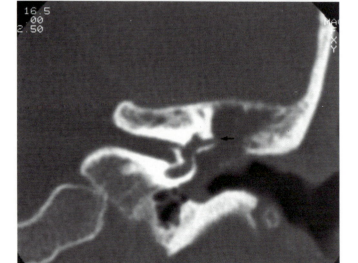

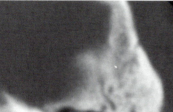

FIGURE 7.13

Acquired attic cholesteatoma. Coronal CT scan. An expansile soft tissue mass (arrow) is seen in the attic with erosion of the scutum and ossicular mass. The ossicular remnant is displaced medially. The Prussak's space is widened.

C

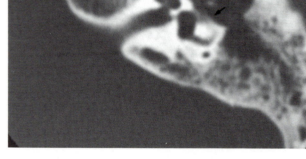

FIGURE 7.14

Acquired cholesteatoma with labyrinthine fistula. 52-year-old man with recurrent left ear infections. (**A**) Coronal CT scan at the level of the cochlea shows an expansile soft tissue mass in the left attic. The scutum and ossicles (arrowhead) are eroded. The tegmen tympani is dehiscent. (**B**) Coronal CT scan at the level of the vestibule reveals erosion of the lateral semicircular canal resulting in a labyrinthine fistula (arrow). (**C**) Axial CT scan at the level of the IAC shows an expansile soft tissue mass. Note the ossicular remnant (arrowhead) and erosion of the lateral semicircular canal (arrow).

A

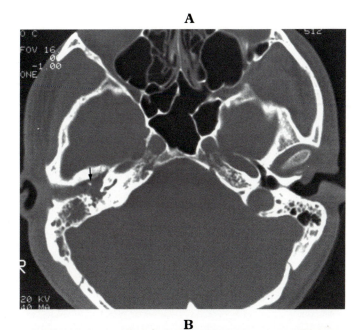

C

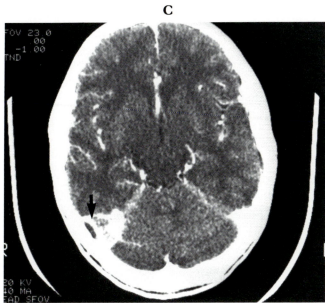

B

FIGURE 7.15

Infected cholesteatoma complicated by epidural abscess. 22-year-old man presented with a draining ear, neck rigidity and fever. (**A**) Axial CT scan shows an expansile soft tissue mass in the right middle ear cavity with ossicular erosion (arrow). The mastoid air cells are opacified. The external ear canal is also filled with soft tissue debris. (**B**) Coronal CT scan also demonstrates the expansile soft tissue mass and erosion of the ossicles and scutum. The constellation of findings is consistent with an acquired cholesteatoma. (**C**) Contrast enhanced axial CT scan of the brain shows an enhancing epidural abscess (arrow).

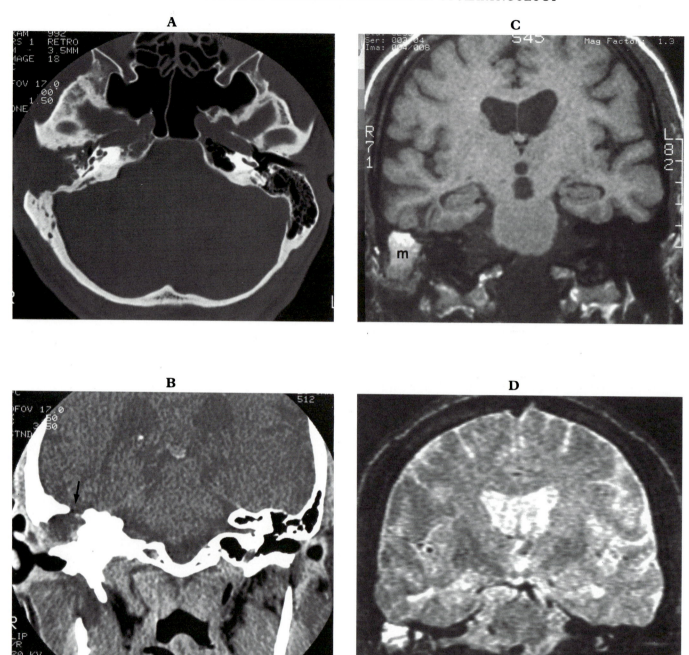

FIGURE 7.16

Recurrent cholesteatoma. 84-year-old man status post right mastoidectomy. (**A, B**) Axial (bone windows) and coronal scans (soft tissue windows). A large soft tissue mass is noted in the mastoidectomy cavity. The middle ear is opacified. Note dehiscence of the tegmen (arrow). Differential diagnosis included recurrent cholesteatoma versus acquired meningoencephalocele. (**C, D**) Coronal T1- and T2-weighted MR images clearly excluded brain herniation and confirmed this mass to be a recurrent cholesteatoma. The mass (m) shows intermediate to high signal on both T1- and T2-weighted images.

A

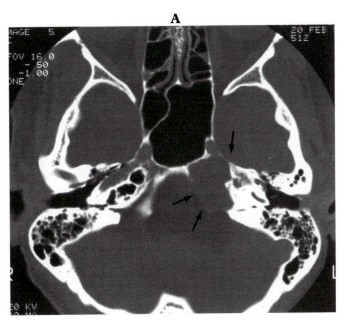

C

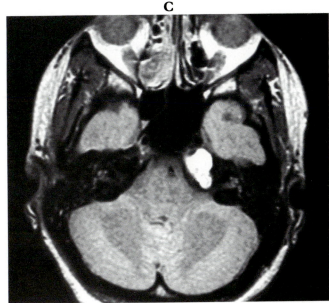

B

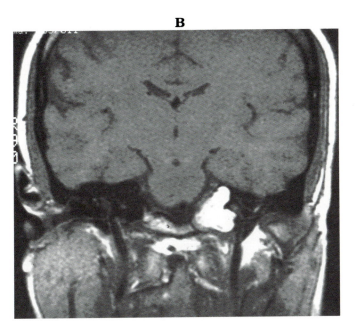

D

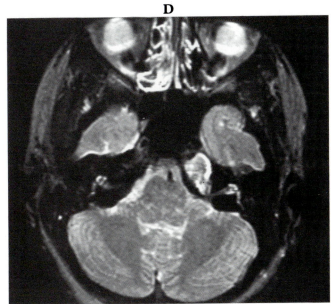

FIGURE 7.17

Giant cholesterol cyst. (**A**) Axial CT scan shows an expansile mass in the left petrous apex abutting the sphenoid sinus (arrows). The middle ear cavity and the mastoid air cells are normal. (**B**) Coronal T1-weighted MR image (TR=450 ms, TE=11 ms). The mass is slightly inhomogeneous and shows high signal intensity. (**C, D**) Axial double-echo, proton density and T2-weighted MR images (TR=2300 ms, TE=30, 90 ms). The mass is inhomogeneous but predominantly of high signal intensity on both images. The middle ear and mastoid cells are normal. The high signal is predominantly secondary to the blood products in this lesion. Incidentally noted is right ethmoid inflammatory disease.

A

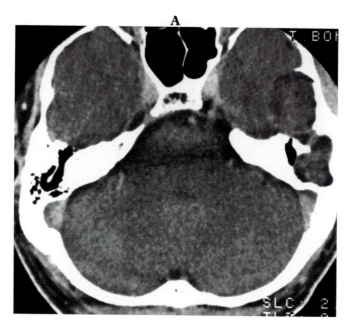

C

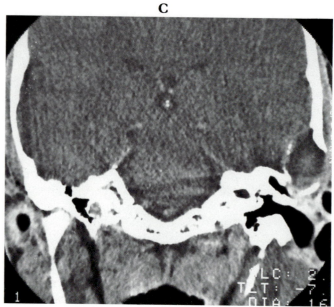

B

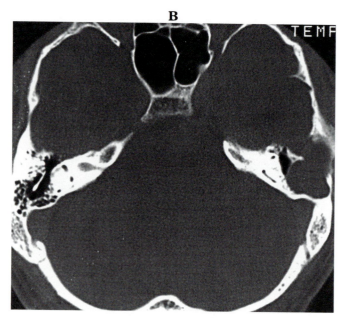

D

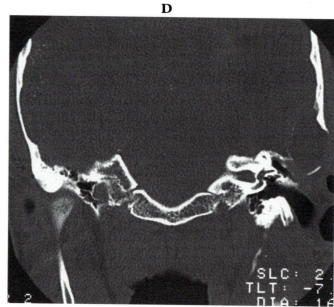

FIGURE 7.18

Congenital cholesteatoma. (**A, B**) Axial CT scans (soft tissue and bone window) show a large expansile mass in the left mastoid and the squamosal portion of the left temporal bone. The mass shows low attenuation. (**C, D**) Coronal CT scans (soft tissue and bone windows). The soft tissue mass in the mastoid and the squamous portion of the temporal bone has expanded and eroded bone. The dura is intact. The middle ear is normal. There was no history of previous ear infections.

A

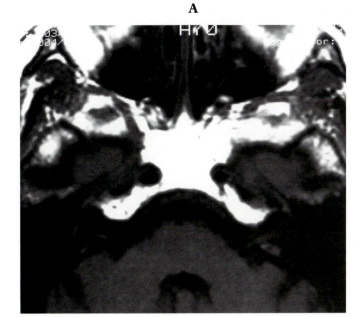

C

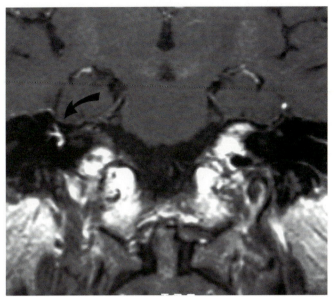

B

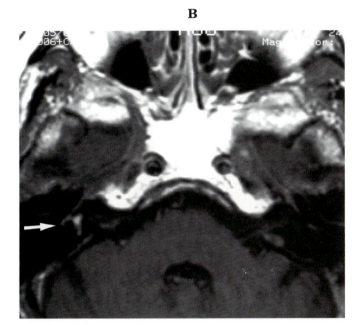

FIGURE 7.19

Labyrinthitis. (**A, B**) Axial T1-weighted MR images (TR=450 ms, TE=12 ms) before and after gadolinium administration. Note enhancement of the right labyrinth, specifically the vestibule, lateral semicircular canal and the posterior semicircular canal (arrow). (**C**) Coronal T1-weighted postgadolinium MR image (TR=450 ms, TE=12 ms) shows enhancement of the vestibule, superior and lateral semicircular canal (arrow).

A

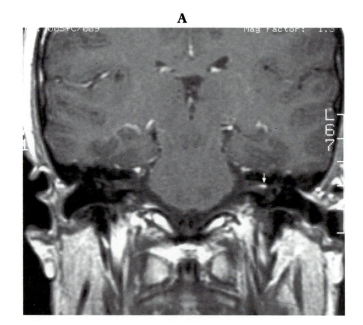

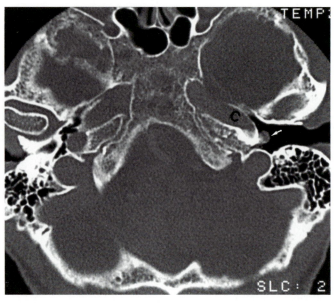

B

FIGURE 7.21

Glomus tympanicum. Axial scan shows a well-defined soft tissue mass in the middle ear cavity (arrow). The horizontal position of the carotid canal is intact (C).

FIGURE 7.20

Bell's palsy. (**A, B**) Axial and coronal T1-weighted postgadolinium MR images (TR=450 ms, TE=11 ms) reveal enhancement of the intracanalicular (at the apex of the IAC) (arrow), labyrinthine, genu and the tympanic portions of the left facial nerve (double arrow).

A
C

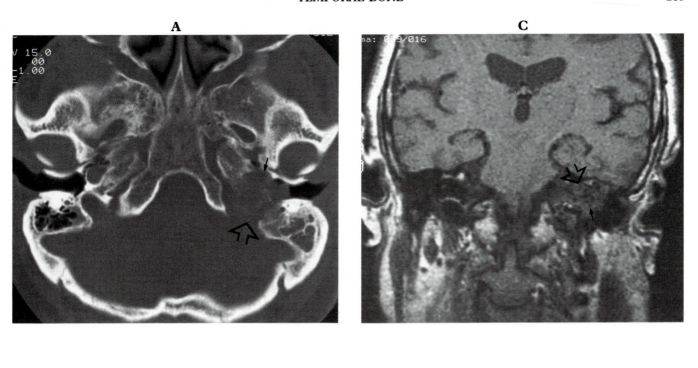

B
D

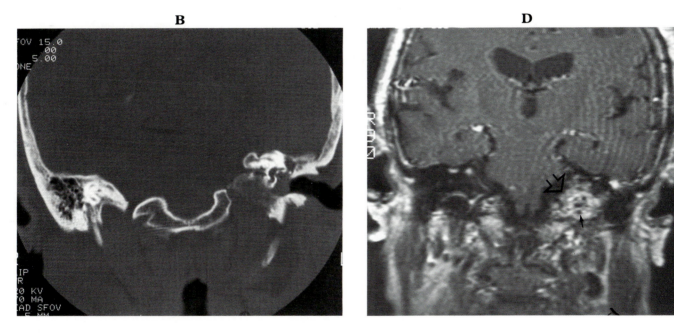

FIGURE 7.22

Glomus jugulare. Unenhanced CT scans in axial (**A**) and coronal (**B**) planes reveal a large soft tissue mass eroding the left jugular fossa (open arrow) with extension into the middle ear cavity. There is erosion of the carotid canal (small arrow) and the inferior aspect of the petrous bone. (**C, D**) T1-weighted MR images (TR=600 ms, TE=20 ms) before and after gadolinium enhancement. The mass (open arrow) in the left jugular fossa reveals intermediate signal intensity with several areas of signal void (small arrow) indicating its vascular nature. The mass enhances intensely.

A

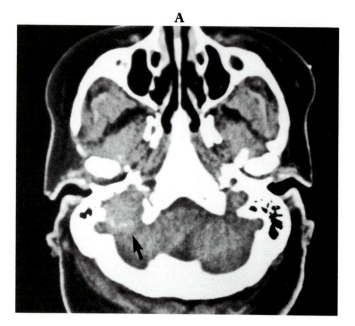

C

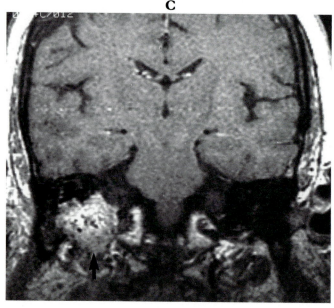

B

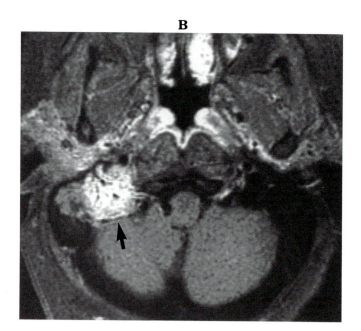

FIGURE 7.23

Glomus jugulare. (**A**) Contrast-enhanced axial CT scan. A large enhancing soft tissue mass causing erosion of the right jugular fossa is seen (arrow). Axial (**B**) and coronal (**C**) T1-weighted MR images (TR=500 ms, TE=20 ms) reveal an enhancing mass in the right jugular fossa (arrow). Note the signal void areas giving the 'salt and pepper' appearance.

A

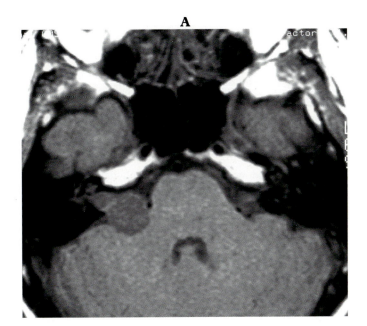

C

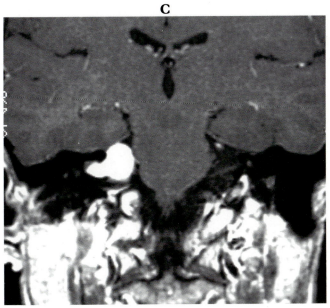

B

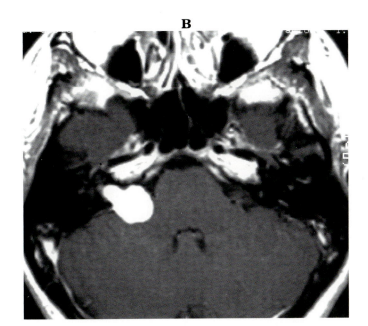

FIGURE 7.24

Acoustic schwannoma. (**A**) Axial T1-weighted MR images (TR=450 ms, TE=12 ms). The right internal auditory canal is enlarged by a soft tissue mass which has a large component extending into the cerebellopontine angle cistern. The mass has intermediate signal intensity. Axial (**B**) and coronal (**C**) T1-weighted MR images following gadolinium administration reveal homogeneous intense enhancement of the mass.

A

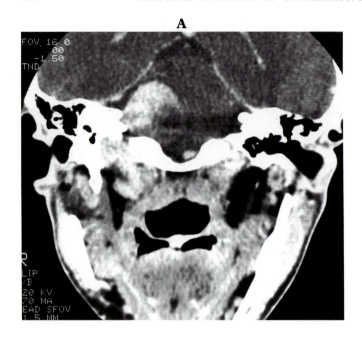

FIGURE 7.25

Cystic acoustic schwannoma. (**A**) Contrast-enhanced coronal CT scan demonstrates a large inhomogeneous enhancing mass in the cerebellopontine angle cistern. The enhancing mass extends into the IAC. (**B, C**) Coronal T1-weighted images (TR=600 ms, TE=20 ms) before and after gadolinium administration show an inhomogeneously enhancing mass in the right IAC and cerebellopontine angle. Note the mass effect on the brain stem.

B

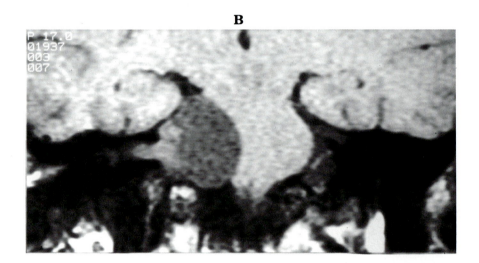

C

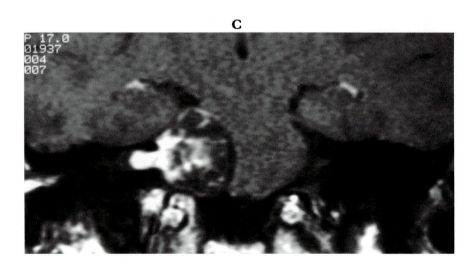

A

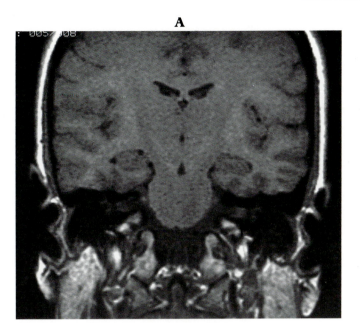

C

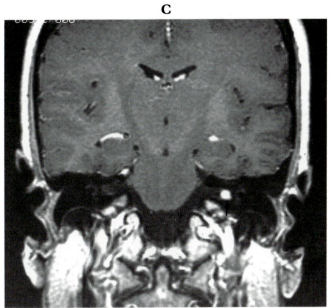

B

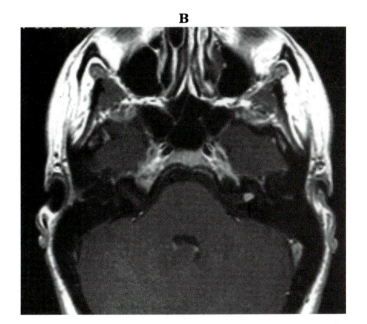

FIGURE 7.26

Intracanalicular acoustic schwannoma. (**A**) Coronal T1-weighted MR image (TR=450 ms, TE=11 ms) reveals minimally high signal along the 7th and 8th nerve complex in the fundus of the IAC (arrow). Axial (**B**) and coronal (**C**) T1-weighted images following gadolinium administration reveal an enhancing mass (arrow) in the fundus of the left IAC.

A

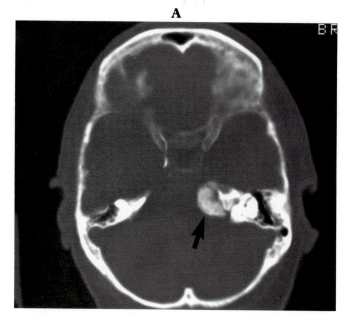

C

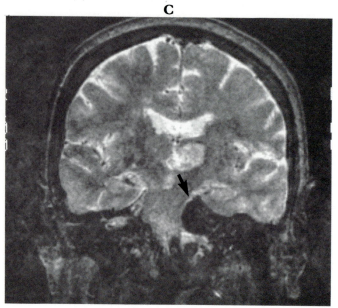

B

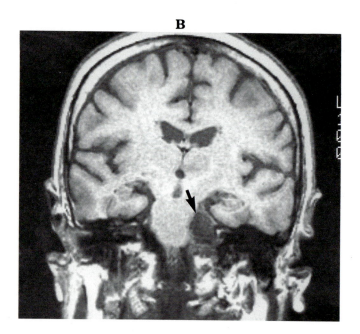

FIGURE 7.27

Meningioma. (**A**) Axial CT scan (bone windows) shows an extraaxial, densely calcified mass (arrow) at the left petrous apex extending into the CPA. (**B, C**) Coronal T1-weighted (TR=600 ms, TE=20 ms) and T2-weighted (TR=2000 ms, TE=80 ms) MR images. The mass (arrow) is of intermediate signal intensity on the T1-weighted image and of lower signal intensity on the T2-weighted image. Note the mass effect on the brain stem.

A

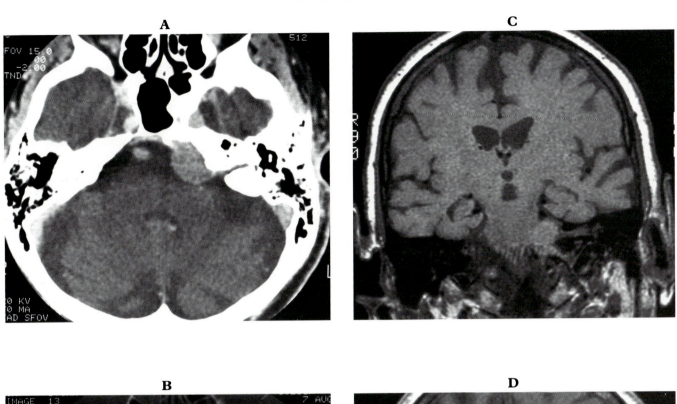

C

B

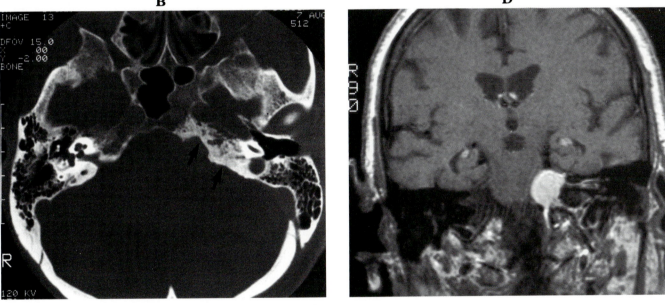

D

FIGURE 7.28

Meningioma. (**A, B**) Contrast-enhanced axial CT scans (soft tissue and bone windows) reveal an intensely enhancing extraaxial mass in the left CPA. Note the hyperostosis at the left petrous apex on image (**B**) (arrows).

(**C, D**) Coronal T1-weighted MR images (TR=800 ms, TE=20 ms) before and after gadolinium administration. The mass is of intermediate signal intensity precontrast and shows intense enhancement (**D**).

continued

E

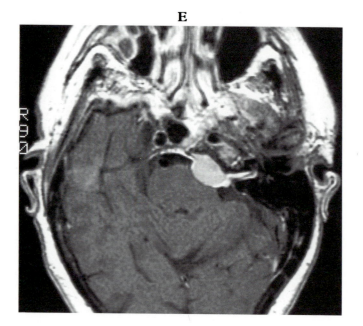

FIGURE 7.28 *(continued)*

(**E**) Axial T1-weighted postgadolinium MR image reveals enhancement in the IAC without enlargement of the nerve complex. A linear area of enhancement is also present anteriorly which is more clearly visualized on image (**D**) and represents the 'dural tail' sign which is described with meningiomas.
(**F**) Axial T2-weighted MR image demonstrates the meningioma to be of low to intermediate signal intensity.

F

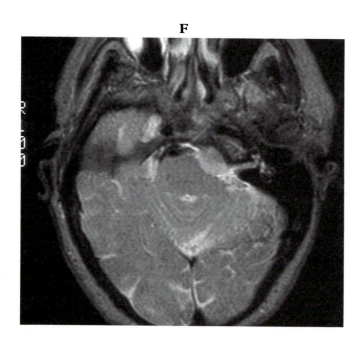

A

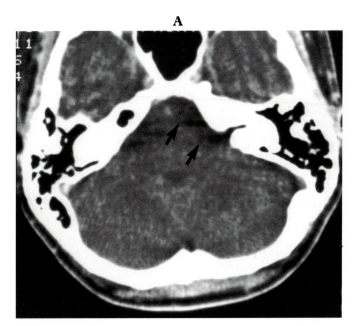

C

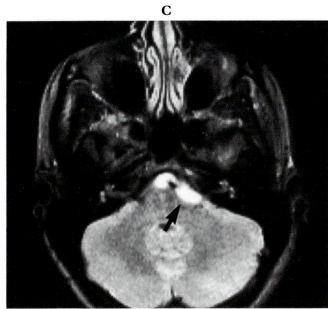

B

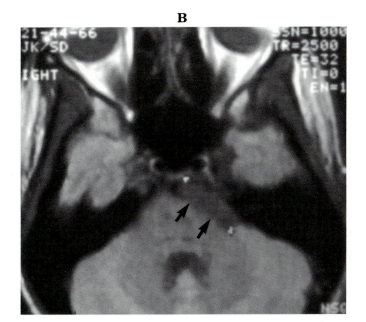

FIGURE 7.29

Epidermoid. (**A**) Axial CT scan demonstrates a low attenuation mass (arrows) in the left CPA extending to the prepontine region. (**B, C**) Axial proton density and T2-weighted MR images. The mass (arrows) reveals long T2 relaxation and shows very high signal intensity on the T2-weighted images.

A

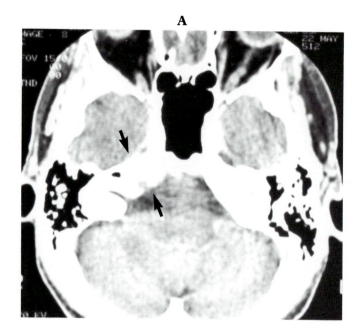

B

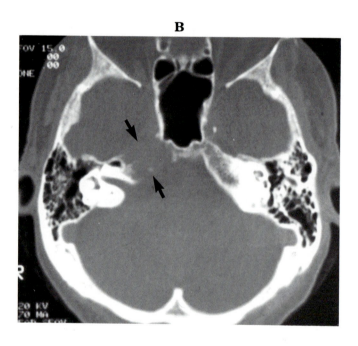

FIGURE 7.30

Metastases. 62-year-old woman with breast carcinoma presented with 5th nerve symptoms on the right. (**A, B**) Contrast-enhanced axial CT scans at soft tissue and bone windows show an enhancing metastatic mass (arrows) which erodes the right petrous apex.

A

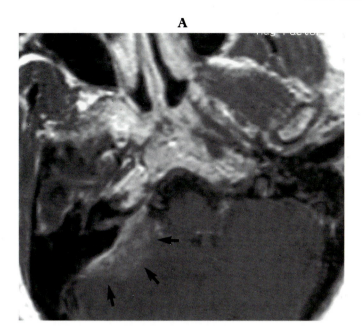

C

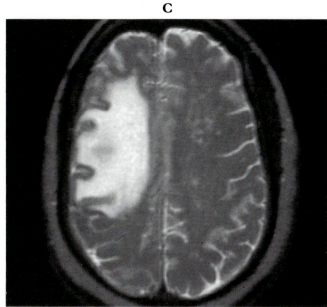

B

FIGURE 7.31

Metastases. 61-year-old woman with lung carcinoma. (**A, B**) Axial and coronal T1-weighted MR images (TR=450 ms, TE=12 ms) following gadolinium administration. A large enhancing dural-based metastatic lesion (arrows) is noted in the right posterior fossa and CPA, mimicking a meningioma. The margins of the mass, however, are irregular, which makes meningioma less likely. Also note the intracanalicular enhancement on the right. The coronal image reveals a second dural-based metastatic lesion (curved arrow) in the right parietal region with inhomogeneous enhancement and is accompanied by extensive surrounding edema (low signal intensity; open arrow). This patient's MRI of the brain done 9 months earlier was completely normal. (**C**) T2-weighted MR image (TR=2300 ms, TE=90 ms) confirms the parietal edema with high signal intensity.

A

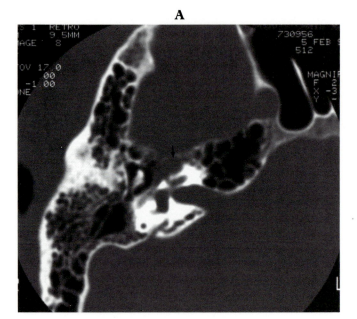

C

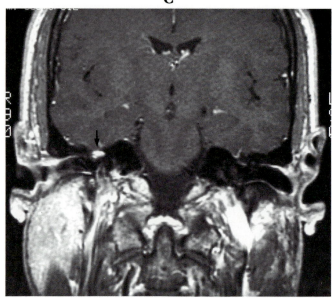

B

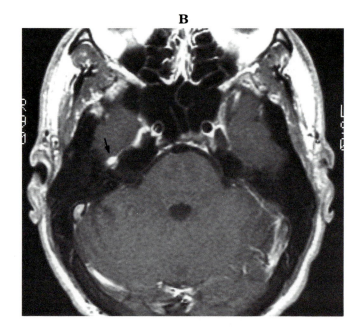

FIGURE 7.32

Facial schwannoma. (**A**) Axial CT scan (bone window) reveals an expansile soft tissue mass at the genu of the right facial nerve (arrow). Axial (**B**) and coronal (**C**) T1-weighted postgadolinium MR images (TR=500 ms, TE=11 ms) show an enhancing mass (arrow) predominantly at the genu of the facial nerve and in the superior compartment of the internal auditory canal fundus.

A

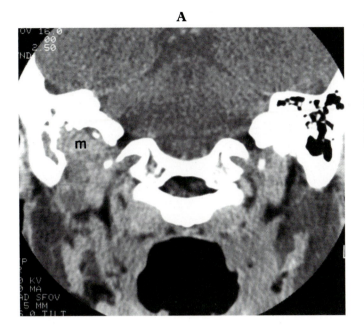

C

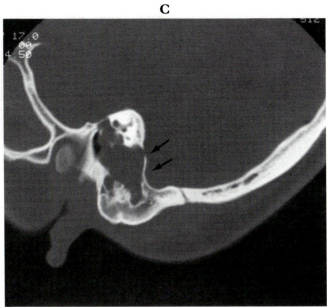

B

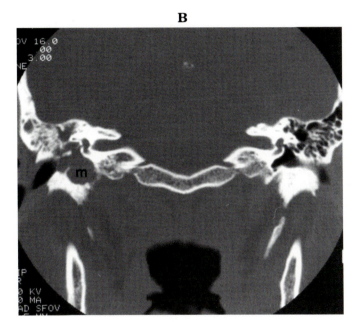

FIGURE 7.33

Facial schwannoma. (**A, B**) Contrast-enhanced coronal CT scans (soft tissue and bone windows). A large, lobulated, fusiform, inhomogeneously enhancing mass (m) is noted along the tympanic and vertical portion of the facial nerve with erosion of the facial nerve canal. (**C**) Sagittal CT scan. The expansile mass is along the vertical portion of the facial nerve (arrows).

continued

D

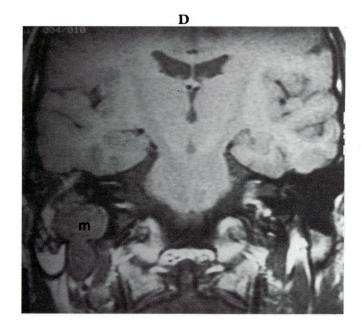

F

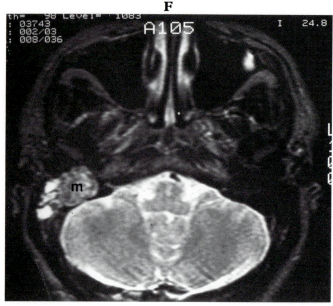

E

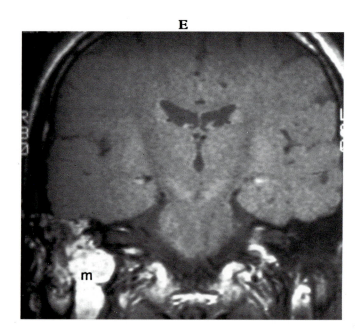

FIGURE 7.33 *(continued)*

(**D, E**) Coronal T1-weighted pre- and postgadolinium MR images (TR=800 ms, TE=20 ms) demonstrate intense enhancement of the mass (m). The IAC is normal. Also note opacification of mastoid air cells by fluid. (**F**) Axial T2-weighted MR image (TR=2500 ms, TE=80 ms) demonstrates the facial neuroma (m) to be of intermediate signal intensity. The fluid in the mastoid air cells is of high signal intensity.

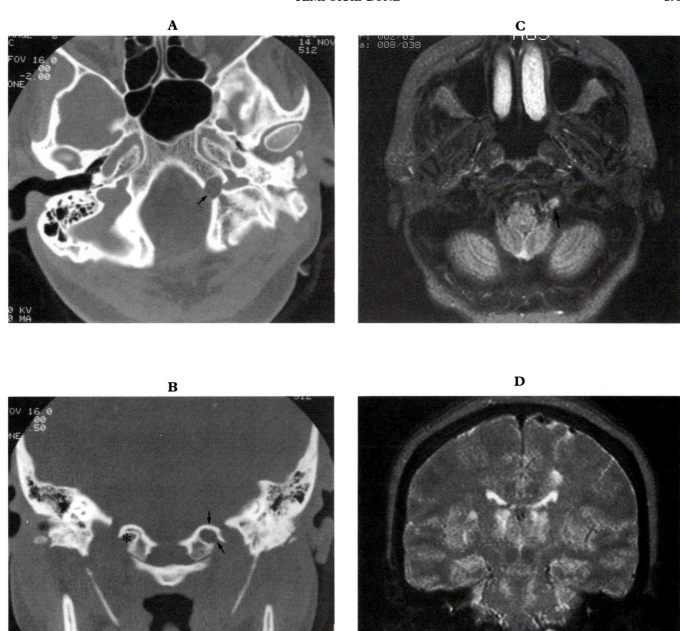

FIGURE 7.34

Hypoglossal schwannoma. (**A, B**) Axial and coronal CT scans reveal smooth enlargement of the left hypoglossal canal (arrows). The normal right hypoglossal canal (∗) is seen in the coronal image

(**B**). (**C, D**) Axial and coronal T2-weighted MR images (TR=2400 ms, TE=80 ms). The hypoglossal schwannoma is of high signal intensity (arrow).

A

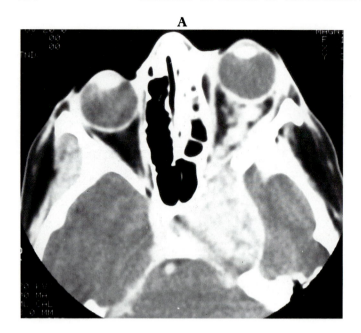

C

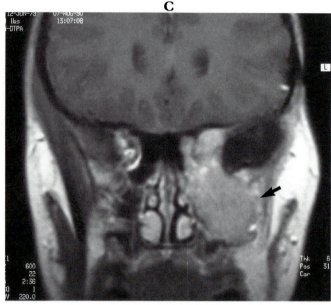

B

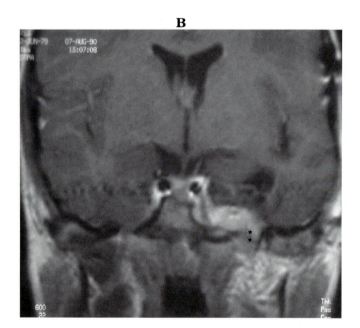

FIGURE 7.35

Trigeminal plexiform neurofibroma. 9-year-old girl with neurofibromatosis type II. (**A**) Contrast-enhanced axial CT scan shows a very large, inhomogeneous, intensely enhancing mass at the Meckel's cave which extends anteriorly along all three divisions of the 5th nerve. There is widening of the superior orbital fissure and inferior orbital fissure at the orbital apex. (**B,C**) Coronal T1-weighted postgadolinium MR images (TR=600 ms, TE= 22 ms). The large enhancing plexiform neurofibroma widens the foramen ovale (✶✶). The orbital apex is expanded by the large mass which extends into the infratemporal fossa (arrow). (Courtesy of Robert A. Zimmerman, MD, Philadelphia.)

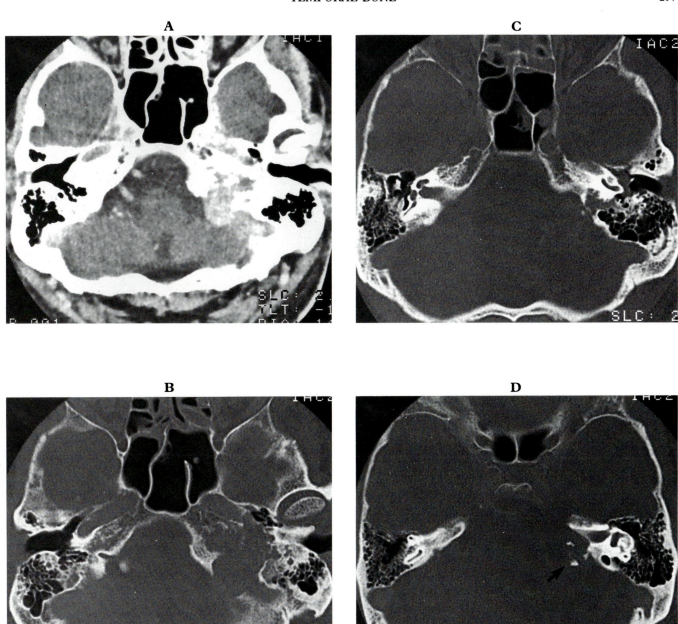

FIGURE 7.36

Chondrosarcoma. 68-year-old man with a mass in the middle ear. (**A–C**) Axial contrast-enhanced CT scans (bone and soft tissue windows) show a large enhancing destructive mass at the skull base, eroding the jugular fossa, petrous bone, otic capsule and extending into the middle ear cavity, mimicking a jugulotympanic glomus tumor. (**D**) Axial CT scan at the level of the IAC reveals a chondroid matrix (arrow) which helps to differentiate this tumor from a paraganglioma.

A

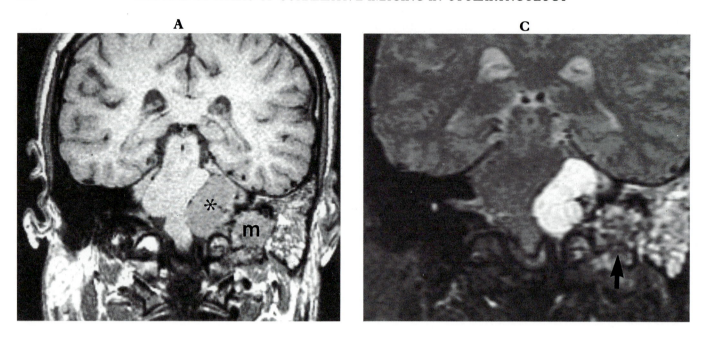

C

B

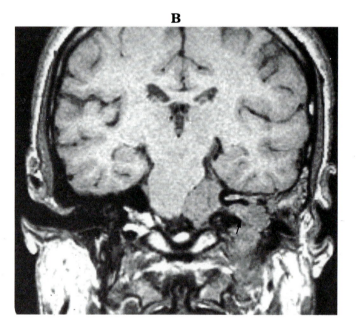

D

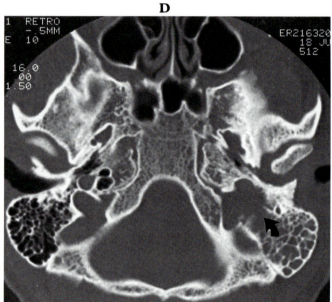

FIGURE 7.37

Osteosarcoma accompanied by arachnoid cyst. (A, B) Coronal T1-weighted MR images (TE= 600 ms, TE=20 ms). There is a mass (m) at the skull base in the region of jugular fossa and a large mass in the left CPA (*). The mastoid air cells are opacified. The mass extends into the middle ear and the internal auditory canal (arrows). The petrous bone is eroded by this tumor. (C) Coronal T2-weighted MR image (TR=2500 ms, TE=80 ms). The mass in the CPA shows very high signal and represents an arachnoid cyst. The mass at the skull base (osteosarcoma) shows intermediate signal intensity (arrow). The mastoid air cells show high signal secondary to fluid. (D) Axial CT scan demonstrates aggressive bony erosion at the skull base involving the jugular fossa and carotid canal (curved arrow).

A

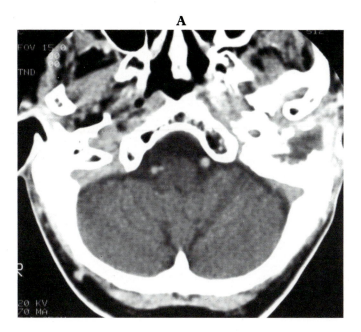

C

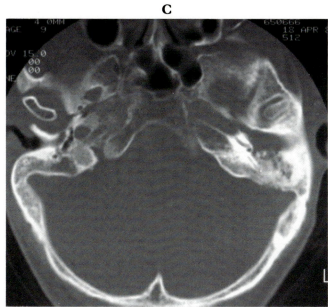

B

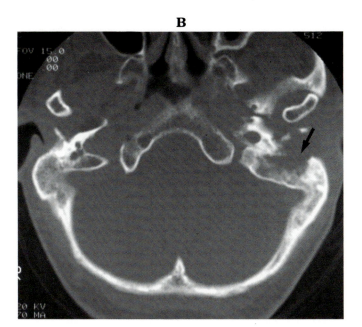

FIGURE 7.38

Squamous cell carcinoma of the external auditory canal. (**A**) Contrast-enhanced axial CT scan reveals an enhancing mass in the left external auditory canal and middle ear cavity with a central area of low attenuation secondary to necrosis. (**B, C**) Axial CT scans (bone windows) reveal extensive erosion of the bony external canal and mastoid (arrow). The soft tissue mass completely opacifies the middle ear cavity.

A

C

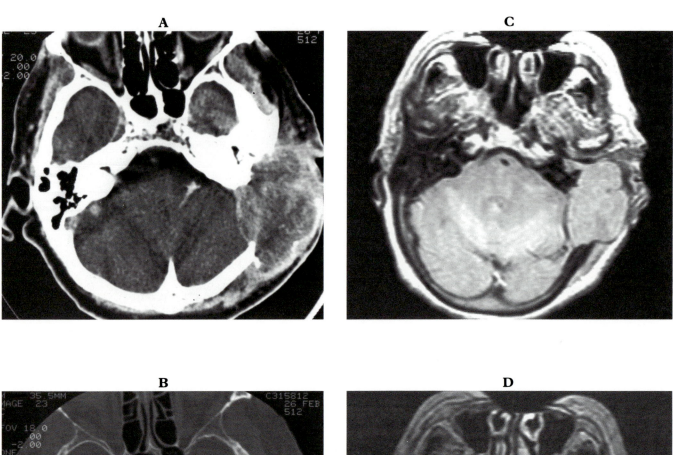

B

D

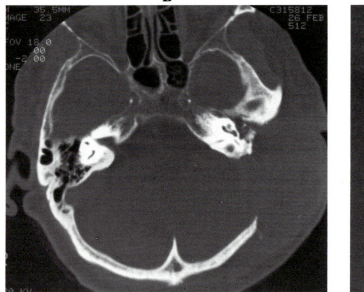
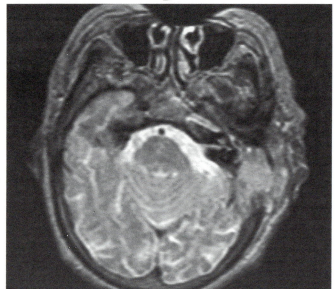

FIGURE 7.39

Squamous cell carcinoma arising from the mastoid complex. (**A, B**) Contrast-enhanced axial CT images (soft tissue and bone windows). A large expansile mass with patchy enhancement is noted in the left mastoid process with complete erosion of the mastoid complex and external ear canal. The soft tissue completely opacifies the middle ear cavity. (**C, D**) Axial proton density (TR=2000 ms, TE= 30 ms) and T2-weighted (TR=2000 ms, TE=80 ms) MR images demonstrate a large mass in the left mastoid complex with extension into the external and middle ear cavities. The mass is of intermediate

continued

E

A

F

B

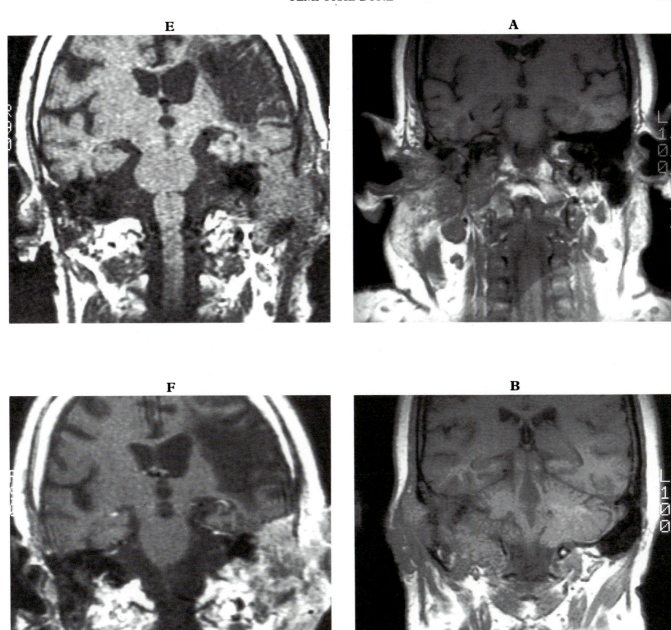

FIGURE 7.39 *(continued)*

signal intensity on both T1- and T2-weighted images. (**E, F**) Coronal T1-weighted pre- and postgadolinium MR images (TR=500 ms, TE=20 ms) demonstrate inhomogeneous enhancement. Note the intradural extension of tumor in the middle cranial fossa. An old infarct in the left MCA distribution is also seen.

FIGURE 7.40

Muco-epidermoid carcinoma. 60-year-old woman with a two-year history of 'Bell's palsy', hearing loss and jaw pain. (**A, B**) Coronal T1-weighted MR images (TR=600 ms, TE=11 ms) show a mass of intermediate signal intensity in the deep portion of the parotid gland with complete erosion of the external auditory canal, middle ear, the petrous bone and the mastoid bone. The mass extends intracranially into the posterior fossa. Laterally, the mass extends to the skin surface.

continued

C   A

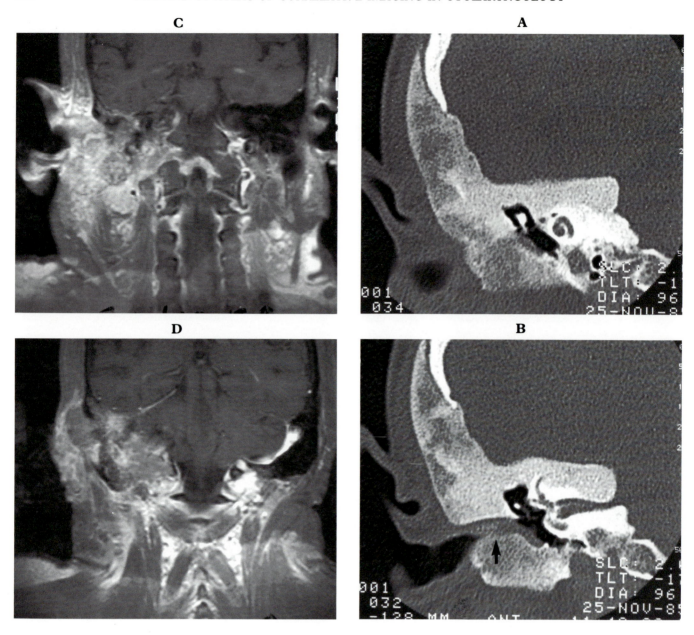

D   B

FIGURE 7.40 *(continued)*   **FIGURE 7.41**

(**C, D**) Coronal T1-weighted postgadolinium MR   Fibrous dysplasia. (**A, B**) Coronal CT scans at the
images (TR=600 ms, TE=11 ms). There is diffuse   level of cochlea and IAC, respectively. The temporal
enhancement of the mass. Intracranial (intradural)   bone is diffusely enlarged. The external auditory
extension of the tumor is well demonstrated in the   canal shows marked narrowing (arrow). The middle
posterior and middle cranial fossa.   ear and inner ear structures are normal.

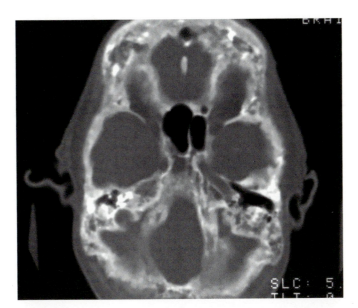

A

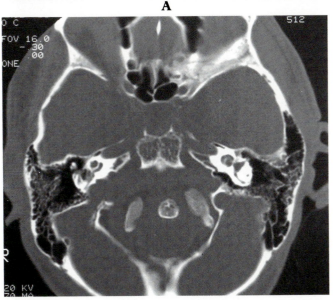

B

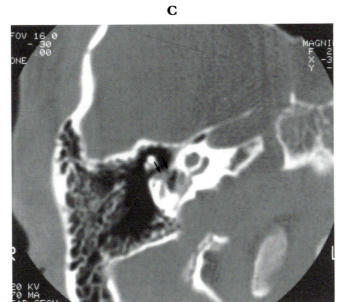

C

FIGURE 7.42

Paget's disease. Axial CT scan shows diffuse extensive demineralization of the calvarium, skull base and the temporal bones bilaterally by Paget's disease. Note expansion of the diploic space and the typically described 'cotton wool' appearance.

FIGURE 7.43

Osteogenesis imperfecta tarda. 42-year-old woman. (**A**) Axial CT scan shows extensive bilateral foci of demineralization in the otic capsule that surrounds the cochlea, vestibule, round and oval windows. (**B, C**) Magnified views of the right temporal bone demonstrate foci of demineralization at the round (single arrow) and oval (double arrows) windows.

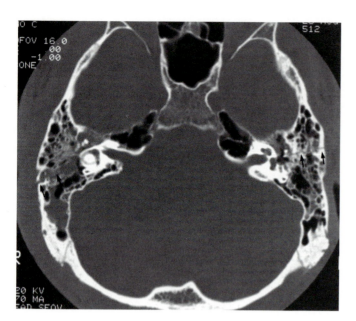

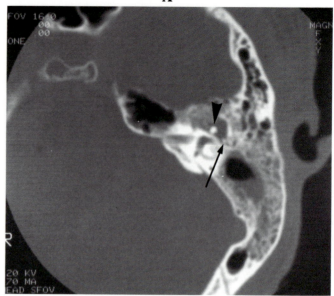

A

FIGURE 7.44

Bilateral longitudinal fractures of the temporal bone.
Axial CT scan demonstrates bilateral longitudinal
fractures (arrows). Opacification of the middle ear
cavity and mastoid air cells is noted bilaterally but
more so on the right side. The ossicles are intact.

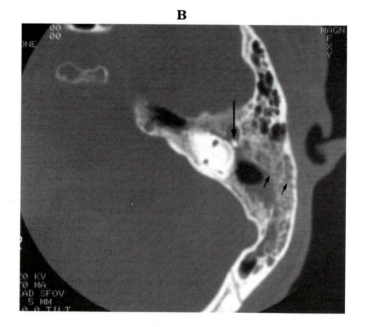

B

FIGURE 7.45

Longitudinal fracture with ossicular disruption.
(**A**, **B**) Axial CT scans show a longitudinal fracture
of the left temporal bone (small arrows).
Opacification of the mastoid air cells and an air
blood level is noted in the antrum. Note the
ossicular disruption. The incus (long stem arrow) is
dislocated superiorly in image (**B**). The head of the
malleus is visualized (arrowhead) with disruption of
the normal 'ice cream cone' appearance.

A

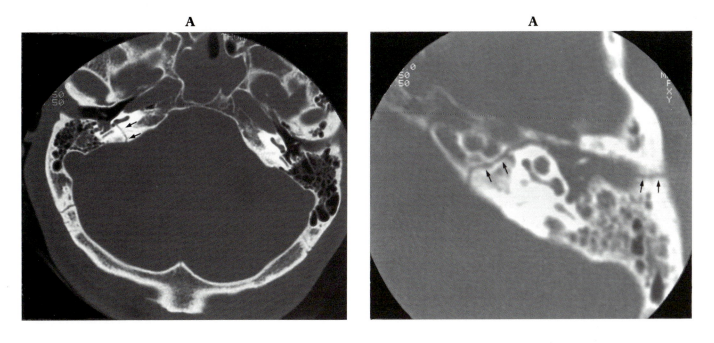

B

A

B

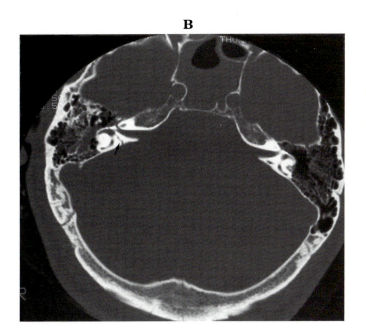

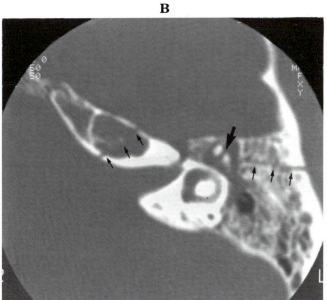

FIGURE 7.46

Transverse fracture of the temporal bone. (**A, B**) Axial CT scans shows a lateral type of transverse fracture (arrows) extending across the basal turn of cochlea (**A**) and across the vestibule (**B**). Also note soft tissue density in the mastoid antrum secondary to hemorrhage.

FIGURE 7.47

Complex fracture with ossicular disruption. (**A, B**) Axial CT scans reveal almost total opacification of the tympanic cavity and mastoid air cells. The fracture line follows an oblique course with a longitudinal component laterally and transverse component medially (small arrows). The otic capsule is spared. The ossicles are abnormal. There is increased distance between the long process of the malleus and the long process of the incus. The incudomallear joint is disrupted (large arrow).

CHAPTER 8

ORBIT

The bony orbit houses the visual apparatus. The eyeball, by virtue of its exterior location, is readily accessible to direct inspection, but the retrobulbar space and the majority of the contents of the bony orbit remain hidden. The eyeball is a natural acoustic window, allowing for detailed sonographic evaluation of its structure and characterization of intraocular lesions. Cross-sectional imaging methods (computed tomography and magnetic resonance imaging) have placed the radiologist in a pivotal role in the diagnosis of ophthalmologic disorders. Computed tomography (CT) and magnetic resonance imaging (MRI) exploit the tissue contrasts in the orbit while revealing fine anatomic details. Formerly, small, en-plaque lesions in the globe were visible only through ophthalmoscopy or ultrasound. With the development of high-resolution surface coil methods and gadolinium-DTPA there has been a marked increase in the diagnostic power of MRI in ophthalmologic imaging. Magnetic resonance imaging has the additional benefit in providing the most detailed in vivo study of the entire visual apparatus, from the globe to the visual cortex. The extraordinary depiction of the visual pathways that MRI provides has changed the practice of neurophthalmology.

Anatomic considerations

Bony orbit

The paired orbits are conical structures, surrounded by bone, containing the eyeballs, optic nerves, extraocular muscles and an abundance of orbital fat (Figs 8.1 and 8.2). Several foramina transmit key vascular and neural structures from the bony orbit to the middle cranial fossa. The entire visual pathway is unique in that it traverses nearly the entire antero-posterior dimensions of the cranial compartment; from eyeball anteriorly, to occipital cortex posteriorly. The relatively large area covered by the visual apparatus dictates that imaging should be tailored to address specific pathologies at specific locations.

The bony orbit is constructed from seven skull bones; the frontal, zygomatic, palatine, ethmoid, sphenoid, lacrimal and maxillary bones. The orbital roof is formed anteriorly by the orbital part of the frontal bone. The apex of the orbit is formed by the lesser wing of the sphenoid bone. The optic canal perforates this structure. Laterally, the orbital wall is composed of the zygomatic process of the frontal bone anteriorly, the greater wing of the sphenoid bone posteriorly and a portion of the zygomatic bone in between. At the orbital apex, the inferior and superior orbital fissures are bordered by the greater wing of the sphenoid bone. Contributions to the medial wall of the orbit come from many separate bones, some of which are very thin. These include the frontal process of the maxilla, the orbital process of the palatine bone, the lacrimal bone and ethmoid bone (lamina papyracea). The lamina papyracea is very thin and incompletely ossified. Neoplastic or inflammatory processes of the ethmoid sinus can spread to the orbit through dehiscence of the thin lamina papyracea.[1] The mucous membranes of the ethmoid sinuses come in direct contact with the periorbita and subperiosteal space.[1,2] Finally, the orbital floor is defined by the orbital part of the maxilla. This bone is traversed by the infraorbital groove. The orbit is completely lined by periosteum, which is also referred to as the periorbita. The periorbita becomes continuous with the dura at the optic foramen and the superior orbital fissure. The anterior part of the periorbita is continuous with the thin, fibrous orbital septum.[2–4]

Extraocular muscles

There are six extraocular muscles, four of which are arranged in opposing pairs; the superior/inferior rectus and the medial/lateral rectus. All four rectus muscles arise from a tendinous ring near the optic foramen called the *annulus of Zinn*. These groups control primarily upward/downward and medial/lateral gaze, respectively. The lateral rectus muscle is innervated by the abducens (VI) nerve. The remainder of the recti and the inferior oblique muscle are innervated by the oculomotor nerve (III). The oblique muscles (superior/inferior) are primarily responsible for intorsion and extorsion of the globe. The inferior oblique is the only muscle not to arise at the orbital apex. It originates from a depression in the orbital plate of the maxilla. The superior oblique muscle is innervated by the trochlear (IV) nerve. The levator palpebrae superioris muscle functions in the elevation of the eyelid rather than in motion of the eyeball.[3,4]

Each muscle is surrounded by a fascial sheath. Extensions of the sheaths form a perimeter around the muscles known as the *intermuscular septum*. This discontinuous layer demarcates the muscle cone and the intraconal space.

Neural/vascular structures

The small nerves of the orbit are branches of the four cranial nerves that innervate the orbital structures; oculomotor nerve (III), trochlear nerve (IV), abducens nerve (VI) and trigeminal nerve (V). Other portions of the visual apparatus include the optic chiasm, optic tracts, optic radiations and the calcarine cortex of the occipital lobe. The lateral geniculate bodies, the superior colliculi, the medial longitudinal fasciculus and the extraocular muscle cranial nerve nuclei make up portions of the visual relay stations within the brainstem.

The vascular supply to the choroid and retina is provided by the ophthalmic artery which is the first branch arising from the supraclinoid internal carotid artery. Small perforating arteries from the circle of Willis nourish portions of the optic chiasm and tracts. The remainder of the visual system is supplied by branches of the vertebrobasilar system. The calcarine division of the posterior cerebral artery supplies the calcarine cortex.

The eye

The eyeball consists of three primary layers: the outer layer or *sclera*, the vascular, pigmented middle layer known as the *uvea*, and the sensory *retina*.[5] The spherical configuration of the eyeball is maintained by the fibrous collagenous structure of the sclera and cornea. Localized weakening or ectasia of the scleral covering of the eye can result in an anomalous shape to the globe known as a staphyloma (Fig. 8.3).[6] The cornea is transparent, allowing light to enter only the anterior portion of the globe. The tear film that moistens the cornea surface provides most of the refracting power of the eye. The cornea merges with the sclera at the *scleral limbus*. The sclera makes up nearly 80% of the surface of the globe and it is thickest at the insertion of the recti muscles. The surface of the sclera is known as the *episclera*. The globe is invested in a thick, fibrous membrane known as *Tenon's capsule*. This cuff of tissue lies superficial to the episclera and is discontinuous at the insertions of the recti and at the optic nerve head.[4] The *uveal tract* is the middle layer of the wall and is located between the sclera and the retina. The uvea consists of the *iris, ciliary body* and *choroid*.[7]

The anterior chamber is the portion of the globe between the cornea and the iris. The very thin posterior chamber is demarcated by the iris anteriorly and the lens posteriorly. It is filled with *aqueous humor*. The epithelium of the ciliary body secretes the aqueous humor which is resorbed in the drainage network of the iridocorneoscleral angle. The lens is an avascular structure, biconvex in shape, composed primarily of fibroelastic elements.[4] The lens and anterior chamber are easily identifiable on both CT and MR studies.[4]

The *vitreous humor* is also produced by the epithelium of the ciliary body. It fills approximately two-thirds the volume of the globe, or approximately 4 ml.[5] The vitreous is 98% water, the remainder is made up of collagen and hyaluronate. Hyaluronate gives vitreous its gel-like properties. The vitreous is anchored to the inner surface of the globe at the optic disc, the ora serrata and fovea.[4] Any insult to the vitreous body produces a fibroproliferative reaction which may result in a tractional retinal detachment.[5]

The vitreous is normally transparent and conducts light to the photoreceptors of the retina. Thus, the retina can be inspected directly through the vitreous. Disease processes that produce opacity of the vitreous interrupt the normal red-reflex of the retina, resulting in a white reflex known as leukocoria. Some of the causes of leukocoria include: retinoblastoma, cataracts, retrolental fibroplasia, Coat's disease, persistent hyperplastic primary vitreous (PHPV) and sclerosing endophthalmitis. Retinoblastoma is the only potentially lethal cause of leukocoria and therefore it is important to be aware of the radiologic features of this neoplasm.[6]

Retina

The retina is the sensory receptor of the eye. It is a complex tissue with ten identifiable cellular layers. The external surface of the retina contacts the choroid and the internal surface is contiguous with the vitreous. The sensory retina is part of the inner layer and contains the light-sensitive rods and cones as well as neurons and neuroglial elements of the retina. The outer layer of the retina is known as the retinal pigment epithelium (RPE) which lies adjacent to the basal lamina of the choroid.[5] Light crosses eight of these layers to reach the photoreceptors, the rods and cones. The rods are most sensitive to light and predominate in the peripheral retina. The cones function best in bright light, are distributed more centrally, and are responsible for color vision. At its thickest portion the retina is only about 0.4 mm thick, therefore it is normally not resolvable by MRI and CT.[4,5] The anterior-most extent of the retina is known as the ora serrata.

Choroid

The retina rests upon the pigmented vascular layer known as the choroid. The choroid's primary function is to provide nourishment for the retina.

The choroid is divided into the basal lamina (Bruch's membrane), choriocapillaris and stromal layer. Blood vessels supplying this layer are derived from the ophthalmic artery. Degenerative diseases of the microvasculature of the choroid can produce deposition of dystrophic calcifications in the choroid. These calcifications can be benign as in optic drusen (Fig. 8.4), or they can be more extensive as in cases of phthisis bulbi (Fig. 8.5). The most clinically significant lesions that produce calcifications in the choroid are the retinoblastoma and choroidal osteoma.

Optic nerve

The term optic nerve is a misnomer. It does not share any similar characteristics to the peripheral nerves, rather, it is a bundle of axons that extend from the brain substance. The optic nerve originates from the bipolar layer of the retina. Axons from the ganglia aggregate near the optic cup and exit the globe as a solitary structure. As the optic nerve courses posteriorly to the orbital apex, it is angled parallel to the hard palate. The nerve is protected by a covering of meninges: dura, arachnoid and pia. These layers merge with the surface of the globe at the point of insertion. Retinal fibers in the periphery of the globe are located peripherally in the nerve while macular fibers are located centrally and make up approximately one-third of the nerve's cross-sectional diameter. Once the nerve has traversed the optic canal, it becomes an intracranial structure lying medial to the carotid artery. The *optic chiasm* is located below the anterior floor of the third ventricle. Study of the optic nerve and tracts is exceptionally demonstrated with MRI, particularly the intracanalicular and chiasmatic portions which are obscured by bone artifacts with CT. The nerve is isointense with respect to white matter on all pulse sequences. The orbital segment of the optic nerve is 3–4 mm in diameter and 20–30 mm in length. The intraorbital segment of the optic nerve is covered with all three layers of meninges (dura, arachnoid and pia). These layers eventually fuse to the sclera of the globe.

Imaging strategies

Both CT and MRI provide high-resolution images of the orbital contents. Magnetic resonance has not completely supplanted CT in orbital imaging for several reasons. Computed tomography has distinct advantages over MR in resolving the bony orbit, in detecting calcification and fractures and it is less sensitive to eye motion.[8,9] Computed tomography exposes the lens to ionizing radiation and iodinated contrast agents are often needed for evaluating intraocular pathology.[10]

Magnetic resonance is ideally suited for the study of the intraocular pathology. Magnetic resonance offers multiplanar evaluation of the orbit and visual apparatus and better characterization of fluid and hemorrhage. The retrobulbar/intraconal structures are demonstrated with high resolution. The lack of signal within bony structures as depicted with MRI allows for detailed evaluation of the orbital apex and the entire course of the optic nerve.[9–11] Magnetic resonance is a relatively insensitive technique for detecting calcifications; this presents potential diagnostic pitfalls when evaluating perioptic meningiomas and retinoblastomas.[9]

Computed tomography

For routine CT study of the orbits, 3 mm contiguous sections in the axial and coronal planes are required as a minimum. Ideally, 1.5 mm axial images should be obtained to resolve small areas of abnormality and to allow for reformations in other planes of interest. Axial images should be performed from the level of the upper maxillary sinuses, extending superiorly through the orbital roofs and into the anterior cranial fossa. Angulation is chosen to approximate the orbital axis, at −10 degrees to the orbital–meatal line (Reid's baseline). Obtaining images parallel to the orbital axis places the entire optic nerve in the plane of section. Some authors advocate having the patient maintain an upward gaze during axial imaging to straighten the course of the nerve. Intravenous injection of iodinated contrast is beneficial in delineating intraocular pathology. In special cases, direct sagittal images can be acquired.

Coronal images should be obtained from the anterior margin of the orbit to the anterior clinoids posteriorly. If an abnormality is suspected in the visual pathways, coronal images can be extended through the cavernous sinus region. In neuro-ophthalmologic disorders, study of the remainder of the visual pathway is mandatory. This can be accomplished with 5 mm axial images of the occipital and posterior temporal lobes to incorporate the optic radiations.

Magnetic resonance imaging

The direct advantages of using MR in preference to CT include lack of ionizing radiation, multiplanar acquisition, superior tissue contrast and superior visualization of the visual pathways.[10] Magnetic resonance imaging of the orbit requires stringent attention to technique. Patient instruction and cooperation are a critical part of successful imaging. In general, acquisition times are longer than required for CT and random eye motion tends to produce more artifact.[8,9] Chemical shift artifacts can obscure portions of the globe.[9–11] Interpretation of MR images must be approached with caution in that the signal patterns on conventional spin-echo imaging often do not permit easy differentiation of benign from malignant masses.[9] Reliance on clinical information and the morphologic appearance of the abnormality remain the best tools in orbital diagnosis.

Use of orbit surface coils is mandatory when imaging the globe.[8–10] We utilize a pair of tuned-coupled three inch surface coils that are designed for temporomandibular joint imaging; however, dedicated orbit coils are available. While providing excellent signal-to-noise properties and spatial resolution in the anterior orbit, there is a marked drop-off of signal in the posterior orbit with surface coils. Lesions in the orbital apex and chiasm are better imaged in the head coil.[10] A field-of-view between 12 and 16 cm is appropriate, depending upon the area of interest; the smaller fields are useful for visualization of intraocular disease. Because random eye motion is present even when the eyes are closed, the patient is often instructed to fix his gaze in one position during image acquisition.[10] Axial T1-weighted (repetition time TR = 800 ms, echo delay time TE = 20–40 ms) and T2-weighted (TR = 1800–2000 ms, TE = 30/80 ms) images should be obtained from the upper margin of the maxillary sinus extending superiorly to the frontal lobes. Image thickness should be no greater than 3 mm with a 1 mm interslice gap. Coronal T1-weighted images should also be obtained with a similar slice thickness and field-of-view. For complete evaluation of the optic nerves, the coronal images should extend posteriorly to include the chiasm and the optic tracts. Additional axial and coronal sections (5 mm thick) of the remainder of the brain, brainstem and visual pathways should also be obtained for any neurophthalmologic disorder.

Gadolinium has been shown to be useful in the diagnosis and characterization of intraocular tumors, intraconal and extraconal neoplasia, intracanalicular tumors, inflammatory or demyelinating diseases and other neurophthalmologic disorders. The use of fat suppression in conjunction with gadolinium administration allows for improved definition of disease by narrowing the inherent dynamic range of the image.[10,12] In addition, fat suppression tends to reduce artifacts induced by random eye motion.

Pathology

Traumatic

Subperiosteal hematoma

The subperiosteal space may fill with blood as the result of trauma. A patient presents with painful, unilateral proptosis. Spontaneous hemorrhage may occur as the result of blood dyscrasias: leukemia, thromboctyopenia and hemophilia. The periorbita is loosely attached in children, therefore, this entity is most commonly reported in pediatric age groups. On CT, the acute subperiosteal hematoma appears as a high-density, well-defined, extraconal mass with a broad base of attachment to the bony orbit, usually the orbital roof. A hematic cyst can result when the blood products are incompletely resorbed and the cyst remains surrounded by a fibrous pseudocapsule. The CT appearance is that of a nonenhancing, well-defined extraconal mass in the superior orbit with a broad base of attachment to the orbital roof and bony erosion/remodeling of the orbital roof. The differential diagnosis includes cyst, epidermoid, teratoma, cholesteatoma, cholesterol granuloma, eosinophilic granuloma, encephalocele and mucocele.[2]

Computed tomography is the initial imaging modality of choice for blunt or penetrating trauma to the bony orbit and contents.[6] Computed tomography provides superior definition of the osseous structures and therefore is well suited for detection of fractures or foreign bodies. Computed tomography also yields very good definition of the soft tissue structures and is an adequate method for determining integrity of the globe, lens, optic nerve and retrobulbar structures. Magnetic resonance imaging is contraindicated when a ferromagnetic foreign body is present in the orbit. However, MR may have a secondary role in trauma due to it high sensitivity in detecting optic nerve injury and orbital hematoma.[6,10]

One of the most common sequelae of blunt trauma to the orbit is the orbital 'blow out' or 'blow-out' fracture in which the force of trauma against the eyeball is transmitted to the orbital contents and dissipated in the bony orbit. The most fragile areas of the bony orbit are most susceptible to disruption; the lamina papyracea medially and orbital process of the maxillary bone inferiorly. Orbital fat and extraocular muscle may herniate through the bony defect (Fig. 8.6).

Retinal and choroidal detachments

There are three potential spaces within the layers of the globe that can collect fluid, these are: the *posterior hyaloid space* (between the vitreous body and sensory retina), the *subretinal space* (between the sensory retina and the retinal pigment epithelium) and the *subchoroidal space* (between the choroid and the sclera). Collection of fluid in these three potential spaces can result in *hyaloid detachment, retinal detachment* (with subretinal effusion) and *choroidal detachment* (with subchoroidal effusion), respectively.[5,10] Retinal detachments are further classified into rhegmatogenous (most common) or non-rhegmatogenous, depending on whether a hole (rhegma) is present in the secondary retina.[10] Nonrhegmatogenous retinal detachments are often caused by tumors of the choroid (e.g. melanoma, metastases) or proliferative processes of the retina such as Coat's disease.[10]

Liquefaction of the vitreous body produces posterior hyaloid detachment. This occurs usually in adults over the age of 50, but has also been reported in children with persistent hyperplastic primary vitreous (PHPV). Persistent hyperplastic primary vitreous is the result of persistence of the embryonic hyaloid vascular tissue. This tissue produces retraction of the posterior hyaloid membrane and retina resulting in vitreous hemorrhage.[5]

Retinal detachment (RD) results from separation of the sensory retina from the retinal pigmented epithelium (RPE). When damaged, the RPE leaks fluid into the subretinal space. Retinal detachment often occurs because of retraction from a mass or from a vitreoretinopathy of prematurity or diabetes.[5] An exudative retinal detachment is characteristic of Coat's disease, a primary vascular anomaly of the retina. The abnormal vessels leak lipid and serum into the subretinal space. Since the retina itself is beyond the resolving power of most CT or MR scanners, detection of RD is dependent upon the ability to detect the subretinal fluid. Exudative subretinal effusions are more conspicuous than nonexudative effusions due to elevation of protein content in the exudative effusions.[10,13] Malignant melanoma and choroidal hemangioma are the most common tumors to produce RD.[5]

Axial CT or MR images taken at the equator of the globe show that retinal detachment assumes a V-shaped configuration with the leaves of the RD converging to the optic nerve head. The greater the RD and subretinal effusion, the narrower the 'V' appears, with the apex directed towards the optic nerve and the limbs pointed to the ciliary body (Fig. 8.7). Visualization of the RD by CT also depends upon the content of the associated subretinal effusion. Serous subretinal fluid is difficult to detect with CT and MR. The greater the protein content of the fluid, the higher its density and signal intensity when compared to the vitreous body. Magnetic resonance is superior to CT in differentiating serous from exudative subretinal effusions. Exudative and proteinaceous fluid collections exhibit hyperintensity on T1- and T2-weighted images while serous collections remain hypointense on T1-weighted sequences.[5,13]

Serous choroidal detachment is a nonhemorrhagic accumulation of fluid in the subchoroidal space,

often caused by surgery, penetrating trauma or inflammation. Inflammation of the choroid secondary to a scleritis and chorioretinitis can result in leakage of proteinaceous fluid into the subretinal space. The inflamed choroid may appear thickened and will abnormally enhance with infusion of contrast material. While the classic configuration of a retinal detachment (RD) is V-shaped, a choroidal detachment is less well defined. The choroid is anchored by the short ciliary arteries and nerves, therefore, fluid accumulations are restricted. Choroidal detachment and effusion assumes a crescentic shape and follows the peripheral margins of the globe. It is often not possible to differentiate choroidal from retinal detachment with CT or MRI (Fig. 8.7).[5]

Inflammatory diseases

Over one-half of the circumference of the orbits consists of bony partitions that are shared by both orbits and the paranasal sinuses. The close anatomic proximity of the orbits to the sinuses predisposes the orbits to involvement with sinus disease. The discontinuous lamina papyracea allows direct contact of the orbital contents with the ethmoid sinus.[1]

Orbital cellulitis

Orbital cellulitis is characterized clinically by ocular pain, lid edema, chemosis, proptosis and limited ocular movements.[14,15] The patient is acutely ill with fever and an elevated white count. Most cases of bacterial orbital cellulitis are secondary to bacterial sinusitis. The most common pathogens are *Staphylococcus aureus* and *Streptococcus*.[6,14,15] Hematogenous spread of infection is rare.

Imaging is an essential part of the diagnostic work-up of orbital cellulitis in ascertaining the location and extent of the disease. Computed tomography may reveal diffuse thickening and increased density of the eyelid and conjunctiva in the preseptal space.[14,15] Postseptal inflammation may extend from the ethmoid sinus to the subperiosteal region of the orbit with lateral deviation of the medial rectus muscle and anterolateral displacement of the globe (Figs 8.8 and 8.9). The CT findings of orbital cellulitis may appear similar to those of orbital pseudotumor with obliteration of the normal tissue planes and a reticulated infiltration of the retrobulbar fat.[14,15] A discrete abscess may present as an area of low attenuation surrounded by a thick, hyperdense, enhancing rim.[14] Intraconal extension of the inflammation is suspected when there is an ill-defined infiltrate of the retrobulbar fat and obliteration of the normal anatomic structures. The MR findings in orbital cellulitis are nonspecific and may be focal or diffuse. The orbital fat will demonstrate a decrease in signal intensity on the T1-weighted images.[14] Pressure effects may compromise the blood supply to the optic nerve, resulting in blindness. Untreated intraconal cellulitis can result in extension to the facial structures, superior ophthalmic vein or cavernous sinus thrombosis and intracranial abscess formation.[6,14]

Other rarer forms of infection that may secondarily affect the orbit include Wegener's granulomatosis (Fig. 8.10), tuberculosis, mucormycosis, aspergillosis (Fig. 8.11) and sarcoidosis.[1]

Optic neuritis

This entity describes primary inflammation of the optic nerve. The clinical presentation consists of the sudden onset of a central visual deficit accompanied by orbital pain.[6] In most cases, the cause of the inflammation is not identified although contiguous spread of bacterial and fungal infections from the intracranial compartment and paranasal sinuses have been implicated. Many cases are immune mediated in the setting of multiple sclerosis.[6] A CT study may be completely normal in the setting of optic neuritis or there may be diffuse enlargement of the nerve with subtle enhancement after administration of iodinated contrast material. Magnetic resonance is exceptional in its sensitivity to the inflammatory changes of optic neuritis (Fig. 8.12). The nerve is increased in caliber and of high signal intensity on long TR/TE images (T2-weighted). Detection of demyelinating lesions in the nerve is facilitated by the use of inversion recovery or fat suppression techniques and the use the gadolinium.[10] Active lesions will show enhancement.

Orbital pseudotumor

In adults, the most common cause of an intraorbital mass lesion is idiopathic orbital pseudotumor.[10,14]

The concept of orbital pseudotumor is fraught with controversy, not only in the radiologic literature, but in the ophthalmologic and pathologic literature as well. Pseudotumor refers to any inflammatory lesion that mimics a tumor when no neoplasia is actually present. While the etiology of pseudotumor is unknown in most cases, the result is an inflammatory process that can affect many structures in the orbit. Some authors prefer the term idiopathic orbital inflammatory syndrome to pseudotumor in that it implies the true nature of the lesion.[16,17] It is speculated that the inflammatory process is probably immune mediated. The clinical hallmark is that of a unilateral, painful proptosis with a rapid onset, lid swelling, chemosis and decreased ocular motility.[14] Biopsy of the acute inflammatory tissue usually reveals a hypocellular polymorphic infiltrate which is mostly composed of lymphocytes. During the acute phase, the disease is very responsive to steroid therapy. When pseudotumor is suspected, a proven response is steroid therapy often used as confirmation of the diagnosis.[14,18] Cases which do not show a dramatic response to steroid therapy may require biopsy. There is supportive evidence that chronic orbital pseudotumor predisposes to orbital lymphoma.[18]

Pseudotumor often demonstrates multifocal involvement of the orbital structures, and the disease is often characterized based upon the structure(s) involved.[14] *Myositis* is characterized by inflammation of one or more of the extraocular muscles. It presents with a painful proptosis and pain with eye movement. On CT scanning, the margins of the muscles appear indistinct and there is enlargement of both the muscle belly and its tendinous insertion (Fig. 8.13).[6] The enlargement of the tendon distinguishes pseudotumor from Graves' disease, in which only the muscle belly is enlarged. Another distinguishing factor between Graves' ophthalmopathy and myositic pseudotumor is that the former is usually a bilateral process, while pseudotumor exhibits bilateral manifestations in only 10–15% of cases.[14] Metastases to the extraocular muscles often exhibit hyperintensity on the T2-weighted images which may distinguish this etiology from benign causes such as Graves' disease or pseudotumor.[9] *Perineuritis* is inflammation of the optic nerve sheath. On imaging, the nerve is diffusely enlarged with irregular borders. There may be reticulation of the surrounding orbital fat. Decrease in visual acuity and exacerbation of pain with retropulsion of the globe are characteristic symptoms. *Dacryoadenitis* refers to inflammatory involvement of the lacrimal gland. Diffuse enlargement of the gland is present on CT or MR. *Periscleritis* is involvement of the fascial tissues covering the sclera of the eyeball (Tenon's capsule). On CT, there is marked thickening of the wall of the globe with irregular, ragged margins. Marked enhancement occurs with the use of the iodinated contrast. Reticulation of the adjacent orbital fat is also present. *Tumefactive* or diffuse pseudotumor is characterized by infiltration of the orbital fat. However, this term has also been used to describe cases in which many structures are involved simultaneously. Diffuse pseudotumor is often subdivided into anterior and posterior.

Computed tomography or MR reveals diffuse infiltration of the orbital fat with obliteration of anatomic landmarks. On CT the normal hypodense orbital fat reverts to hyperdensity (Fig. 8.14).[14,16,18] This infiltration of the orbital fat produces decreased signal intensity on the T1-weighted MR images. A characteristic feature of chronic pseudotumor on MRI is low signal intensity on the T2-weighted images while other entities such as metastatic lesions exhibit high signal intensity on the T2-weighted image.[9,10,14]

Graves' ophthalmopathy

Dysthyroid ophthalmopathy or Graves' disease is the most common cause of proptosis.[14,15] Although this condition is linked to disorders of the thyroid gland, there is poor correlation between the ophthalmologic disorder and the hormonal disturbance. The disease is more common in women by a factor of four. Orbital manifestations can precede the hormonal disease or can occur after the hormonal disorder has been corrected.[6,14] The hyperthyroid state is most often implicated as a cause, although an autoimmune mechanism is probably also responsible. Hyperthyroidism can cause ophthalmologic symptoms distinct from those of Graves' disease including lid lag and stare which are due to failure of the lid muscles to relax; a true proptosis is not present. Bilateral, painless proptosis is the clinical presentation of Graves' disease. Vision is usually not affected unless muscle enlargement encroaches upon the optic nerve at the orbital apex.

On CT, the characteristic appearance is bilateral enlargement of multiple extraocular muscles. The inferior and medial rectus muscles are most commonly involved (Fig. 8.15).[14] Typically, the muscle bellies are enlarged while the muscle tendons are spared.[6] Coronal images are especially helpful in determining which muscles are involved. The involved muscles will enhance following administration of contrast material.[14] Increased volume of fat in the retrobulbar space and the eyelids is also characteristic of dysthyroid ophthalmopathy.[6,14] The fat is of normal density. The muscle enlargement is well depicted on the coronal T1-weighted images. The signal characteristics are nonspecific.

Neoplasia

There are essentially four orbital spaces that can be used to describe the location of orbital masses. These are: Tenon's space, the central orbital space (intraconal space), the peripheral orbital space (the area between the muscle cone and the orbital periosteum) and the subperiosteal space. Both the periosteal space and Tenon's space are potential spaces. Tenon's space and the central orbital space are both intraconal in location. The differential diagnosis of lesions by location are given in Tables 8.1–8.3.

Benign neoplasia

Developmental orbital cysts

The most common developmental orbital cysts are the dermoid, epidermoid and teratoma. These are inclusion cysts of ectodermal elements that are incorporated into the orbit during embryologic development. All three forms have a fibrous capsule. The contents of the cysts differ; the epidermoid is lined by keratinized squamous epithelium, the dermoid contains sebaceous glands and/or hair follicles and teratomas contain tissue derived from primitive ectoderm, endoderm and mesoderm. Teratomas are usually present at birth and are cystic on gross inspection. The dermoid and epidermoid cyst is commonly found in the superior temporal quadrant of the orbit.[2,6,15]

Table 8.1

Lesions in the subperiosteal space (adapted from ref. 2, p. 536).

Inflammation
Hematoma
Hematic cyst
Dermoid cyst
Extension of sinus neoplasia/infection
Lacrimal gland tumor
Meningioma
Plasmacytoma
Lymphoma
Fibrous histiocytoma

On CT, these cysts may contain both cystic and solid components (Figs 8.16 and 8.17). Erosion and remodeling of the orbital roof is characteristic. The lesion itself is typically well defined, of low density, extraconal in location and nonenhancing. Calcification is not uncommon. The fatty component is usually evident on CT. On MR, the fatty component is typically hyperintense on T1-weighted images, isointense to orbital fat (Figs 8.18 and 8.19).[2]

Lesions intrinsic to the lacrimal gland are also located in the superior-temporal quadrant of the orbit and can be differentiated with CT or MRI from the cyst-like or fat-containing dermoid cyst. One-half of the primary tumors of the lacrimal gland consist of epithelial tumors and the remainder are of lymphoid or inflammatory origin. One-half of the epithelial tumors are of the benign mixed variety (pleomorphic adenoma) (Fig. 8.20), while the other half are malignant tumors.

Table 8.2

Peripheral orbital (extraconal) lesions (adapted from ref. 2, p. 541).

Dermoid cyst
Capillary hemangioma
Pseudotumor
Lymphoma
Sarcoidosis
Inflammatory/neoplastic sinus disease
Cavernous hemangioma
Lymphangioma
Hemangiopericytoma
Vascular leiomyoma
Hemangiosarcoma
Vascular leiomyosarcoma
Fibrous histiocytoma
Lacrimal gland tumors
Wegener's granuloma
Benign reactive lymphoid hyperplasia
Plasmacytoma
Epithelial tumors

Table 8.3

Intraconal orbital lesions (adapted from ref. 2, pp. 550–1).

Optic nerve meningioma
Optic nerve glioma
Cavernous hemangioma
Lymphangioma
Orbital varix
Hemangiopericytoma
Pseudotumor
Orbital lymphoma
Schwannoma
Neurofibroma
Leukemia
Necrobiotic xanthogranuloma
Hematocele
Optic nerve sheath cyst
Colobomatous cyst
Alveolar sarcoma

Capillary hemangioma

This uncommon tumor usually presents in infants within the first year. It increases in size for 6 to 10 months and spontaneously regresses.[6,14,15] The tumor is made up of endothelial cells and capillary spaces and can bleed profusely.[14] The capillary hemangioma is most commonly found in the extraconal space; it can transgress the optic canal, superior orbital fissure or orbital roof and extend intracranially. Computed tomography of capillary hemangioma reveals a poorly marginated, irregularly enhancing mass in the superior nasal quadrant of the orbit.[14,15] The morphologic characteristics on MR are similar to those observed with CT (Fig. 8.21).

Lymphangioma

Orbital lymphangioma is also a tumor of children and young adults and are less frequent than either capillary or cavernous hemangioma.[14] In contrast to the capillary hemangioma, the lymphangioma progressively enlarges with time and does not undergo spontaneous regression.[14] Lymphangiomas are composed of dilated lymphatic channels surrounded by lymphoid tissue that invade the surrounding fat and connective tissue.[6,14,15] A common feature of lymphangioma and capillary hemangioma is the lack of a defined capsule. Typical features of this vascular lesion is infiltration of the adjacent tissues of the orbit and spontaneous hemorrhage. Symptoms from lymphangioma consist of lid swelling, exophthalmus, diplopia and decreased visual acuity. The intrinsic lymphatic tissue in the lymphangioma may enlarge during viral illnesses.[14] They may occur in the conjunctiva, eyelid or retrobulbar region.[6,14] Lymphangiomas are not amenable to complete surgical resection and recurrence is common.[2]

Computed tomography studies reveal a poorly circumscribed lobulated lesion of increased attenuation in the intra- or extraconal space.[14] Internal calcification is rare and contrast enhancement is variable. However, enhancement is usually less than observed with hemangiomas.[14] This tumor may be both intraconal and extraconal in location. Cystic structures with peripheral enhancement are characteristic.[14]

Magnetic resonance imaging depicts lymphangiomas as nodular tumors with variable signal intensity which is dependent upon the amount of intra-

tumoral hemorrhage. The internal signal characteristics may be hypo- to isointense relative to orbital fat on the T1-weighted image and hyperintense on the T2-weighted image.[14,15] Lymphangiomas may be distinguished from other orbital tumors on MR due to their indistinct borders and evidence of internal hemorrhage (Fig. 8.22).[2,14,15]

Cavernous hemangioma

The cavernous hemangioma occurs most frequently in adults from the second and fourth decades. It is the most common benign tumor of the orbit.[6,14] In contrast to the capillary hemangioma, the cavernous hemangioma progressively enlarges with time and is not exceptionally vascular. The cavernous hemangioma is composed of large vascular spaces and is enveloped by a fibrous pseudocapsule which produces distinct tumor margins on imaging studies.[14] The well-defined capsule allows for complete surgical resection. The vast majority (83%) occur within the muscle cone, although they can occur anywhere in the orbit.[14] Gradual enlargement compresses the extraocular muscles or optic nerve causing diplopia or papilledema.[14] These tumors are soft and malleable and tend to respect the globe and adjacent tissues. Spontaneous hemorrhage of a cavernous hemangioma may simulate rapid tumor enlargement.[2]

Computed tomography of the cavernous hemangioma shows a well-marginated, homogenous, ovoid or lobulated soft tissue mass which can calcify and produce bone erosion. Uniform enhancement may be demonstrated with iodinated contrast material.[14] By comparison, capillary hemangioma exhibit rapid circulation time and enhance dramatically on dynamic contrast CT studies (Fig. 8.23).[2]

On MRI cavernous hemangiomas appear as well-circumscribed intraconal masses that are hypointense relative to fat and isointense relative to muscle on the T1-weighted images and revert to hyperintensity on the T2-weighted images.[10,14] There is prominent enhancement with gadolinium (Figs 8.24 and 8.25).

Orbital varix

Orbital varices are congenital venous malformations characterized by an abnormal proliferation of venous elements. They may be associated with intraorbital or intracranial arteriovenous communications.[14] Usually, one or more veins is massively dilated due to a congenital weakness in the wall of the vessels.[2,14] Enormous distention of these abnormal veins occurs with increased venous pressure such as during laughing, coughing or with the valsalva maneuver. Distention of the varix produces intermittent proptosis and visual loss.[2,6,10]

Computed tomography or MR imaging demonstrates a tubular soft tissue mass in the superior orbit oriented towards the orbital apex.[6,14] Coronal CT images should be obtained while the patient performs the valsalva manuever or in the prone position with the neck in hyperextension to facilitate increased venous pressure and distension of the varix. As with any venous structure, there is enhancement with infusion of intravenous contrast material.[14] Complex flow patterns within the varix may be demonstrated on spin-echo MR imaging ranging from a true flow void to flow related enhancement.[14] Flow-related enhancement can be exploited with gradient echo imaging and the use of gadolinium (Fig. 8.26).[2,10]

Orbital schwannoma and neurofibroma

Schwannomas (a.k.a. neuroma, neurilemmoma) are benign nerve sheath tumors that can arise anywhere in the orbit, yet are most commonly found in the intraconal space. Orbital schwannomas originate from the branches of the cranial nerves in the orbit; oculomotor, abducens and trigeminal. These are slow growing neoplasms and they account for up to 6% of all orbital tumors in some series.[2] The schwannoma exhibits distinct margins and has a thin, fibrous capsule.

Neurofibromas, on the other hand, are poorly encapsulated, less cellular and are more difficult to separate from neural tissue. Neurofibromas usually occur in the setting of van Recklinghausen's disease (neurofibromatosis type I) or they may occur as an isolated finding. The plexiform type of neurofibroma is pathognomonic of neurofibromatosis and is often demonstrated in association with dysplasia of the sphenoid wing and floor of the middle cranial fossa.[14] The clinical presentation ranges from proptosis, diplopia and strabismus to papilledema and optic nerve atrophy.[2]

Imaging of schwannoma or isolated neurofibroma with CT shows a well-circumscribed oval or fusiform hyperdense lesion, usually in the intraconal space. There is moderate to marked contrast enhancement (Figs 8.27 and 8.28).[14] Isolated neurofibromas may contain calcification. In contrast, the plexiform neurofibroma appears as an ill-defined, infiltrative, enhancing mass associated with dysplasia of the greater wing of the sphenoid bone.[14] The MR signal characteristics are nonspecific; low signal on T1-weighted images and hyperintense on T2-weighted images.[14] The differential diagnosis of the isolated schwannoma or neurofibroma is cavernous hemangioma, meningioma and hemangiopericytoma (Table 8.2).[2]

Optic nerve tumors

The differential diagnosis for tumors of the optic nerve is limited, consisting primarily of glioma and meningioma. The most common clinical presentation of an optic nerve tumor is decreased visual acuity and papilledema. Loss of peripheral vision is the most common visual field defect. A clinical hallmark for optic nerve tumors is a significant visual impairment associated with a low grade proptosis.[19] Other orbital masses produce a visual deficit proportional to the degree of proptosis. Although the clinical presentation is similar for optic nerve glioma and meningioma, the age of presentation is markedly different; optic gliomas occur most often in the first decade while optic nerve meningioma occurs in middle-aged females. The loss of visual acuity may be less with a meningioma than a glioma due to the exophytic growth of meningiomas.[19,20]

The optic nerve can enlarge when an intraocular melanoma or retinoblastoma extends into the distal optic nerve. There are rare primary tumors of the optic nerve which include hemangioblastoma, hemangiopericytoma and choristoma (Table 8.4).[20]

Optic nerve meningioma

Optic nerve meningioma occur most often in middle-aged women. When they occur in children, they are often histologically more aggressive than in adults. Cases are also reported in association with neurofibromatosis. Meningiomas arise from arachnoid rest cells. With the exception of the optic nerve

Table 8.4

Causes of optic nerve enlargement (adapted from ref. 2, pp. 574–9).

Optic nerve meningioma
Optic nerve glioma
Schwannoma
Hemangioblastoma
Hemangiopericytoma
Choristoma
Lymphoma
Sarcoid
Toxoplasmosis
Tuberculosis
Syphilis
Optic neuritis
Traumatic edema or hematoma
Pseudotumor
Graves' disease
Increased intracranial pressure

sheath, it is rare for meningiomas to arise de novo in the orbit. Usually, the tumor develops from the dura surrounding the optic nerve or as an extension of an intracranial meningioma which protrudes into the orbit through a foramen.[19]

Thin section axial and coronal CT is an excellent method of demonstrating optic nerve meningioma when performed both with and without contrast material. In most cases, there is a well-defined eccentric thickening of the optic nerve. Fusiform enlargement is evident in about one-fifth of cases. Stippled or ring-shaped calcifications are also common within the enlarged optic nerve (Fig. 8.29). Sclerotic changes at the orbital apex may also be observed.[19] When the optic nerve meningioma has irregular margins, it suggests that it has transgressed the optic nerve sheath. Computed tomography is superior to MR in its ability to demonstrate discrete calcifications associated with meningioma.[8]

The advantage of using MRI is that it provides superior definition of the optic nerve, especially the intracanalicular portion, without the bony artifacts

commonly encountered with CT (Figs 8.29–8.31).[10] Meningiomas demonstrate varying signal intensities on MRI, presumably due to differing proportions of calcification.[10] While CT has the advantage in demonstrating small calcified lesions, MRI with gadolinium is extremely sensitive for detecting enplaque noncalcified meningiomas.

Optic nerve glioma

Optic nerve glioma is a tumor of childhood. Fifty percent of cases are diagnosed by age 5. Optic nerve glioma is benign, well differentiated and slow growing. Outward expansion of this tumor is limited by the dural covering of the nerve. The nerve is enlarged in a fusiform configuration. Anterior growth produces proptosis while posterior extension through the optic canal produces enlargement of the optic foramen.[15] In rare cases tumor invades the tissues of the brain or eyeball.[21] Optic nerve glioma is reported with increased frequency in neurofibromatosis. Fifteen percent of patients with optic glioma show evidence of neurofibromatosis. When the glioma is bilateral, it is almost always in the setting of neurofibromatosis (Fig. 8.32).[15] If left untreated, progressive visual loss results from compression of the optic nerve. In the adult, optic glioma is often malignant, leading to rapid blindness and death.

Computed tomography shows a well-defined, fusiform enlargement of the optic nerve. The thickened nerve appears to buckle along its course in the orbit.[2,19] When large, the optic glioma can mimic any solid intraconal tumor such as hemangioma.[19] With infusion of contrast material, the optic glioma exhibits intense enhancement. Areas of cystic degeneration may develop in the tumor when it reaches a large size.

Magnetic resonance imaging demonstrates the enlarged optic nerve with optic glioma exceptionally well.[6] The tumor is isointense to white matter on the T1-weighted images and is isointense to moderately hyperintense on the T2-weighted images (Figs 8.33–8.35).[17] Magnetic resonance provides superior definition of the intracanalicular, chiasmatic and retrochiasmatic portions of the optic nerves. Visualization of the intracanalicular and intracranial segments is aided by the lack of bone artifacts.

Retrochiasmatic involvement is usually hyperintense on the T2-weighted images. Arachnoidal hyperplasia associated with optic nerve glioma is hyperintense on the long TR/TE images allowing for differentiation from the nerve itself.[11]

Malignant neoplasia

Melanoma

Primary and metastatic lesions to the eye usually involve the vascular component of the eyeball, the choroid. The most common ocular neoplasm in adults is melanoma. Uveal melanoma involves whites more than blacks by a factor of fifteen. Clinical detection of uveal melanoma is usually quite sensitive and accurate, however, direct visualization may be hampered by associated hemorrhage or cloudy vitreous. On rare occasions, choroidal hemorrhage has been mistaken for malignant melanoma with disastrous clinical consequences.[7,13]

Uveal melanomas appear as well marginated, hyperdense elevations of the choroid that exhibit a moderate degree of enhancement with intravenous contrast material on CT.[13] When an associated retinal detachment is present, intravenous contrast material is necessary to distinguish enhancing tumor from subretinal fluid.[10] The pigmentation in melanoma (melanin) is unique in that it has natural paramagnetic properties. Relative to other malignant tumors of the eye, uveal melanoma exhibits relatively short T1 and T2 relaxation characteristics.[10,13] Melanotic melanomas exhibit a characteristic appearance with MRI; the melanotic tumors are relatively hyperintense (relative to vitreous) on the T1-weighted images and mildly hypointense on the T2-weighted images (Figs 8.36 and 8.37). This differs from the appearance of other choroidal lesions such as hemangioma (Fig. 8.38), metastases (Fig. 8.39) and amelanotic melanoma (Fig. 8.40), which are lower in signal intensity on T1-weighted images and hyperintense on the T2-weighted images.[13] The degree of relaxation enhancement appears to be related to the amount of melanotic pigmentation. Choroidal hemangioma exhibits the greatest amount of contrast enhancement on CT or MR when compared to melanoma.[13] Magnetic resonance is superior to CT in the depiction of associated retinal detachment and scleral invasion (Fig. 8.41).[7] Despite the improved tissue characterization of tumors with MRI, other ocular lesions such as choroidal hemangioma, choroidal metastasis, choroidal hematoma, inflammatory uveitis, choroidal effusion, macular degeneration, retinal gliosis and retinal detachment can be mistaken for uveal melanoma.[13]

Lymphoid tumors

Lymphoid tumors account for up to 15% of all orbital masses and are the third most common cause of proptosis in the adult.[14,22] Many authors subdivide lymphoid tumors of the orbit into three separate categories: (1) malignant lymphoma; (2) atypical/intermediate lymphoid hyperplasia; and (3) benign reactive lymphoid hyperplasia. Overlap exists between certain chronic forms of pseudotumor and types of lymphoid hyperplasia. In the pediatric orbit, lymphoma is usually secondary to Hodgkin's disease.[6] Chronic types of pseudotumor have been linked to orbital lymphoma. Concurrent systemic lymphoma is present in 75% of patients with malignant orbital lymphoma and up to 25% with reactive lymphoid hyperplasia.[23,24]

Lymphoma of the orbit presents in older patients with a unilateral, painless, progressive proptosis or swelling of the eyelids.[14,24] In contrast to the clinical presentation of orbital pseudotumor, pain and inflammatory changes are not present in orbital lymphoma. orbital lymphomas are usually made up of the B-cell type (non-Hodgkin's); T-cell lymphoma in the orbit is rare.[14,24]

Imaging reveals a wide range of findings which may range from well-defined tumor mass which molds to the contours of the adjacent normal tissues (Figs 8.42 and 8.43) to a diffusely infiltrative process.[14,24,25] The mass may occupy portions of the lacrimal gland (Fig. 8.43), extraocular muscles, eyelids and conjunctiva.[6,14,24,25] On MRI, lymphoma is of low signal intensity relative to orbital fat on the T1-weighted images and iso- to hyperintense on the proton density and T2-weighted images.[14] Differentiation between true lymphoma, leukemic infiltrates (chloroma) (Fig. 8.44) and forms of benign reactive hyperplasia may not be possible with imaging alone. Biopsy is necessary in many instances.[25]

Orbital metastases

Orbital metastases (hematogenous and direct extension) account for approximately 10% of all orbital tumors.[14] Primary tumors of the breast and lung are the most common lesions to metastasize to the orbit, followed by genitourinary and gastrointestinal primaries in adults.[14] In children, neuroblastoma, Ewing sarcoma (Fig. 8.45) and Wilms' tumor are the most common sources of metastatic disease.[6,14] Metastases to the globe are rare in children.[6,25] An orbital metastases from lung, kidney, prostate, testicle, pancreas and stomach may be the first clinical presentation of a primary malignancy. A patient may present with sudden onset of diplopia, visual loss, ptosis, proptosis and lid swelling. Scirrhous carcinoma of the breast can induce a fibrotic reaction that results in enophthalmos.[14] Metastases can occur anywhere in the orbit, including the globe, extraocular muscles and lacrimal gland (Figs 8.39, 8.45–8.51).

With CT, most intraorbital metastases are poorly marginated soft tissue masses that are moderately hyperdense relative to the muscles.[14] With the use of contrast material, a mild degree of enhancement is noted. In general, the appearance of lesion varies, depending upon the area of the orbit that is affected. In contrast to melanotic melanomas, most metastastic lesions on MRI have long T1 and long T2 characteristics relative to orbital fat (Figs 8.46 and 8.50) and are therefore hypointense and hyperintense on the T1- and T2-weighted images, respectively.[13,14]

When metastases implant on the vascular choroid of the globe, this is often accompanied by retinal detachment and subretinal effusions (Figs 8.39 and 8.50). It is difficult to differentiate the lesion from the effusion on CT. With MR, differential signal characteristics can be appreciated between the tumor and the effusion. If the effusion contains sufficient protein or hemorrhagic breakdown products, it may be hyperintense on the T1-weighted images.[13] A moderately hyperintense lesion may contrast with the effusion on either the T1- or T2-weighted sequence. Often the effusion is hyperintense relative to the lesion itself. Gadolinium is particularly useful in that the tumor nidus will preferentially enhance on the T1-weighted images.

Metastases can also implant in the extraocular muscles causing a segmental area of widening of the muscle belly, an irregular border and adjacent fat infiltration (Figs 8.47–8.49).[14] It may be difficult to distinguish this lesion from myositic pseudotumor, lymphoma or dysthyroid ophthalmopathy. An unusual pattern of muscle involvement or bony destruction is suggestive of muscle metastasis.[14] The involved muscle may be hyperintense on the T2-weighted images and can exhibit abnormal enhancement patterns with administration of gadolinium. Metastatic deposits can infiltrate the intraconal and extraconal space simultaneously.

Retinoblastoma

Retinoblastoma is the most common malignant primary intraocular tumor in the pediatric population. This tumor occurs spontaneously in approximately one of 17 000 births. Ten percent of retinoblastomas are familial and up to 25% are multifocal within the same eye or are bilateral. The tumor is derived from neuroectoderm in the retina and usually produces a calcified, nodular mass in the posterior globe (Figs 8.52 and 8.53). In rare cases, retinoblastoma is uncalcified. Bilateral retinoblastomas are sometimes associated with a pineal neuroectodermal tumor and is known as trilateral retinoblastoma (Fig. 8.53). Approximately 1% of retinoblastomas spontaneously regress without treatment.[6]

Rhabdomyosarcoma

Rhabdomyosarcoma is the most common malignant tumor of the orbit in the pediatric population yet it is only one-tenth as common as retinoblastoma. Ten percent of all pediatric rhabdomyosarcomas occur primarily in the orbit and another 10% invade the orbit secondarily (Fig. 8.54). The average age of onset is in a child 8 to 10 years, presenting with a rapidly progressive proptosis.[6,14]

Paraorbital and miscellaneous conditions

Mucoceles

Since the most common location for mucoceles is in the frontal and ethmoid sinuses, orbital swelling and displacement of the globe are common clinical findings. Frontal sinus mucoceles produce inferior displacement of the globe as they expand the roof of the orbit and produce swelling of the upper eyelid. Ethmoid sinus mucoceles produce proptosis and lateral displacement of the globe as the medial wall of the orbit is expanded. Although they are rare, mucoceles in the sphenoid sinus can have devastating clinical consequences. The close proximity of the sphenoid sinus to the cavernous sinus can result in blindness or multiple cranial nerve palsies as the mucocele expands.[1]

Computed tomography is an excellent method for evaluating mucoceles and bony remodeling. A hypodense soft tissue mass fills the involved paranasal sinus with expansion, remodeling and erosion of the bony margins. Frank destruction of the sinus or orbital wall is not characteristic of a mucocele and more aggressive processes should be considered in these cases (See Chapter 1, Paranasal Sinuses). Although the bony changes are not as well demonstrated with MRI, the signal properties of the mucocele can help in distinguishing this from neoplastic processes of the paranasal sinus. The signal intensity of the proteinaceous components of mucous secretions may exhibit both a shortened T1 and prolonged T2.

Miscellaneous conditions

Meningiomas occurring outside of the bony orbit can affect the visual apparatus or optic pathways by direct invasion of the orbit or by displacement or compression of the optic nerves, chiasm and optic tracts (Figs 8.55–8.58). Although most meningiomas are parasagittal, others can develop closer to the skull base, specifically arising from the olfactory groove, tuberculum sella, lesser wing of the sphenoid, sella turcica and cavernous sinus. Tuberculum sella meningiomas usually produce unilateral visual loss, headache and optic atrophy. Meningiomas arising near the cavernous sinus may produce dysfunction of cranial nerves III, IV, V and VI. Meningiomas are usually most conspicuous on CT due to the presence of calcifications. The relaxation times of meningiomas on MRI often approximate those of brain parenchyma and therefore they may be difficult to demonstrate without contrast material. For this reason, gadolinium is essential for the evaluation of meningiomas.

The close proximity of the optic chiasm to the sella turcica makes it susceptible to compression from large intrasellar/suprasellar tumors such as pituitary macroadenomas and craniopharyngiomas. While pituitary microadenomas tend to produce endocrine abnormalities by elaborating hormones (for example, prolactin, growth hormone and adrenocorticotropic hormone) macroadenomas (that is greater than 10 mm in size) produce symptoms by compressing adjacent structures. Enlargement of the sella turcica and extension into the suprasellar cistern are characteristic imaging findings. Direct sagittal and coronal images are useful for assessing the degree of compression on adjacent structures. When the tumor is very large, it can compress the optic chiasm against the base of the brain (Fig. 8.59), which produces the characteristic visual symptoms of bitemporal hemianopsia. Pituitary macroadenomas will enhance with gadolinium and iodinated contrast material when using MRI and CT, respectively. The appearance of a macroadenoma can vary on MR depending upon the presence of internal hemorrhage, calcification or cystic degeneration.[26]

Aneurysms of the circle of Willis may be responsible for visual symptoms. The most common location of an aneurysm to produce visual symptoms is the internal carotid artery at the origin of the ophthalmic artery (Fig. 8.60). If the aneurysm is large enough it can compress the optic nerve, optic chiasm or optic tract. Aneurysms of the posterior communicating artery and posterior circulation typically will compress the cranial nerves that innervate the extraocular muscles. While angiography is the most sensitive imaging modality for the detection of cerebral aneurysms, CT and MRI offer critical diagnostic information about the relationship of the aneurysm to the adjacent structures.[26]

Disease processes that can affect the optic tracts as they lead to their termination at the occipital poles include primary neoplasms of the brain, cerebrovascular accidents and demyelinating disease. The most common demyelinating disease to affect the optic pathways is multiple sclerosis (MS). Multiple sclerosis affects patients between 10 and 50 years of age and is more common in females. Nearly one-half of all patients with multiple sclerosis exhibit clinical signs of optic nerve involvement and one-fifth elicit symptoms of isolated optic neuritis (Fig. 8.12) during initial presentation. Magnetic resonance imaging has supplanted CT in the diagnosis and evaluation of MS. The MS plaques that were formerly elusive to CT are easily demonstrated with MRI as areas of confluent hyperintensity on proton-density and T2-weighted images. Activity of a lesion may be inferred by focal enhancement of plaques with gadolinium (Fig. 8.61).[26]

References

1. WEBER AL, MIKULIS DK, Inflammatory disorders of the paraorbital sinuses and their complications, *Radiol Clin North Am* (1987) **25**: 615–30.

2. MAFEE MF, PUTTERMAN A, VALVASSORI GE et al, Orbital space-occupying lesions: role of computed tomography and magnetic resonance imaging, *Radiol Clin North Am* (1987) **25**: 529–59.

3. ZONNEVELD FW, KOORNEEF L, HILLEN B et al, Normal direct multiplanar CT anatomy of the orbit with correlative anatomic cryosections, *Radiol Clin North Am* (1987) **25**: 381–407.

4. LANGER BG, MAFFE MF, POLLACK S et al, MRI of the normal orbit and optic pathway, *Radiol Clin North Am* (1987) **25**: 429–46.

5. MAFEE MF, PEYMAN GA, Retinal and choroidal detachments: role of magnetic resonance imaging and computed tomography, *Radiol Clin North Am* (1987) **25**: 487–507.

6. HOPPER HD, HAAS DK, SHERMAN JL, The radiologic evaluation of congenital and pediatric lesions of the orbit, *Semin Ultrasound CT MR* (1988) **9**: 413–27.

7. PEYMAN GA, MAFEE MF, Uveal melanoma and similar lesions: the role of magnetic resonance imaging and computed tomography, *Radiol Clin North Am* (1987) **25**: 472–86.

8. SULLIVAN JA, HARMS SE, Surface-coil MR imaging of orbital neoplasms, *AJNR* (1986) **7**: 29–34.

9. ATLAS SW, BILANIUK LT, ZIMMERMAN RA et al, Orbit: initial experience with surface coil spin-echo MR imaging at 1.5 T, *Radiology* (1987) **164**: 501–9.

10. ATLAS SW, MR of the orbit: current imaging applications, *Semin Ultrasound CT MR* (1988) **9**: 381–400.

11. BILANIUK LT, ATLAS SW, ZIMMERMAN RA, Magnetic resonance imaging of the orbit, *Radiol Clin North Am* (1987) **25**: 509–28.

12. SIMON J, SZUMOWSKI J, TOTTERMAN S et al, Fat-suppression MR imaging of the orbit, *AJNR* (1988) **9**: 961–8.

13. MAFEE MF, PUKLIN J, BARANY M et al, MRI and in vivo proton spectroscopy of the lesions of the globe, *Semin Ultrasound CT MR* (1988) **9**: 428–42.

14. ARMINGTON WG, BILANIUK LT, The radiologic evaluation of the orbit: conal and intraconal lesions, *Semin Ultrasound CT MR* (1988) **9**: 455–73.

15. WELLS RG, STY JR, GONNERING RS, Imaging of the pediatric eye and orbit, *Radiographics* (1989) **9**: 1023–44.

16. CURTIN HD, Pseudotumor, *Radiol Clin North Am* (1987) **25**: 583–99.

17. JAKOBIEC FA, MCLEAN I, FONT RL, Clinicopathologic characteristics of orbital lymphoid hyperplasia, *Ophthalmology* (1979) **86**: 948–66.

18. FLANDERS AE, MAFEE MF, RAO VM et al, CT characteristics of orbital pseudotumors: our experience and a review of the literature, *Comput Assist Tomogr* (1989) **13**: 40–7.

19. JAKOBIEC FA, DEPOT MJ, KENNERDELL JS et al, Combined clinical and computed tomographic diagnosis of orbital glioma and meningioma, *Ophthalmology* (1984) **91**: 137–55.

20. AZAR-KIA B, NAHEEDY MH, ELIAS DA et al, Optic nerve tumors: role of magnetic resonance imaging and computed tomography, *Radiol Clin North Am* (1987) **25**: 561–81.

21. BILANIUK LT, SCHENCK JF, ZIMMERMAN RA et al, Ocular and orbital lesions: surface coil MR imaging, *Radiology* (1985) **156**: 669–74.

22. TEWFIK HH, PLATZ EE, CORDER MP et al, A clinico-pathologic study of orbital and adnexal non-Hodgkin's lymphoma, *Cancer* (1979) **44**: 1022–8.

23. NUGENT RA, ROOTMAN J, ROBERTSON WD et al, Acute orbital pseudotumors: classification and CT features, *AJR* (1981) **137**: 957–62.

24. FLANDERS AE, MAFEE MF, MARKIEWICZ DA et al, Orbital lymphoma: role of CT and MRI, *Radiol Clin North Am* (1987) **25**: 601–13.

25. PEYSTER RG, SHAPIRO MD, HAIK BG, Orbital metastasis: role of magnetic resonance imaging and computed tomography, *Radiol Clin North Am* (1987) **25**: 647–62.

26. ARMINGTON WG, ZIMMERMAN RA, BILANIUK LT, Imaging of the visual pathways. In: Som PM, Bergeron RT, eds, *Head and Neck Imaging* (Mosby-Year Book Inc.: St Louis 1991) 829–73.

A

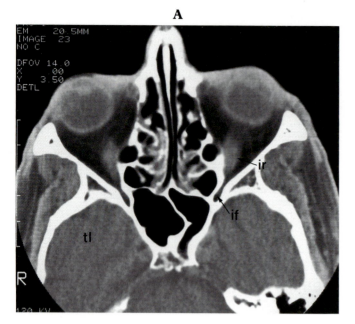

C

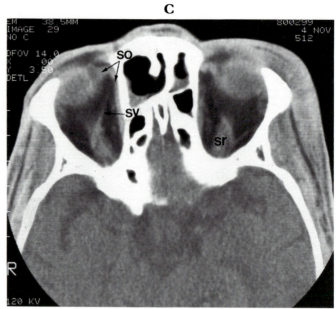

B

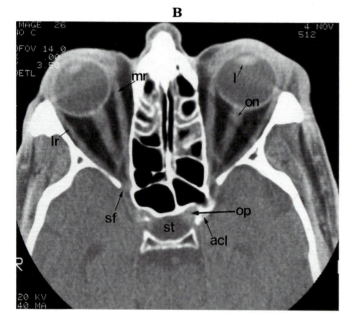

D

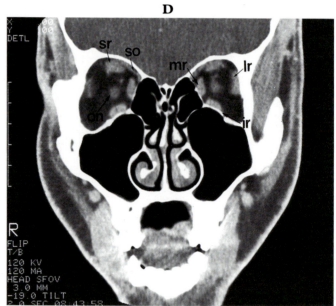

FIGURE 8.1

Normal CT anatomy of the orbit. (**A**) Axial CT image through the inferior orbit. (**B**) Axial CT image of the midorbit.

(**C**) Axial CT image of the superior orbit.
(**D**) Coronal CT image of the midorbit.

continued

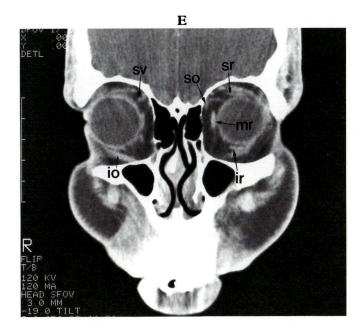

Key:

ac, anterior chamber; acl, anterior clinoid; ca, caudate nucleus; cb, ciliary body; ch, choroid (enhancing); cl, clivus; co, cornea; cs, cavernous sinus (lateral margin); ic, internal carotid artery; if, inferior orbital fissure; io, inferior oblique muscle; ir, inferior rectus muscle; l, lens; lg, lacrimal gland; lr, lateral rectus muscle; mr, medial rectus muscle; oa, ophthalmic artery; oc, optic chiasm; on, optic nerve; op, optic canal; p, pituitary gland; s, sclera; sf, superior orbital fissure; so, superior oblique muscle; sr, superior rectus/levator palpebrae muscles; st, sella turcica; sv, superior ophthalmic vein; tl, temporal lobe; 3, oculomotor nerve (branches).

FIGURE 8.1 *(continued)*

(**E**) Coronal CT image of the anterior orbit.

A

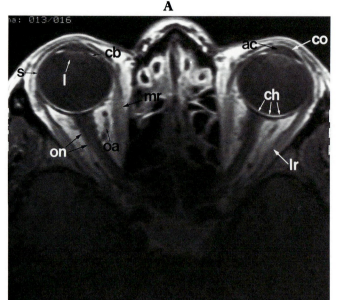

C

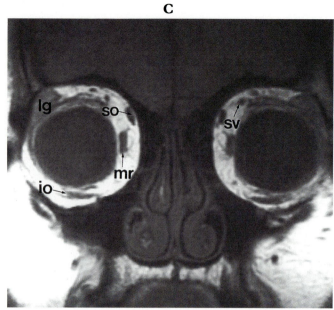

B

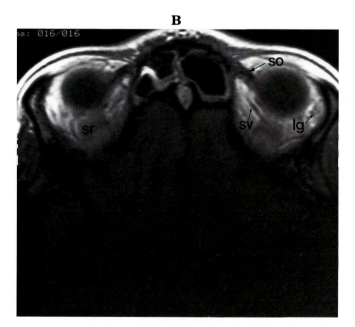

D

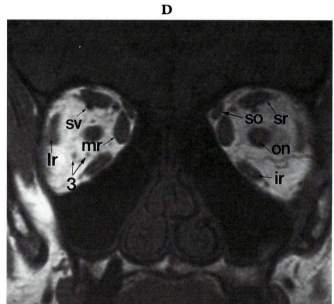

FIGURE 8.2

Normal MR anatomy of the orbit. (**A**) T1-weighted axial image (TR = 600 ms, TE = 25 ms) with gadolinium, obtained at the level of the midorbit. (**B**) T1-weighted axial image (TR = 600 ms, TE = 25 ms) obtained through the upper orbit.

(**C**) T1-weighted coronal image (TR = 400 ms, TE = 14 ms) of the anterior orbit. (**D**) T1-weighted coronal image (TR = 400 ms, TE = 14 ms) of the retrobulbar space.

continued

E

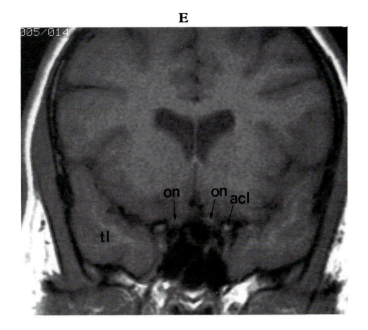

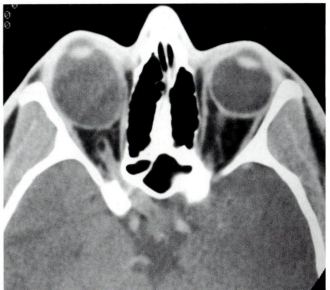

F

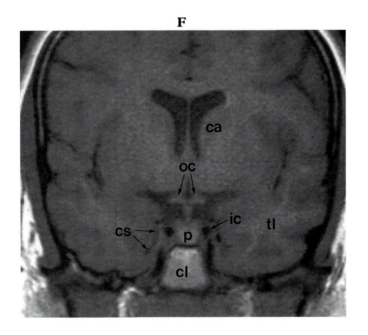

FIGURE 8.3

Staphyloma. A noncontrast axial CT image shows that the right globe has an abnormal configuration due to weakening of the posterior sclera which results in protrusion of the vitreous body. Also of note is abnormal thickening of the right optic nerve, presumably secondary to an optic sheath meningioma.

FIGURE 8.2 *(continued)*

(**E**) T1-weighted coronal image obtained immediately posterior to the optic foramen. (**F**) T1-weighted coronal image obtained through the optic chiasm. See Figure 8.1 for key.

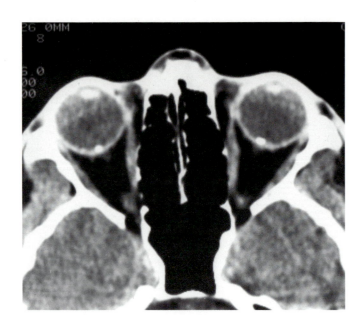

FIGURE 8.4

Optic nerve drusen. An axial CT image reveals punctate calcifications at the approximate location of the optic disk or insertion of the optic nerve head. These benign calcifications are discrete and there is no association with a mass lesion. Bilateral choroidal osteomas may demonstrate a similar CT appearance.

A

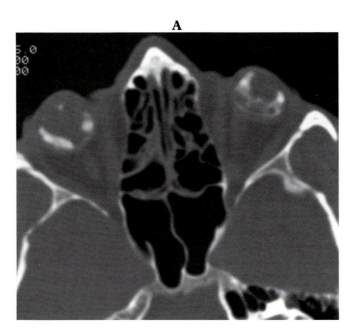

B

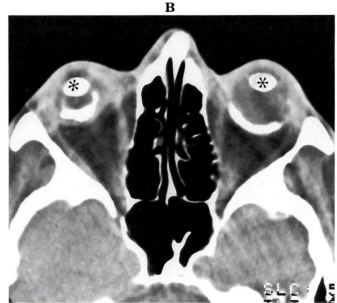

FIGURE 8.5

Phthisis bulbi. (**A**) An axial CT image filmed at a wide window shows that there is bilateral microphthalmia with extensive calcification in the choroid and extent into the vitreous cavity. These dystrophic changes may have been the result of prior infection.

(**B**) An axial CT image in another patient shows thick calcifications in the posterior globe bilaterally. Microphthalmia is present on the right and there are calcified cataracts demonstrated bilaterally (*).

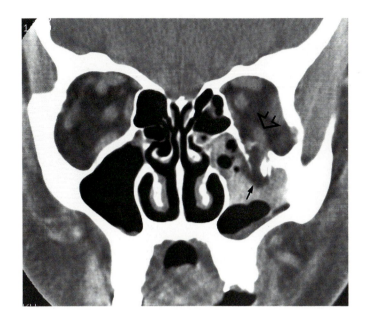

FIGURE 8.6

Blow-out fracture. There is disruption of the floor of the left orbit as depicted on this coronal CT image. Orbital fat is prolapsed through the bony defect (arrow). The inferior rectus is displaced inferiorly (open arrow).

A

B

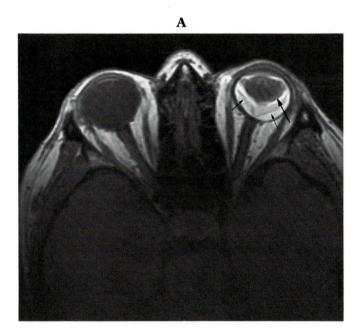

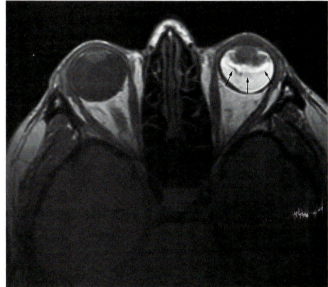

FIGURE 8.7

Choroidal, subhyaloid and subretinal hemorrhage. (A) The contents of the left globe are markedly hyperintense on this T1-weighted axial image (TR = 500 ms, TE = 20 ms). The relatively hypointense retina is elevated in the characteristic 'V-shaped' configuration due to attachments at the optic disk (short arrows) and is contrasted posteriorly by the

hyperintense subretinal hemorrhage. The intact vitreous body is compressed anteriorly (long arrow). (B) Another axial view taken 4 mm below (a) shows the choroid (short arrows) outlined ventrally by subhyaloid hemorrhage and dorsally by choroidal hemorrhage.

continued

C

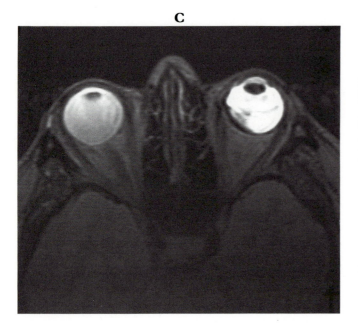

E

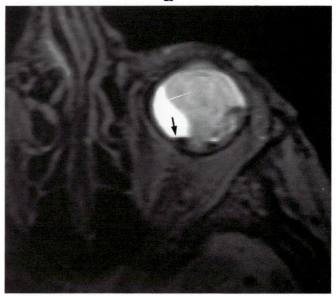

D

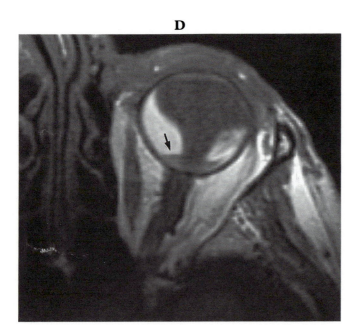

FIGURE 8.7 *(continued)*

(**C**) The normal vitreous reverts to hyperintensity on the T2-weighted images (TR = 2000 ms, TE = 80 ms) and intraocular detail is lost. (**D**) A T1-weighted axial image (TR = 400 ms, TE = 23 ms) in another patient shows subacute hyperintense hemorrhage in the characteristic 'V-shaped' configuration of the subretinal space. Note that the collections extend radially from the optic disk. Hypointense deoxyhemoglobin layers in the dependent portion (arrow). (**E**) On a T2-weighted axial image (TR = 1800 ms, TE = 80 ms) (same patient as (**D**)), the subacute hemorrhage in the subretinal space on the right remains hyperintense (methemoglobin) while the acute component (deoxyhemoglobin) in the dependent portion of the globe (arrow) remains hypointense.

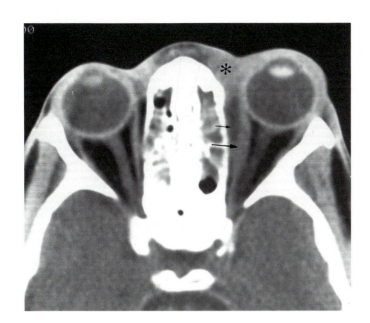

FIGURE 8.8

Orbital cellulitis secondary to pansinusitis with subperiosteal abscess. A non contrast axial CT image shows a well defined inflammatory mass occupying the preseptal compartment of the medial conjunctiva (*) left orbit. There is thickening of the conjunctiva and eyelid on the left. Infiltration of the extraconal fat is demonstrated (short arrow), as is inflammatory thickening of the left medial rectus muscle (long arrow). Note, by comparison, the size of the muscles on the right and the density of the extraconal fat. Opacification of the ethmoid air cells is also noted; a probable source for this infection.

A

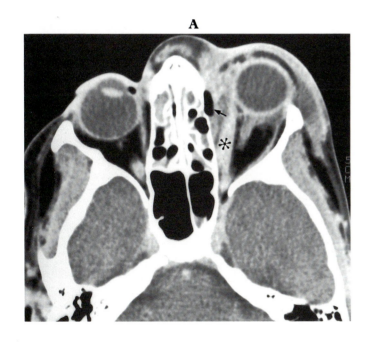

B

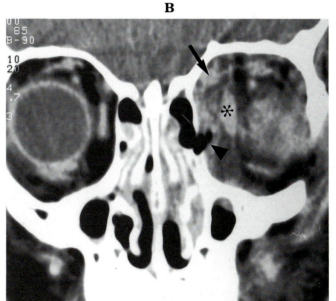

FIGURE 8.9

Advanced orbital cellulitis secondary to ethmoid sinusitis. (**A**) There is severe edema of the eyelid and conjunctiva of the left eye on this postcontrast axial CT image. Air has ruptured into the medial orbit (arrow) from the infected ethmoid air cells and induced an inflammatory reaction within the subperiosteal space as well as in the extraconal fat. Note the thickening and abnormal enhancement of the medial rectus muscle (*). (**B**) A coronal CT image of the retrobulbar space shows the extensive inflammatory reaction with increased density of the orbital fat medially and edema of the medial rectus muscle (*) and superior oblique muscle (arrow). The communication between the ethmoid air cells and the orbit is well demonstrated (arrowhead).

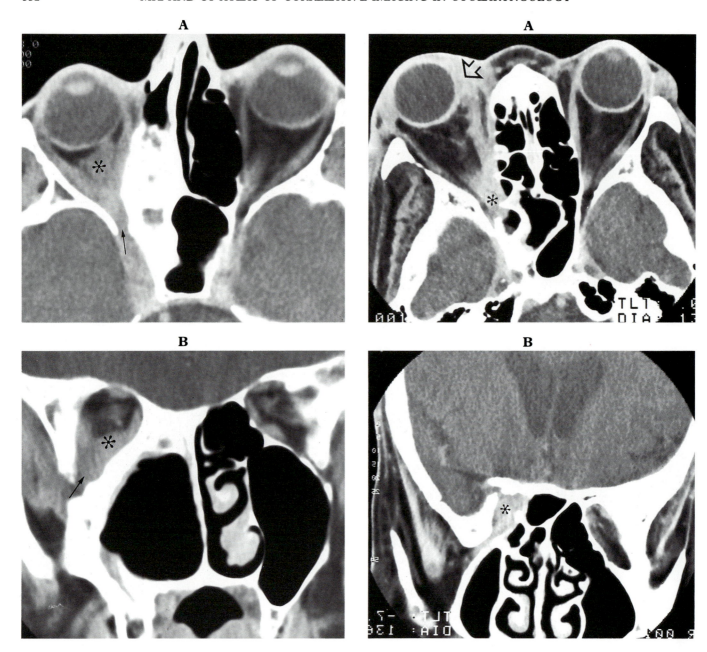

FIGURE 8.10

Wegener's granulomatosis. (**A**) A soft tissue mass is present intraconally on the right (*) which extends into the orbital apex and replaces the orbital fat (arrow). There is also mild thickening of the rectus muscles. (**B**) In the coronal plane, tissue is present primarily in the inferior aspect of the intraconal space of the right orbit (*). Note that there is extension of the process into the inferior orbital fissure (arrow). Surgical changes are evident in the right maxillary sinus and nasal cavity from a prior episode of the same process.

FIGURE 8.11

Orbital cellulitis and subperiosteal abscess from aspergillosis. (**A**) Postcontrast axial CT image shows an inflammatory mass in the preseptal compartment of the right orbit medially that involves the muscle belly and tendinous insertion of the medial rectus muscle (open arrow). The subperiosteal space and extraconal fat are infiltrated adjacent to the medial rectus and the infection extends posteriorly to involve the orbital apex (*). (**B**) Coronal CT image through the orbital apex shows hyperdense infiltration of the orbital fat (*) in the apex of the right orbit with obliteration of normal structures.

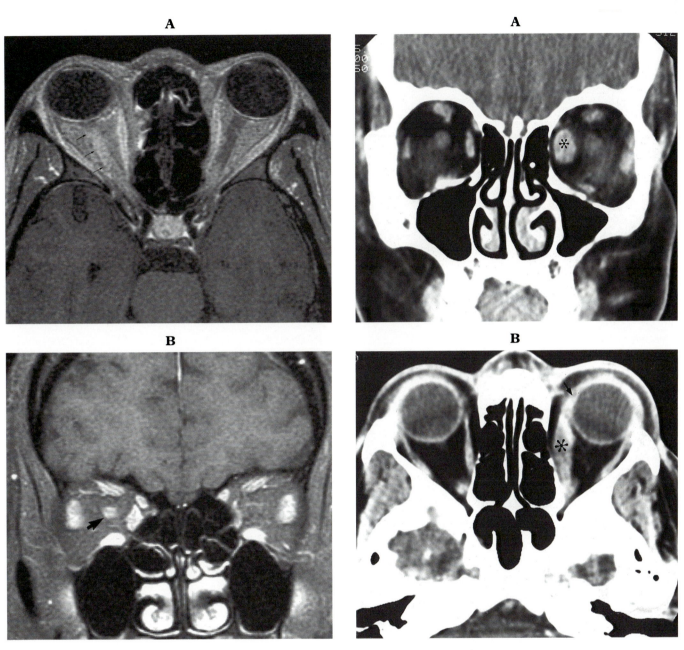

FIGURE 8.12

FIGURE 8.13

Optic neuritis. (**A**) A postcontrast T1-weighted axial image (TR = 400 ms, TE = 10 ms) which utilizes fat suppression reveals diffuse enhancement of the right optic nerve (arrows) compared to the normal nerve on the left. (**B**) A coronal image on the same patient again shows enhancement of the right optic nerve (arrow) compared to the normal left optic nerve. Note the extensive (normal) enhancement of the extraocular muscles when a fat suppression technique is used in conjunction with gadolinium.

Orbital pseudotumor (myositic type). (**A**) This postcontrast coronal CT study demonstrates focal enlargement of the medial rectus muscle (*) in the left orbit. Note that there is no involvement of the adjacent orbital fat and the margins around the muscle are distinct. (**B**) Axial image from the same study reveals enlargement of the entire muscle (*) *including* the tendinous insertion on the globe (arrow). Note the lack of inflammatory changes in the orbital fat and the normal ethmoid air cells. The absence of any related inflammatory condition and involvement of the muscle tendon is suggestive of pseudotumor.

A

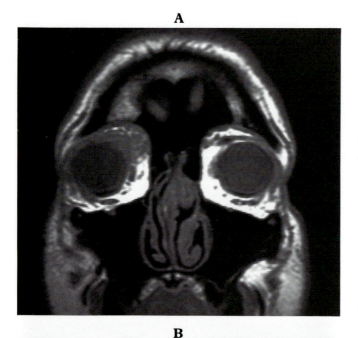

C

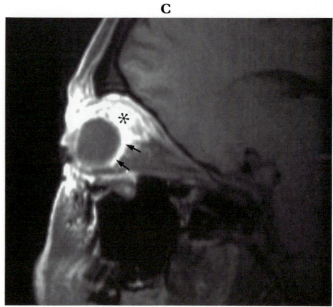

B

FIGURE 8.14

Orbital pseudotumor (tumefactive type). (**A**) Coronal T1-weighted image (TR = 600 ms, TE = 20 ms), obtained through the midportion of the globes shows a hypointense mass in the superomedial compartment of the right orbit. The mass is adjacent to the globe and effaces the orbital fat. (**B**) Fat-suppressed postcontrast T1-weighted image (TR = 600 ms, TE = 20 ms) at the same location as (A) shows intense enhancement of the mass (*) which surrounds the globe, yet does not invade or deform it. (**C**) Parasagittal postcontrast T1-weighted image (TR = 600 ms, TE = 20 ms), with fat suppression reveals the intraconal portion of the mass (*) and the enhancement of the posterior sclera, that is, posterior scleritis (arrows).

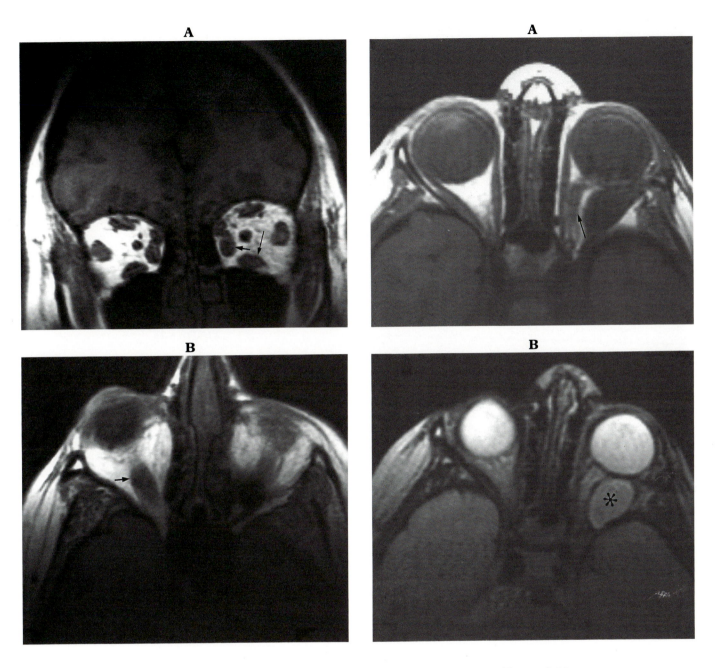

FIGURE 8.15

Thyroid ophthalmopathy in Graves' disease. (**A**) Coronal T1-weighted image (TR = 500 ms, TE = 12ms) through the middle of the muscle cone shows bilateral thickening of the medial rectus muscles (short arrow) and inferior rectus muscles (long arrow). There is probably enlargement of the other extraocular muscles as well. (**B**) A T1-weighted axial image (TR = 500 ms, TE = 12 ms) obtained through the lower right orbit reveals enlargement of the belly of the inferior rectus muscle (arrow).

FIGURE 8.16

Orbital teratoma in a 3-year-old male. (**A**) A well-defined mass demonstrated in the lateral compartment of the left orbit which is of low signal intensity on this T1-weighted (TR = 600 ms, TE = 20 ms) axial image. Note that the optic nerve is displaced around the mass (arrow). (**B**) The mass reverts to moderate hyperintensity (∗) on the T2-weighted sequence (TR = 2000 ms, TE = 80 ms). There is no evidence of fatty elements within the mass.

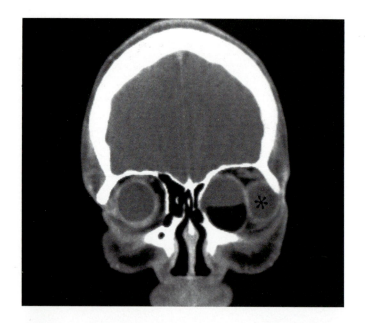

FIGURE 8.17

Cystic dermoid. A coronal CT image shows a large, oval shaped mass in the medial compartment of the left orbit. The globe (*) is displaced laterally by this mass which is larger than the globe itself. The mass contains two discrete components separated by a fluid level. The hypodense material in the inferior half of the tumor is fatty in composition, while the upper half is a complex fluid. The fatty material 'floats' above the complex, hyperdense fluid as this image was acquired with the patient supine and the head in extension.

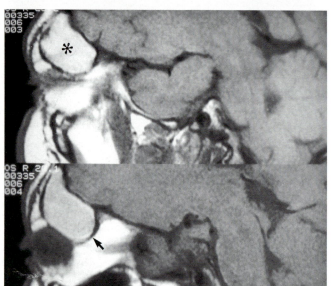

FIGURE 8.18

Dermoid. There is a large, well-defined mass (*) in the superior-lateral quadrant of the right orbit on this sagittal T1-weighted image (TR = 800 ms, TE = 20 ms). The mass is predominantly hyperintense on this pulse sequence secondary to fatty elements. The tumor is surrounded by a capsule of low signal intensity (arrow). The globe is mildly distorted and displaced inferiorly. This is the most common location for a orbital dermoid.

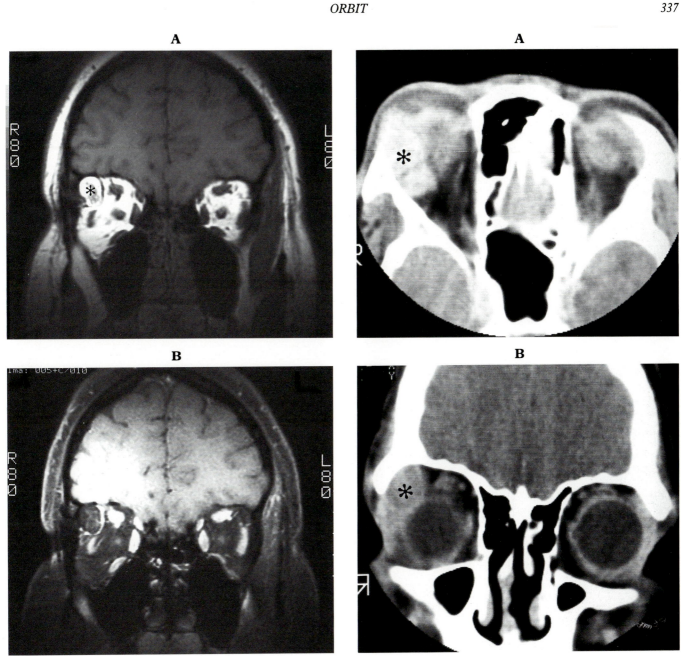

FIGURE 8.19

Dermoid. (**A**) A 1.5 cm hyperintense mass (*) is demonstrated in the superior-lateral quadrant of the right orbit on this T1-weighted coronal image (TR = 600 ms, TE = 20 ms). Note that the mass is isointense to orbital fat and is small enough in size as to not create significant displacement of the adjacent orbital structures. (**B**) Conversion to low signal intensity on this fat-suppressed coronal image (TR = 600 ms, TE = 20 ms) is confirmation of the fatty composition of the mass. Gadolinium produces mild enhancement of the fibrous capsule. Note the normal enhancement of the extraocular muscles.

FIGURE 8.20

Pleomorphic adenoma in the lacrimal gland. (**A**) A well-defined enhancing mass is identified in the superior-lateral quadrant of the right orbit (*) on this postcontrast axial CT image at the level of the upper orbit. (**B**) In the coronal plane, the mass (*) is noted to be in continuity with the lacrimal fossa and is displacing the globe.

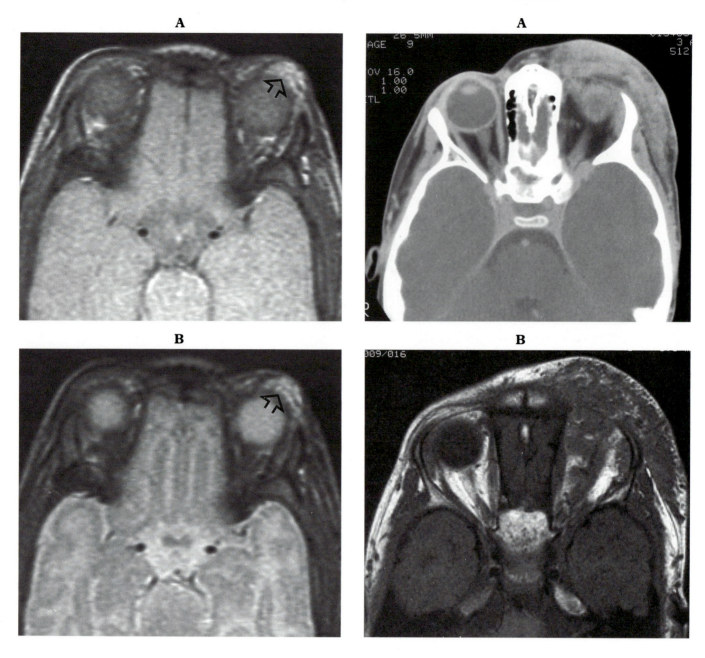

FIGURE 8.21

Capillary hemangioma of the eyelid. (**A**) Newborn male with discoloration and swelling of the left eyelid. First echo of the T2-weighted sequence (TR = 2000 ms, TE = 50 ms) in the axial plane shows an area of high signal intensity localized to the soft tissues of the left eyelid (arrow). The lesion is isointense with subcutaneous fat. (**B**) The hyperintense signal persists in the second echo of the T2-weighted sequence (TR = 2000 ms, TE = 100 ms) (arrow). This type of tumor characteristically regresses with time.

FIGURE 8.22

Lymphangioma. (**A**) 4-year-old male, born with a soft, flocculent mass over the left orbit which has grown slowly. Axial CT image shows a complex, infiltrating soft tissue mass which involves the superficial soft tissues of the eyelid and left temporal region, but also extends into the superior left orbit. (**B**) An axial T1-weighted image (TR = 500 ms, TE = 14 ms) reveals the infiltrating character of this abnormality. The orbital component is seen to better advantage and is noted to be more extensive than as depicted on the CT.

continued

C

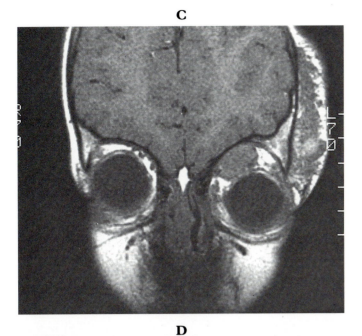

E

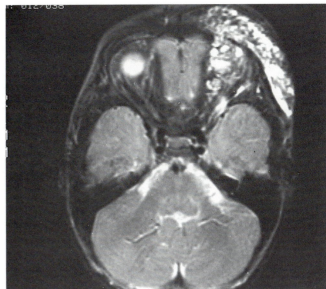

D

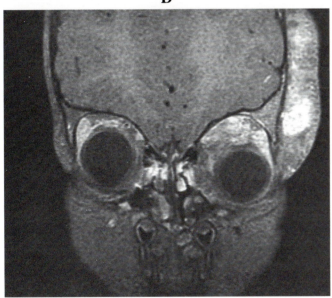

(E) The T2-weighted axial image (TR = 2500 ms, TE = 90 ms) depicts the tumor as multiloculated and of uniformly high signal intensity. The differential diagnosis includes lymphangioma vs hemangioma. The infiltrating character and the lack of uniform enhancement is more suggestive of lymphangioma. Capillary hemangiomas typically regress with time.

FIGURE 8.22 *(continued)*

(C) The T1-weighted coronal image shows a well-defined tissue mass in the superior orbit and infiltration of the temporalis muscle. The globe is depressed and deviated laterally. (D) With gadolinium and fat suppression, there is inhomogeneous enhancement of the tumor with mild enhancement of the intraorbital component.

A

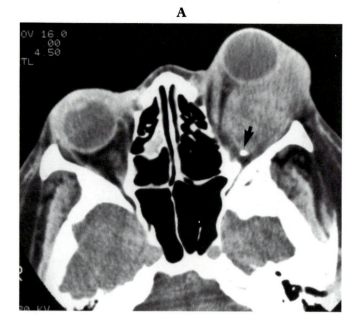

B

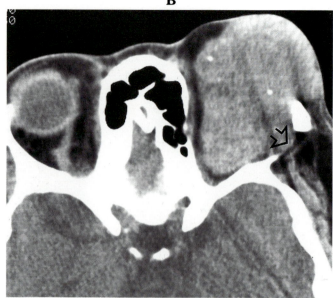

FIGURE 8.23

Cavernous hemangioma (recurrent). (**A**) Precontrast axial CT image shows a large soft tissue mass in the left orbit producing marked displacement of the globe anteriorly. The mass is intraconal, well defined and homogeneous in density. The mass displaces adjacent structures without invasion. Calcification (arrow) is seen scattered throughout the tumor; typical for hemangioma. (**B**) The bulk of the tumor is present in the superior orbit. Note the defect in the orbital wall from a prior lateral orbitotomy (open arrow). While the tumefactive form of orbital pseudotumor can exhibit a similar appearance with respect to density, extent and morphology, intrinsic calcifications are uncommon in pseudotumor.

A

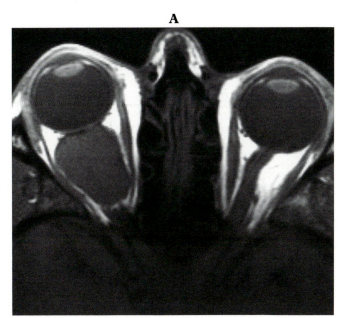

C

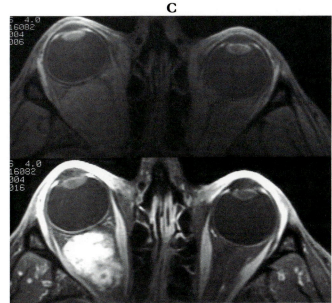

B

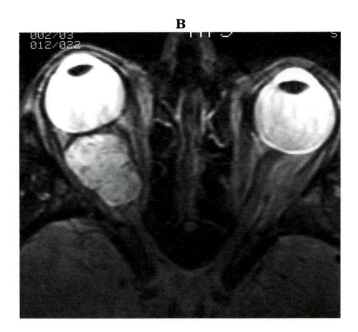

D

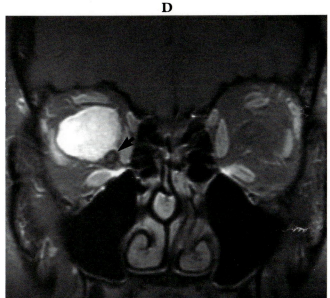

FIGURE 8.24

Cavernous hemangioma. (**A**) A T1-weighted axial image (TR = 500 ms, TE = 13 ms) obtained at the level of the lens shows a large, well-defined, intraconal mass which is producing a moderate degree of proptosis of the right globe. (**B**) The tumor is uniformly hyperintense on the T2-weighted image (TR = 2000 ms, TE = 80 ms) and is encapsulated by a rim of low signal intensity. (**C**) Fat-suppressed, axial T1-weighted images, precontrast (above) and following gadolinium (below) show intense enhancement of the tumor. (**D**) Fat-suppressed, coronal T1-weighted image, following gadolinium infusion confirms the true intraconal location of the tumor. This image also illustrates that the optic nerve is displaced inferiorly by the mass (arrow) rather than surrounded by tumor; a differentiating point between hemangioma and optic nerve/sheath tumors. Other differential considerations include orbital neuroma.

A

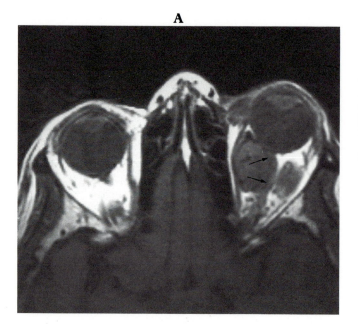

C

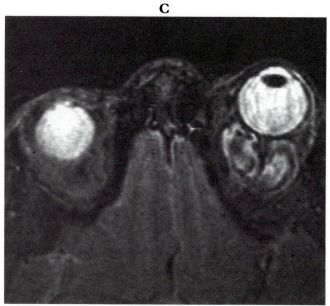

B

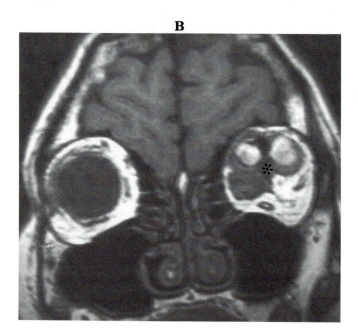

FIGURE 8.25

Lobulated cavernous hemangioma. (**A**) Multiple ovoid masses are present intraconally in the left orbit and the optic nerve (arrows) is draped around the largest of the masses on this T1-weighted axial image (TR = 600 ms, TE = 20 ms). (**B**) The T1-weighted coronal image (TR = 700 ms, TE = 20 ms), confirms the intraconal location of the tumor which surrounds the optic nerve (*). The pockets of high signal intensity within the superior masses represent large internal vascular spaces with stagnant blood flow. (**C**) The tumor is predominantly hyperintense on the T2-weighted (TR = 2000 ms, TE = 80 ms) axial image.

A

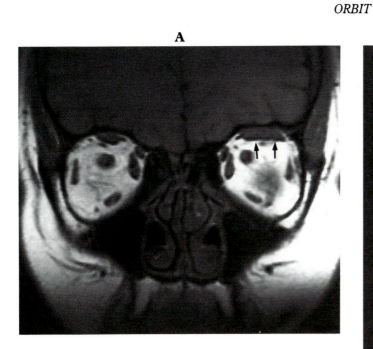

B

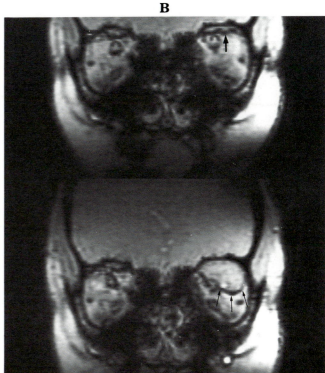

FIGURE 8.26

Orbital varix. (**A**) T1-weighted coronal image (TR = 600 ms, TE = 20 ms) shows a broad, flat structure in the superior aspect of the left orbit which blends in with the superior rectus/levator palpebrae complex (arrows). (**B**) Rapid gradient echo coronal images (TR = 50 ms, TE = 15 ms, 30° flip) of the orbit obtained in normal respiration (above) and with the Valsalva maneuver (below) shows dramatic enlargement of the mass secondary to increased venous pressure (arrows). Application of the Valsalva maneuver was accompanied clinically by proptosis.

A

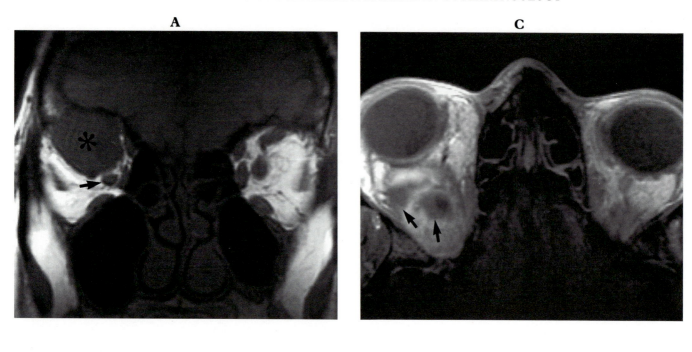

C

B

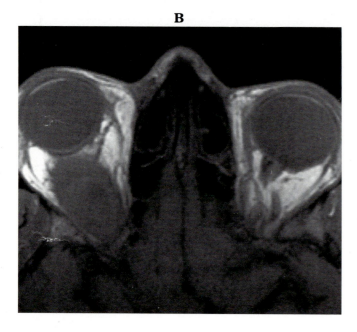

D

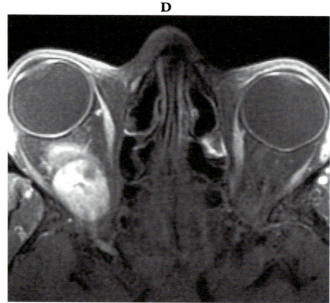

FIGURE 8.27

Schwannoma (neuroma). (**A**) Coronal T1-weighted MR image (TR = 500 ms, TE = 23 ms) shows a large mass filling the superior half of the right orbit (*). The conal and extraconal structures are displaced inferiorly as is the optic nerve (arrow). (**B**) The mass is well defined and occupies a large portion of the orbit, extending from the orbital apex to the globe.

(**C**) There is inhomogeneous enhancement of the mass with infusion of gadolinium. Areas of little or no enhancement suggest internal necrosis (arrows). Note that the margins of the tumor are less well defined with gadolinium alone due to decreased contrast between enhancing tumor and orbital fat. (**D**) Fat suppression with gadolinium offers superb delineation of the tumor borders and intensifies enhancement of the mass by decreasing the dynamic range of the image.

continued

E

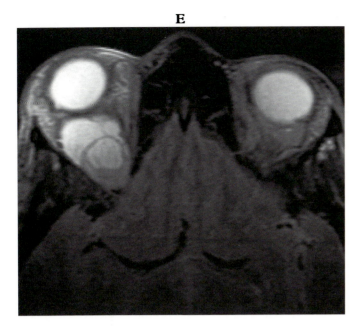

A

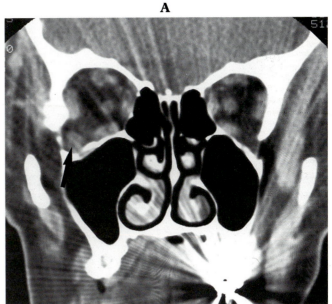

B

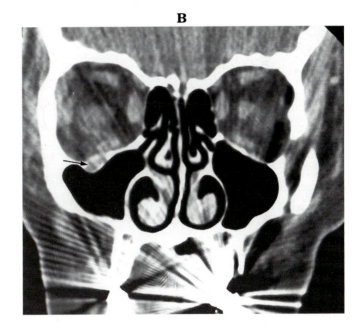

FIGURE 8.27 *(continued)*

(**E**) The tumor is predominantly hyperintense on the T2-weighted image (TR = 1860 ms, TE = 80 ms). The variations in signal intensity are most likely secondary to areas of internal necrosis. Differential considerations in this case include hemangioma versus nerve sheath tumor originating from the first division of the fifth cranial nerve.

FIGURE 8.28

Neuroma of the infraorbital nerve. (**A**) Patient with neurofibromatosis and parathesias in the distribution of the second division of the trigeminal nerve. Coronal CT image shows a extraconal soft tissue density in the inferolateral quadrant of the right orbit (arrow). (**B**) Coronal CT image obtained approximately ten millimeters anterior to (a) shows that the mass continues into the inferior orbital fissure (arrow).

A

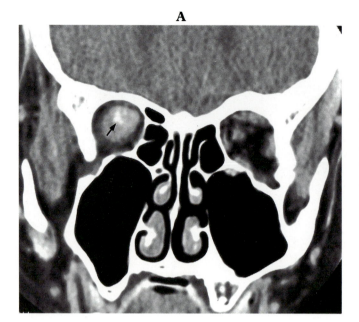

C

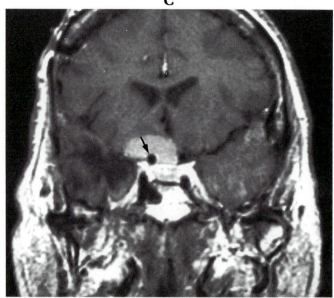

B

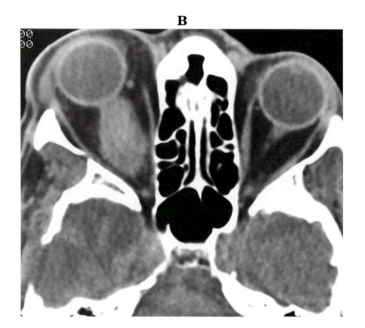

FIGURE 8.29

Optic nerve sheath meningioma with cavernous meningioma. (**A**) A noncontrast coronal CT image reveals a large soft tissue mass which surrounds the right optic nerve and contains a small area of calcification (arrow). (**B**) The corresponding axial CT image shows that the mass is spindle shaped and that it extends from the posterior sclera to the orbital apex. The shape of the mass and the existence of calcification are more compatible with meningioma than optic glioma. (**C**) A postcontrast T1-weighted coronal MR image obtained through the cavernous sinus demonstrates another meningioma in a cavernous location. The enhancing mass encases the supraclinoid internal carotid artery (arrow).

A

B

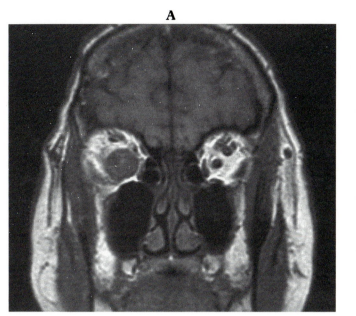
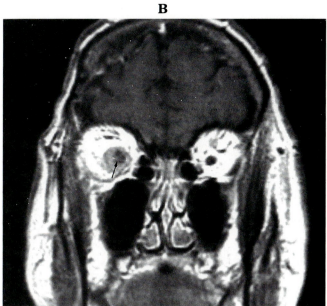

FIGURE 8.30

Optic nerve sheath meningioma. (**A**) A large mass of low signal intensity surrounds the right optic nerve on this T1-weighted (TR = 900 ms, TE = 20 ms), coronal MR image. The optic nerve cannot be distinguished from the tumor itself. (**B**) The intense enhancement of the tumor with gadolinium on this image actually decreases the conspicuity of the tumor itself. Note that the tumor appears smaller in size than on the precontrast image largely due to peripheral enhancement which is isointense to orbital fat. The hypointense optic nerve (arrow) is now visible centrally. Fat suppression in conjunction with gadolinium enhancement would have improved the visualization of this tumor.

A

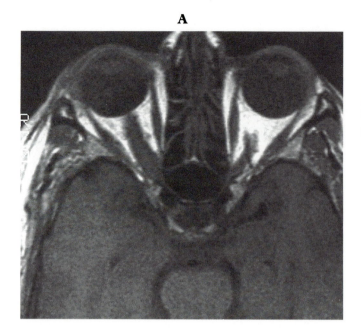

C

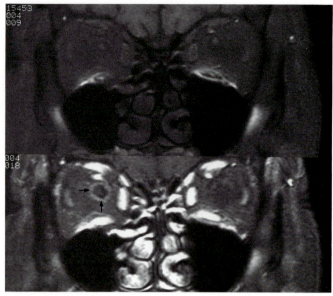

B

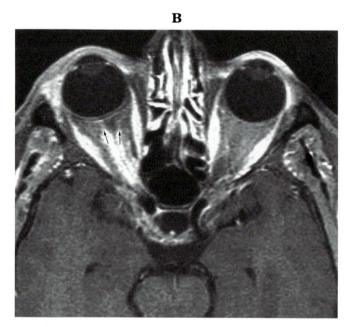

D

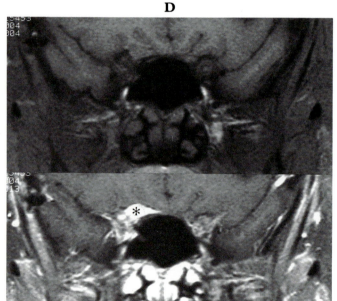

FIGURE 8.31

Optic nerve sheath meningioma. (**A**) Marked
enlargement of the right optic nerve/sheath complex
is demonstrated on this T1-weighted (TR = 500 ms,
TE = 12 ms) axial image. Both optic nerve sheath
meningioma and optic nerve glioma may share this
appearance. (**B**) Use of gadolinium and fat
suppression shows significant enhancement of the
perimeter of the nerve without enlargement/
enhancement of the nerve itself. Note the shell of
enhancement around the nerve anteriorly (arrows).

(**C**) T1-weighted, coronal images of the middle
orbit, with fat suppression. Precontrast (above) and
gadolinium-enhanced (below) show a
morphologically normal optic nerve with peripheral
enhancement (arrows) suggesting that the process
involves the optic nerve sheath exclusively. (**D**) Same
technique as in (C), obtained at the level of the
orbital apex, shows a broad-based enhancing mass
(*) attached to the lesser wing of the sphenoid bone
and anterior clinoid, characteristic of meningioma.

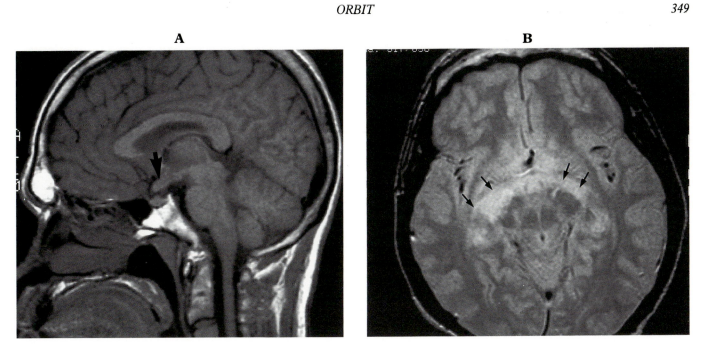

FIGURE 8.32

Neurofibromatosis 1 with optic glioma.
(A) Midsagittal T1-weighted image (TR = 500 ms, TE = 16 ms) shows thickening of the optic tracts (arrow). (B) A proton-density (TR = 2000 ms, TE = 30 ms) axial image at the level of the midbrain shows areas of abnormal signal intensity within the optic tracts and internal capsules (arrows) characteristic of hamartomatous changes of neurofibromatosis versus infiltration by the glioma.

A

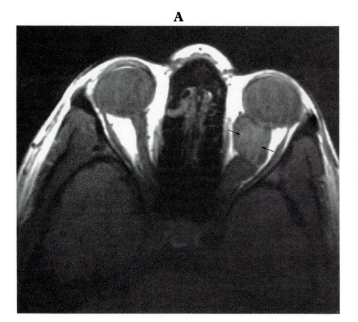

B

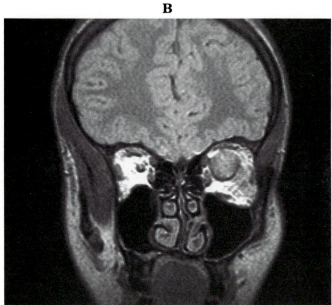

FIGURE 8.33

Optic glioma. (**A**) There is diffuse enlargement of the left optic nerve on this T1-weighted axial image (TR = 600 ms, TE = 25 ms). The enlarged nerve (arrows) is shown within the dilated nerve sheath.

(**B**) A proton density image (TR = 2000 ms, TE = 25 ms) of the glioma in coronal view. This lesion is isolated, limited to the orbit and does not involve the chiasm or the remainder of the visual apparatus.

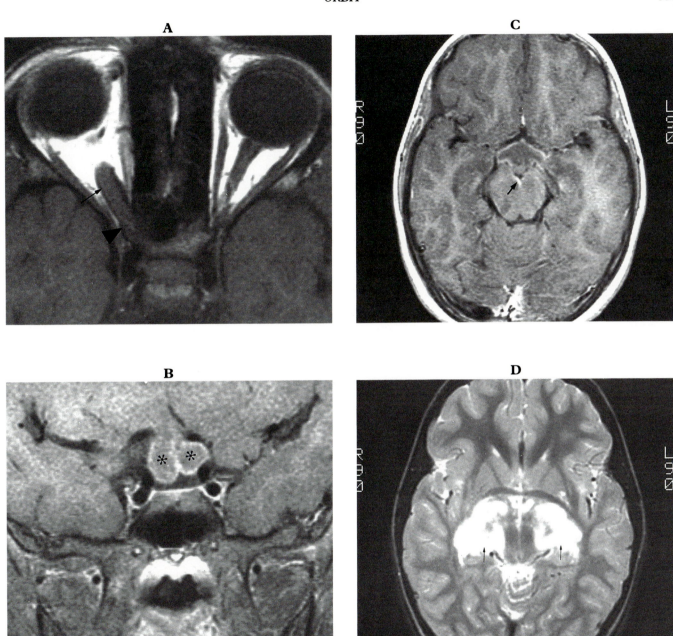

FIGURE 8.34

Optic chiasm/hypothalamic glioma with invasion. (**A**) Axial T1-weighted axial image (TR = 500 ms, TE = 14 ms) shows diffuse enlargement of the right optic nerve (arrow) with extension into through the optic foramen (arrowhead). The left optic nerve appears grossly normal. (**B**) A gadolinium-enhanced, T1-weighted, coronal image, using fat suppression shows bulbous enlargement of the optic chiasm (*) with a mild degree of peripheral enhancement suggesting invasion of the visual apparatus by glioma. (**C**) Invasion of the optic chiasm and optic tracts is confirmed on this post contrast T1-weighted axial image. There is diffuse enlargement of the optic chiasm with enhancement that appears to also involve the ventral margin of the brainstem (arrow). (**D**) The T2-weighted image (TR = 2600 ms, TE = 90 ms) shows the advanced degree of invasion of the visual apparatus and adjacent structures including the lateral geniculate bodies of the thalamus (arrows), the midbrain, the posterior limbs of the internal capsules and hypothalamus.

A

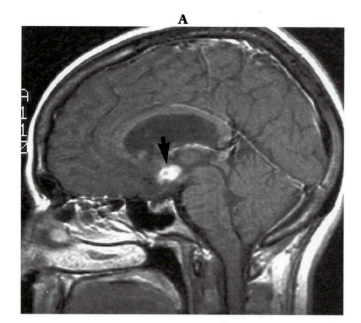

C

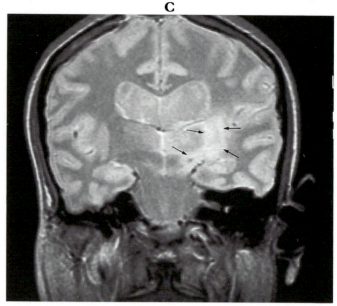

B

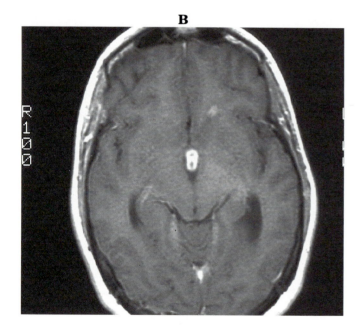

FIGURE 8.35

Hypothalamic glioma with invasion of visual pathways. (**A**) A midsagittal, contrast-enhanced, T1-weighted image (TR = 500 ms, TE = 16 ms), shows a discrete area of enhancement below the posterior third ventricle (arrow). The optic chiasm, nerves and tracts (not shown), show minimal enlargement on the left. (**B**) An axial image obtained at the level of the inferior third ventricle/interpeduncular cistern shows that the area of enhancement is restricted to the midline. (**C**) A proton density, coronal image (TR = 2700 ms, TE = 30 ms), shows a large area of increased signal within the posterior limb of the left internal capsule and left pulvinar/lateral geniculate body (arrows) secondary to infiltration of the optic pathways. The lateral ventricles are enlarged, presumably secondary to partial obstruction of CSF outflow from the third ventricle.

A

B

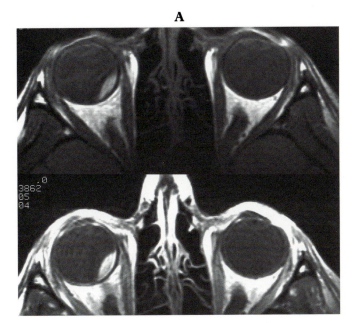

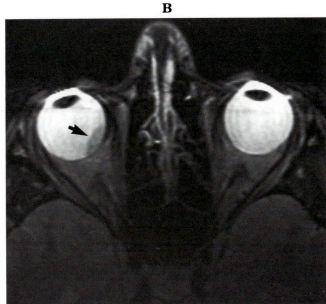

FIGURE 8.36

Melanotic melanoma. (**A**) A crescentic shaped mass is present in the postero-medial choroid of the right globe. The mass is hyperintense on the noncontrast T1-weighted (TR = 650 ms, TE = 23 ms) image (above). The lower image depicts enhancement of the tumor with infusion of intravenous gadolinium. (**B**) An axial T2-weighted image (TR = 2000 ms, TE = 80 ms) shows the typical hypointensity of melanotic melanoma relative to vitreous (arrow).

A

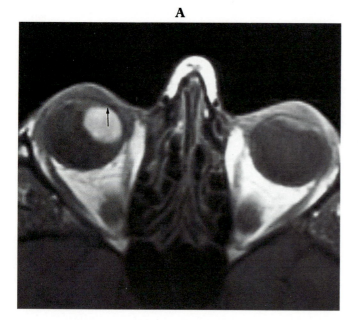

C

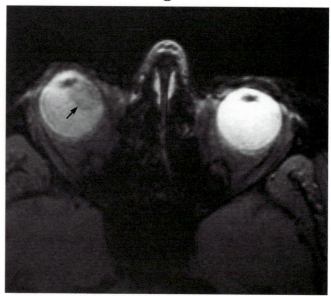

B

FIGURE 8.37

Melanotic melanoma in the ciliary body. (**A**) A T1-weighted axial image (TR = 500 ms, TE = 20 ms) demonstrates a large hyperintense mass in the right globe which abuts the anterior chamber medially (arrow) and probably originates from the ciliary body. (**B**) Fat-suppressed T1-weighted images (TR = 500 ms, TE = 20 ms), without (above) and with (below) gadolinium reveal minimal enhancement of the tumor. (**C**) There is magnetic susceptibility by the tumor as shown by its hypointensity relative to vitreous (arrow) on this gradient echo image (TR = 300 ms, TE = 15 ms, 15° flip).

A

C

B

D

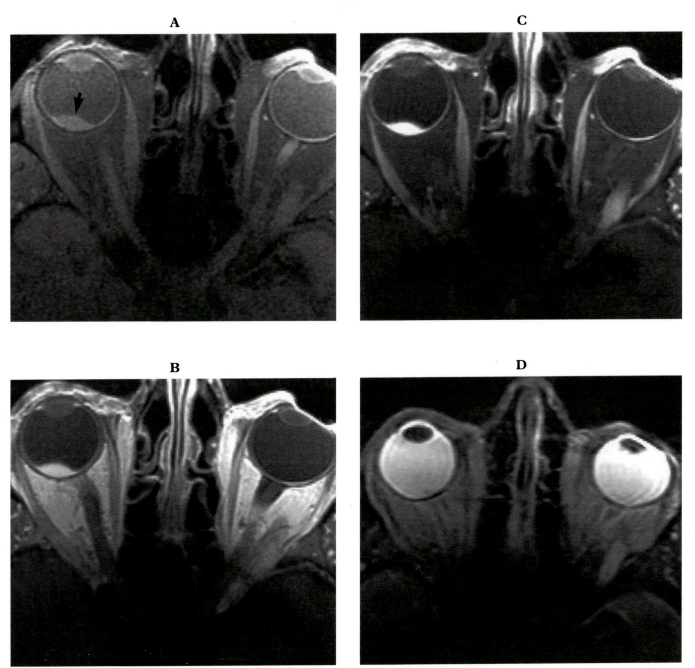

FIGURE 8.38

Choroidal hemangioma. (**A**) A choroidal mass (arrow) is present in the right globe on this fat-suppressed T1-weighted (TR = 500 ms, TE = 23 ms) image. The mass is mildly hyperintense relative to the vitreous body. (**B**) There is intense enhancement of the mass on this postgadolinium T1-weighted axial image (TR = 500 ms, TE = 23 ms).

(**C**) The degree of enhancement is even more pronounced with the use of fat suppression. The excessive enhancement pattern is more typical of hemangioma than of melanoma. (**D**) Unlike melanotic melanoma, the choroidal hemangioma is hyperintense (isointense to vitreous) on the T2-weighted image (TR = 1800 ms, TE = 80 ms).

A

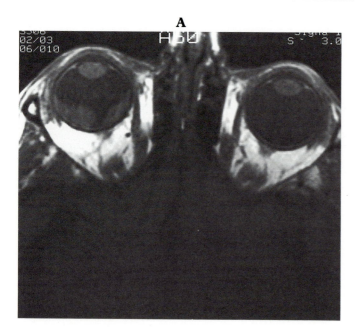

B

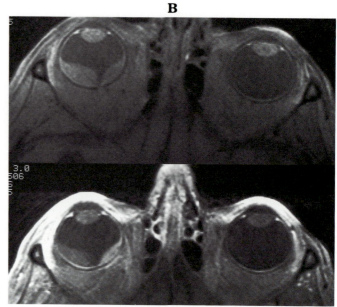

FIGURE 8.39

Breast metastasis to right globe. (**A**) An axial T1-weighted (TR = 500 ms, TE = 16 ms) image shows a mildly hyperintense biconvex mass located medial and lateral to the optic nerve head. (**B**) The lesion is visualized better on the fat-suppressed T1-weighted images (TR = 600 ms, TE = 15 ms). The two lesions are of similar signal intensity relative to vitreous on the noncontrast image (above) and there is differential enhancement on the postcontrast image (below) suggesting that the enhancing (medial) abnormality is the metastatic lesion, while the lateral abnormality represents subretinal fluid.

A

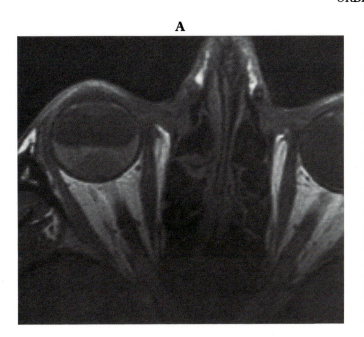

C

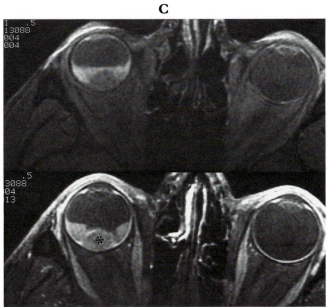

B

FIGURE 8.40

Amelanotic melanoma with choroidal effusion. (**A**) A mound of tissue is present at the level of the optic disk which is slightly hyperintense relative to vitreous on this T1-weighted axial image (TR = 500 ms, TE = 20 ms). Also noted the hyperintense subchoroidal effusion which outlines the choroidal tumor. (**B**) On the T2-weighted image (TR = 2000 ms, TE = 80 ms), the tumor becomes relatively hypointense while the effusion becomes isointense with the vitreous. (**C**) Fat-suppressed T1-weighted (TR = 600 ms, TE = 25 ms) images; precontrast above and postgadolinium below. Fat suppression produces a narrowed dynamic range which tends to improve the contrast differential between the choroidal effusion and the normal vitreous. The melanoma (∗) enhances minimally with gadolinium.

A

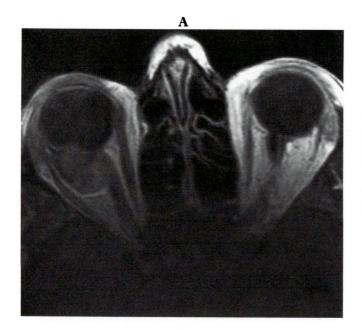

C

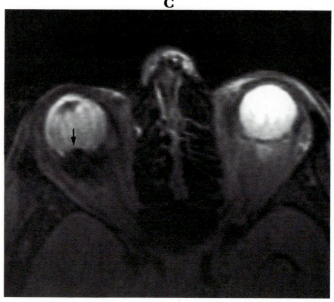

B

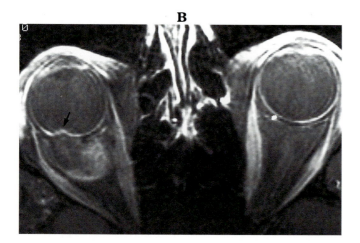

FIGURE 8.41

Melanoma with extraocular extension. (**A**) A contrast-enhanced T1-weighted axial image (TR = 500 ms, TE = 20 ms) shows a lobulated mass attached to the posterior pole of the right eye which protrudes into the retrobulbar region. The mass is heterogeneous in signal intensity and appears to be contiguous with a smaller choroidal mass. The optic nerve is draped over the extraocular tumor. (**B**) The enhancing choroid is buckled by the underlying tumor (arrow) on this fat-suppressed, gadolinium-enhanced image (TR = 800 ms, TE = 25 ms). (**C**) On T2-weighting (TR = 2000 ms, TE = 80 ms), the intraocular and extraocular components of the tumor are both markedly hypointense (arrow).

A

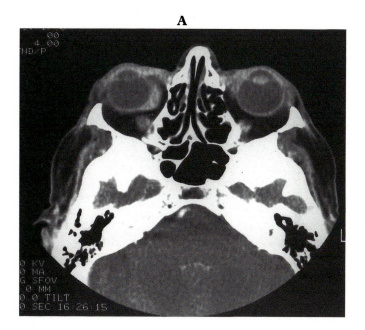

C

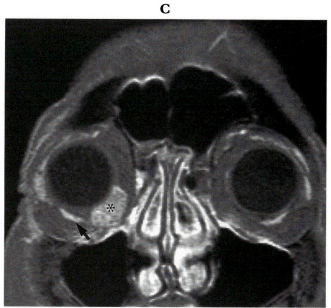

B

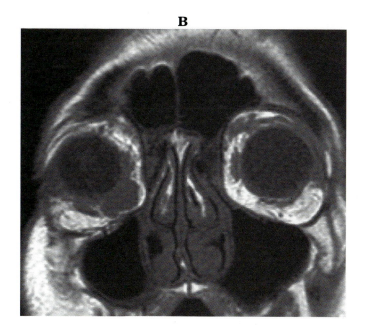

FIGURE 8.42

Orbital lymphoma. (**A**) An enhancing mass is noted along the mesial surface of the right globe on this axial CT image. There is no distortion of the globe or evidence of invasion. (**B**) The mass is of low signal intensity on this T1-weighted (TR = 400 ms, TE = 12 ms) coronal image. It follows the inferior and medial contours of the sclera. (**C**) There is enhancement of the mass (∗) following infusion of intravenous gadolinium on this fat suppressed coronal image. Note that there is no involvement of the adjacent inferior oblique muscle (arrow).

A

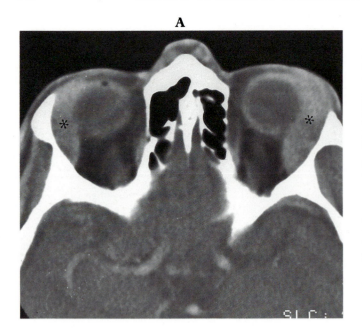

C

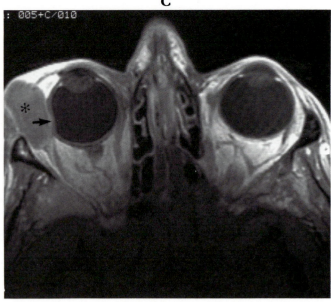

B

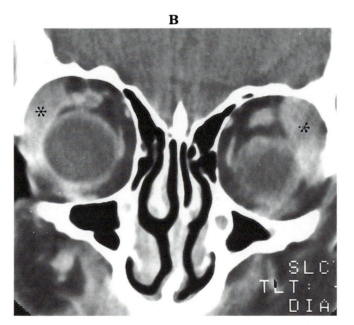

D

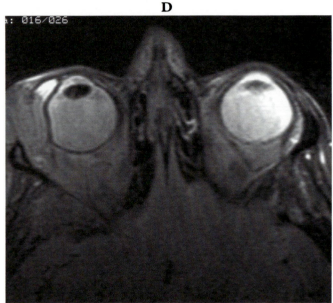

FIGURE 8.43

Orbital lymphoma in the lacrimal region. (**A**) Well-defined masses are demonstrated in the superior-lateral quadrants of the orbits bilaterally (∗). The tumor molds itself to the contours of the globe and extends anteriorly to involve the preseptal space. The extraconal fat is preserved. (**B**) The coronal CT image confirms the characteristic location of the lesions (∗); as an extension of the lacrimal glands. This is the most common location for orbital lymphoma. (**C**) An axial MR image, T1-weighting (TR = 500 ms, TE = 14 ms) with gadolinium in a different patient reveals a lobulated mass (∗) in the temporal quadrant of the right anterior orbit. The mass enhances minimally and indents the lateral aspect of the globe without invasion (arrow). (**D**) With T2-weighting (TR = 1800 ms, TE = 80 ms) (same patient as (**C**)). Unlike other neoplasia, this lymphoma is hypointense relative to vitreous.

continued

E

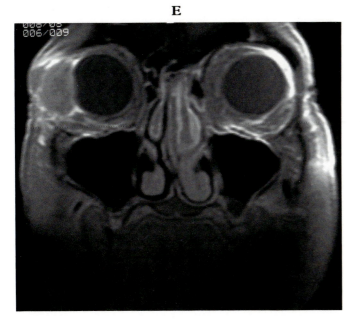

A

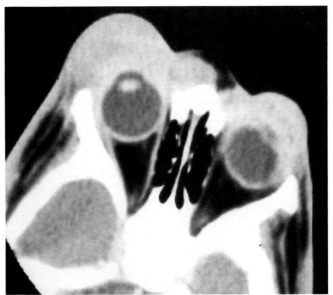

FIGURE 8.43 *(continued)*

(**E**) Same patient as (C) and (D). A fat-suppressed, gadolinium-enhanced, T1-weighted (TR = 650 ms, TE = 13 ms) coronal image.

FIGURE 8.44

Orbital chloroma from acute myelocytic leukemia in an 18-month-old infant. A contrast-enhanced axial CT image shows bulky, homogeneously enhancing masses in the preseptal space, conjunctiva and eyelids bilaterally. Note the absence of deformity of the globes or invasion of the retrobulbar spaces.

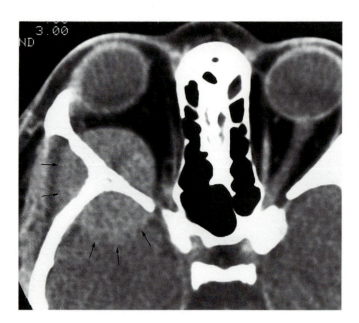

A

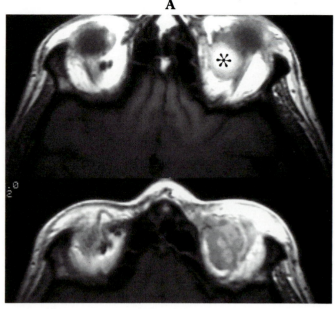

FIGURE 8.45

Ewing sarcoma metastasis to lateral orbit wall. A large soft tissue mass originates from the right sphenoid wing and orbital wall and extends into the lateral extraconal compartment of the orbit, the temporal fossa and middle cranial fossa (arrows).

B

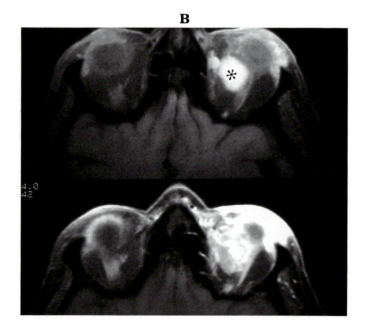

FIGURE 8.46

Metastasis to the superior orbit. (**A**) Gadolinium-enhanced axial T1-weighted images (TR = 500 ms, TE = 20 ms), obtained at the level of the upper orbit, show an enhancing mass (*) in the medial portion of the superior left orbit. This melanoma abuts the globe and the superior rectus muscle. (**B**) Same technique as (A) with fat suppression shows somewhat better contrast definition of the mass (*).

continued

C

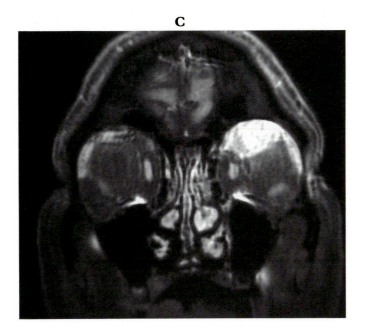

E

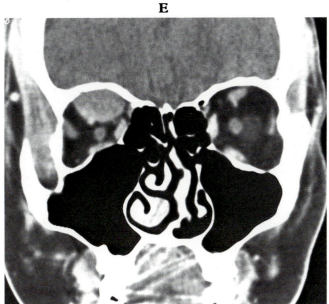

D

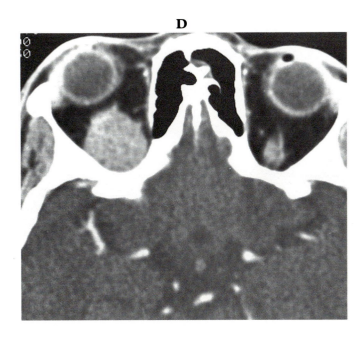

(**E**) The coronal CT image (same patient as (D)) illustrates the extraconal location of the mass. Note that unlike the appearance of a benign extraconal mass, this tumor incorporates the superior rectus muscle rather than displacing it.

FIGURE 8.46 *(continued)*

(**C**) A fat-suppressed, postgadolinium coronal image confirms that the mass is extraconal, abuts the superior orbit and appears to infiltrate rather than displace the extraocular muscles. This infiltrative characteristic is suggestive of an aggressive process. (**D**) A contrast-enhanced axial CT image in a different patient with metastatic breast carcinoma shows a well-defined mass in the superior right orbit.

A

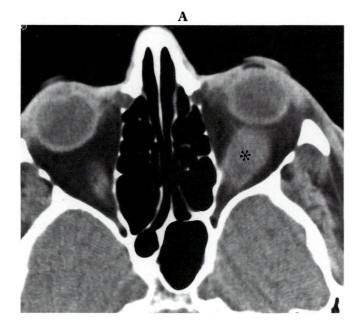

B

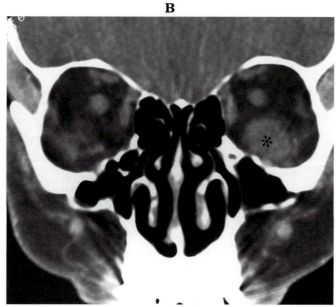

FIGURE 8.47

Melanoma metastasis to the inferior rectus muscle. (**A**) Axial CT image shows an oval shaped mass in the lower left orbit (∗). (**B**) A coronal CT image confirms that the mass (∗) is confined to the left inferior rectus muscle. These findings are nonspecific; metastasis is a diagnosis of exclusion. Graves' ophthalmopathy should be ruled out in any instance of isolated inferior rectus enlargement.

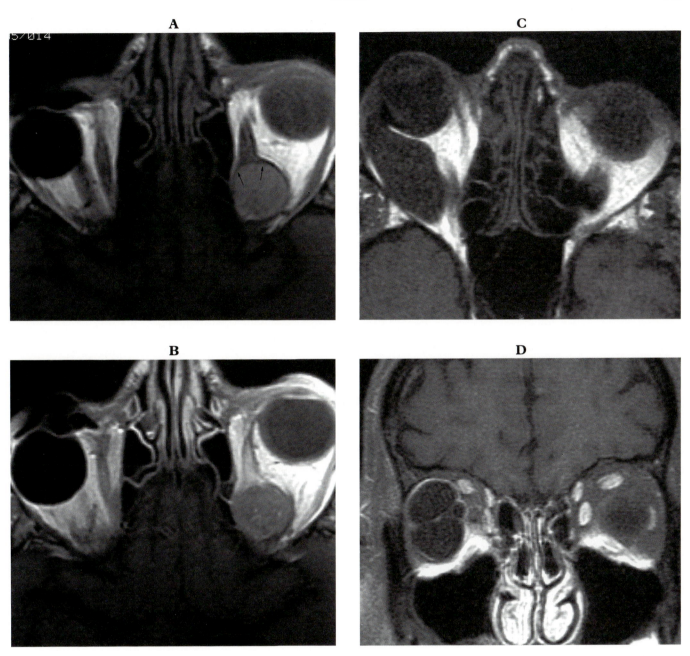

FIGURE 8.48

Isolated rectus muscle enlargement. (**A**) There is bulbous enlargement of the medial rectus muscle in the left orbit by a well-defined hyperintense mass on this T1-weighted (TR = 500 ms, TE = 23 ms) axial image. The mass is situated within the substance of the muscle and the muscle fibers are splayed around the tumor (arrows). (**B**) Same location and technique as (A) with gadolinium reveals minimal enhancement of this melanoma metastasis. Of incidental note is an orbital prosthesis on the right. (**C**) In a different patient, there is massive enlargement of the lateral rectus muscle on the right.

Unlike the metastatic deposit in (A) and (B), this process appears to involve the entire muscle including the tendinous insertion at the globe and is noted to be isointense with respect to the vitreous body. (**D**) Same patient as (C), on a coronal T1-weighted image (TR = 550 ms, TE = 12 ms) with gadolinium, shows peripheral enhancement of a thin capsule with the suggestion of multiple septations. There is no nodular enhancement as expected with a true neoplasm. At surgery, this was found to be a developmental cyst.

A

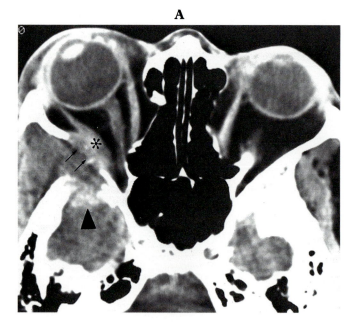

A

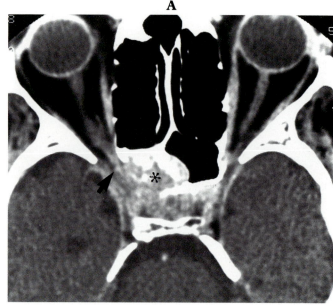

FIGURE 8.50

Prostate metastasis to orbital apex. On a postcontrast axial CT image, a perisellar mass extends into the right cavernous sinus and orbital apex (arrow). Tumor erodes the tuberculum sella and extends into the sphenoid sinus (*).

B

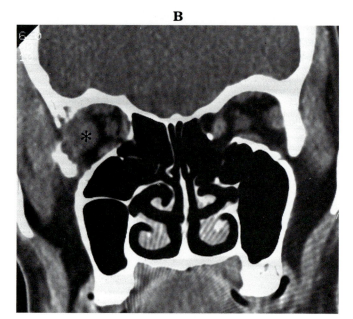

FIGURE 8.49

Lung metastasis to orbital wall and lateral rectus muscle. (**A**) A contast-enhanced axial CT image at the level of the midorbit demonstrates a soft tissue mass which has destroyed the lateral wall of the right orbit (small arrows). There is effacement of the extraconal fat in this location and thickening of the lateral rectus muscle (*). Tumor has also eroded the sphenoid bone and invaded the middle cranial fossa (arrowhead). (**B**) The coronal CT image shows that tumor has infiltrated the extraconal fat and invaded the fascia of the lateral rectus muscle resulting in edema (*).

A

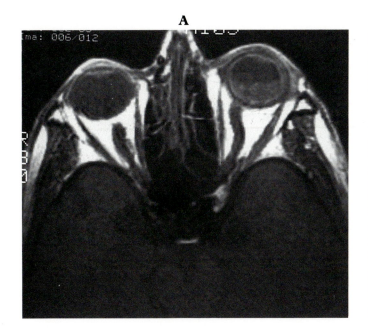

B

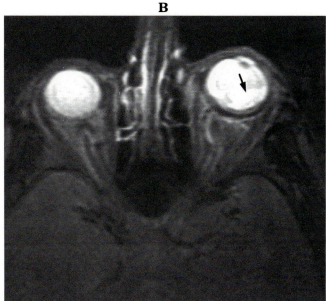

FIGURE 8.51

Adenocarcinoma metastasis to left globe. (**A**) On a noncontrast T1-weighted image (TR = 500 ms, TE = 20 ms) there is a lobulated, mildly hyperintense ocular mass. There is proptosis of the left globe. (**B**) The tumor is somewhat hyperintense (arrow) relative to vitreous on the T2-weighted image (TR = 2000 ms, TE = 80 ms). These signal characteristics differ from those of pigmented melanoma, which is often hyperintense on T1-weighted images and hypointense on T2-weighted images relative to vitreous. Gadolinium is necessary to differentiate tumor from choroidal effusion in this case.

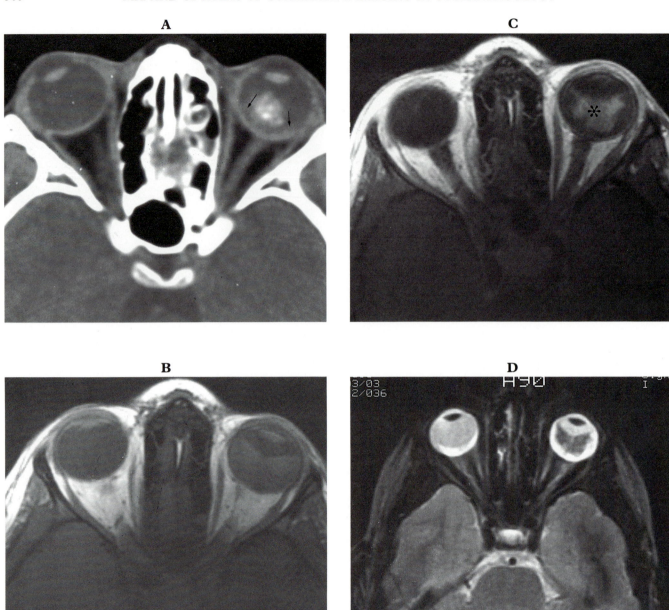

Figure 8.52

Retinoblastoma. (**A**) A calcified mass is present in the left globe which protrudes into the vitreous cavity. The area behind the mass itself is slightly hyperdense suggesting the presence of a proteinaceous choroidal effusion (arrows). (**B**) A T1-weighted axial image (TR = 600 ms, TE = 14 ms) in another patient shows a large hyperintense mass originating from the posterior choroid/retina of the left globe which fills the majority of the globe and approximates the ciliary body anteriorly. (**C**) Same patient as (B). With gadolinium administration there is a moderate amount of central enhancement (*). (**D**) Same patients as (B) and (C). The mass is hypointense relative to vitreous on this T2-weighted (TR = 2400 ms, TE = 90 ms) axial image presumably due to the presence of intrinsic calcification which is characteristic of retinoblastoma.

A

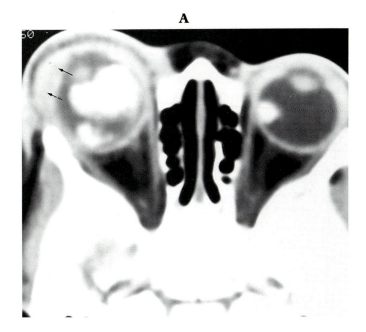

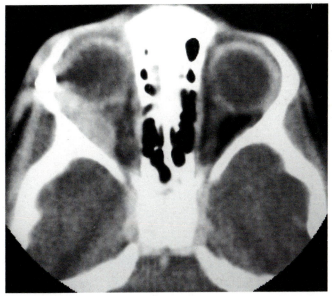

B

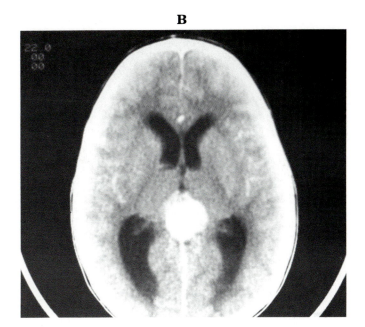

FIGURE 8.54

Orbital rhabdomyosarcoma in a 3-year-old female. A contrast-enhanced axial CT image shows an ovoid mass extraconally in the right orbit which abuts the lateral wall and the globe. The configuration of the mass suggests that it arises from the lateral rectus muscle.

FIGURE 8.53

Bilateral retinoblastoma. (**A**) Calcified intraocular masses are present bilaterally. The immense size of the mass on the right has promoted enlargement of the globe and has produced an intense scleral reaction (arrows). The macrophthalmia results in a proptotic right orbit. (**B**) An axial CT image of the brain in another patient with bilateral retinoblastoma reveals a calcified mass originating from the pineal gland, which fulfills the criteria for trilateral retinoblastoma. The large mass is producing obstructive hydrocephalus.

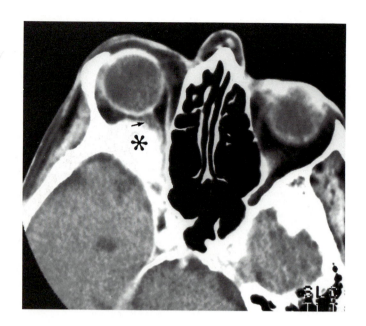

FIGURE 8.55

Meningioma, orbital and extraconal. Contrast-enhanced, axial CT image through the midorbit shows a densely enhancing, well-defined mass in the right lateral orbit (*) which has a broad base of attachment to the lateral orbital wall. Note the optic nerve (arrow) which is draped medially over the mass.

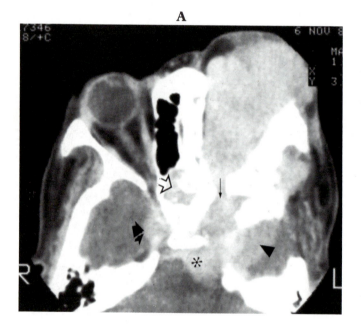

A

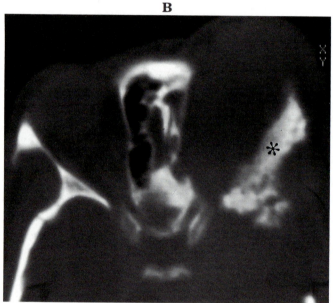

B

FIGURE 8.56

Recurrent orbital meningioma. (**A**) There is a massive, enhancing soft tissue mass filling the entire left orbit. The meningioma has invaded adjacent compartments via the superior orbital fissure (small arrow). Tumor now extends into the left middle cranial fossa (arrowhead) and the prepontine cistern (*) with compression of the brainstem. Tumor also breeches the sphenoid sinus (open arrow) with involvement of the contralateral cavernous sinus

(short solid arrow). Also of note are operative changes in the left middle cranial fossa. (**B**) Axial CT image at the level of the optic foramen photographed at bone windows shows the characteristic hyperostotic changes of the lateral wall of the orbit (*).

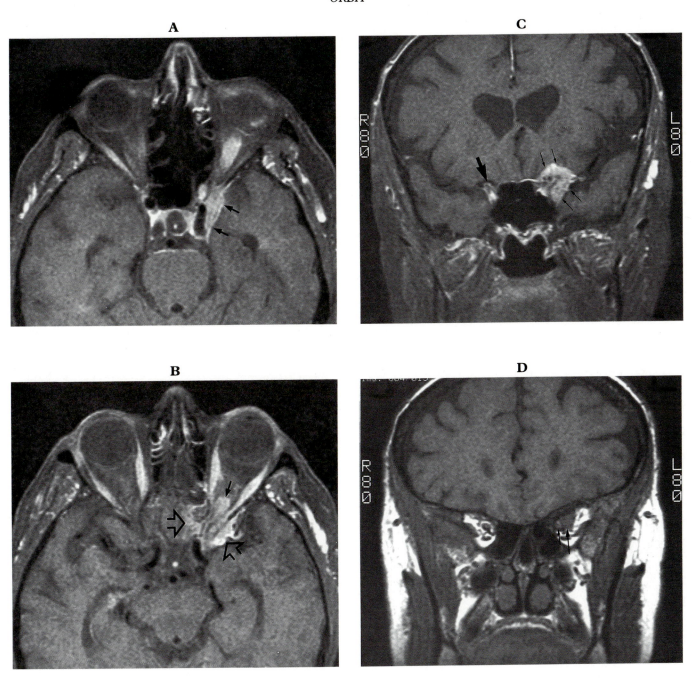

A

B

C

D

FIGURE 8.57

Cavernous meningioma with orbital involvement.
(**A**) Postcontrast axial T1-weighted MR image with fat suppression (TR = 600 ms, TE = 23 ms) shows bulging of the lateral wall of the left cavernous sinus (arrows) which extends anteriorly towards the left orbital apex. (**B**) Axial image obtained 6 mm superior to (A), at the level of the optic foramen, reveals enhancing tissue along the lesser wing of the sphenoid bone which surrounds the orbital apex (open arrows). A tongue of enhancing tumor extends centrally, into the orbital apex (arrow). (**C**) The meningioma has a broad base of attachment to the lesser wing of the sphenoid bone (small arrows) and anterior clinoid process. Note the normal anterior clinoid process on the right (thick arrow). (**D**) The tumor is isointense with respect to the optic nerve and extraocular muscles (long arrow) as shown on this noncontrast T1-weighted coronal image obtained through the orbital apex. The optic nerve (short arrow) is displaced medially around the mass.

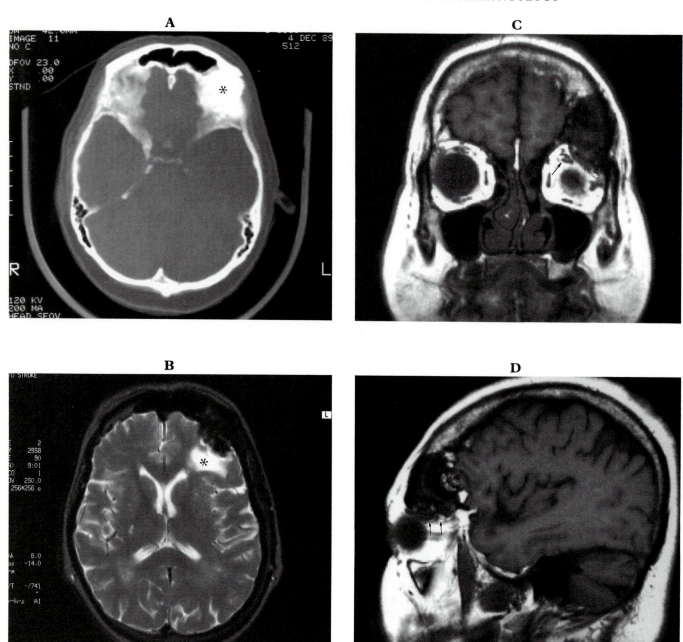

FIGURE 8.58

Meningioma of orbital roof. (**A**) Axial CT image at the level of the lesser wing of the sphenoid bone shows characteristic hyperostotic changes involving the roof of the orbit (∗). (**B**) A T2-weighted axial MR image (TR = 3000 ms, TE = 90 ms) at the level of the frontal lobes shows the hypointense hyperostotic bone protruding into the anterior cranial fossa. Edematous changes are noted in the parenchyma of the left frontal lobe (∗).

(**C**) A coronal T1-weighted image (TR = 500 ms, TE = 15 ms) shows that the predominantly hypointense mass protrudes into the superior orbit with displacement of the extraocular muscles medially (arrow). (**D**) The component of the mass in the superior extraconal space (arrow) is shown on this T1-weighted sagittal image (TR = 550 ms, TE = 15 ms).

A   **B**

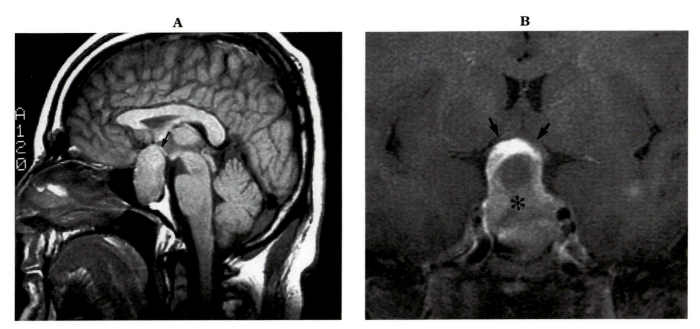

FIGURE 8.59

Pituitary macroadenoma. (**A**) 43-year-old male with bitemporal hemianopsia. A midsagittal T1-weighted image (TR = 500 ms, TE = 16 ms) shows a large intrasellar mass with significant suprasellar extension. The optic tracts (arrow) are displaced and stretched over the tumor. (**B**) A postcontrast coronal T1-weighted image reveals inhomogeneous enhancement of the pituitary tumor (∗) probably due to central necrosis. The optic tracts (arrows) are stretched and flattened against the upper border of the tumor.

A

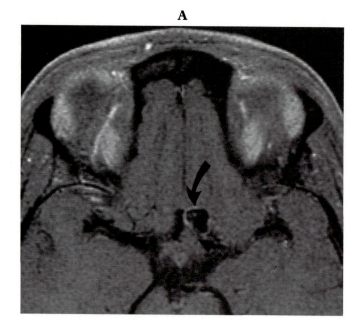

C

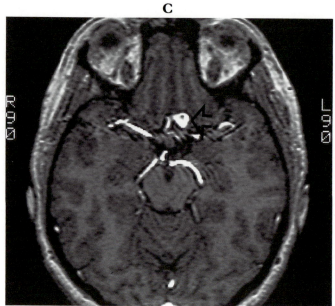

B

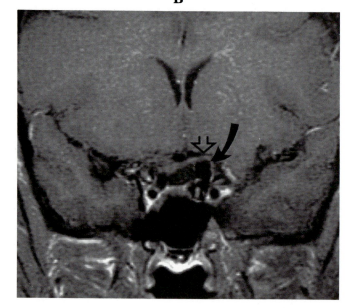

FIGURE 8.60

Aneurysm of the ophthalmic artery. (**A**) 35-year-old female with left orbital pain. A gadolinium-enhanced T1-weighted image (TR = 650 ms, TE = 16 ms) shows a lobulated area of signal void (curved arrow) juxtaposing the left optic nerve (arrowhead). (**B**) On coronal view (TR = 550 ms, TE = 12 ms) the left optic nerve (open arrow) is shown to be elevated and stretched over the aneurysm (curved arrow). (**C**) A gradient echo axial image (TR = 55 ms, TE = 5 ms, 50° flip angle) demonstrates high signal intensity within the abnormality (open arrow) secondary to flow related enhancement, confirming the diagnosis of aneurysm.

A

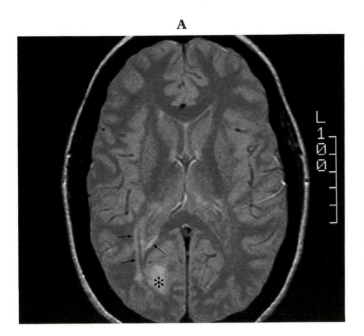

B

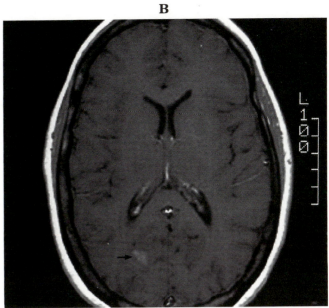

FIGURE 8.61

Multiple sclerosis. (**A**) 46-year-old female with a left homonomous hemianopsia. A proton-density axial MR image (TR = 2500 ms, TE = 30 ms) reveals areas of abnormal signal intensity confined to the optic radiations (arrows) and subcortical white matter of the calcarine region (∗) representing foci of demyelination. (**B**) The discrete focus of enhancement (arrow) within the peripheral lesion on this post contrast T1-weighted image (TR = 400 ms, TE = 11 ms) suggests that this is a region of active inflammation.

INDEX